I0031529

Recent Advances in Anesthesiology

Volume 4

Obstetric Anesthesia: Clinical Updates

Edited by

Eugenio Daniel Martinez-Hurtado
Department of Anesthesiology and Intensive Care
University Hospital Infanta Leonor
Madrid, Spain

Monica Sanjuan-Alvarez & Marta Chacon-Castillo
Department of Anesthesiology and Intensive Care,
University Hospital Severo Ochoa,
Madrid, Spain

Recent Advances in Anesthesiology

Volume # 4

Obstetric Anesthesia: Clinical Updates

Editors: Eugenio Daniel Martinez-Hurtado, Monica Sanjuan-Alvarez & Marta Chacon-Castillo

ISSN (Online): 2589-9392

ISSN (Print): 2589-9384

ISBN (Online): 978-981-5051-84-1

ISBN (Print): 978-981-5051-85-8

ISBN (Paperback): 978-981-5051-86-5

©2022, Bentham Books imprint.

Published by Bentham Science Publishers Pte. Ltd. Singapore. All Rights Reserved.

First published in 2022.

BENTHAM SCIENCE PUBLISHERS LTD.
End User License Agreement (for non-institutional, personal use)

This is an agreement between you and Bentham Science Publishers Ltd. Please read this License Agreement carefully before using the ebook/echapter/ejournal (**"Work"**). Your use of the Work constitutes your agreement to the terms and conditions set forth in this License Agreement. If you do not agree to these terms and conditions then you should not use the Work.

Bentham Science Publishers agrees to grant you a non-exclusive, non-transferable limited license to use the Work subject to and in accordance with the following terms and conditions. This License Agreement is for non-library, personal use only. For a library / institutional / multi user license in respect of the Work, please contact: permission@benthamscience.net.

Usage Rules:

1. All rights reserved: The Work is the subject of copyright and Bentham Science Publishers either owns the Work (and the copyright in it) or is licensed to distribute the Work. You shall not copy, reproduce, modify, remove, delete, augment, add to, publish, transmit, sell, resell, create derivative works from, or in any way exploit the Work or make the Work available for others to do any of the same, in any form or by any means, in whole or in part, in each case without the prior written permission of Bentham Science Publishers, unless stated otherwise in this License Agreement.
2. You may download a copy of the Work on one occasion to one personal computer (including tablet, laptop, desktop, or other such devices). You may make one back-up copy of the Work to avoid losing it.
3. The unauthorised use or distribution of copyrighted or other proprietary content is illegal and could subject you to liability for substantial money damages. You will be liable for any damage resulting from your misuse of the Work or any violation of this License Agreement, including any infringement by you of copyrights or proprietary rights.

Disclaimer:

Bentham Science Publishers does not guarantee that the information in the Work is error-free, or warrant that it will meet your requirements or that access to the Work will be uninterrupted or error-free. The Work is provided "as is" without warranty of any kind, either express or implied or statutory, including, without limitation, implied warranties of merchantability and fitness for a particular purpose. The entire risk as to the results and performance of the Work is assumed by you. No responsibility is assumed by Bentham Science Publishers, its staff, editors and/or authors for any injury and/or damage to persons or property as a matter of products liability, negligence or otherwise, or from any use or operation of any methods, products instruction, advertisements or ideas contained in the Work.

Limitation of Liability:

In no event will Bentham Science Publishers, its staff, editors and/or authors, be liable for any damages, including, without limitation, special, incidental and/or consequential damages and/or damages for lost data and/or profits arising out of (whether directly or indirectly) the use or inability to use the Work. The entire liability of Bentham Science Publishers shall be limited to the amount actually paid by you for the Work.

General:

1. Any dispute or claim arising out of or in connection with this License Agreement or the Work (including non-contractual disputes or claims) will be governed by and construed in accordance with the laws of Singapore. Each party agrees that the courts of the state of Singapore shall have exclusive jurisdiction to settle any dispute or claim arising out of or in connection with this License Agreement or the Work (including non-contractual disputes or claims).
2. Your rights under this License Agreement will automatically terminate without notice and without the

need for a court order if at any point you breach any terms of this License Agreement. In no event will any delay or failure by Bentham Science Publishers in enforcing your compliance with this License Agreement constitute a waiver of any of its rights.

3. You acknowledge that you have read this License Agreement, and agree to be bound by its terms and conditions. To the extent that any other terms and conditions presented on any website of Bentham Science Publishers conflict with, or are inconsistent with, the terms and conditions set out in this License Agreement, you acknowledge that the terms and conditions set out in this License Agreement shall prevail.

Bentham Science Publishers Pte. Ltd.
80 Robinson Road #02-00
Singapore 068898
Singapore
Email: subscriptions@benthamscience.net

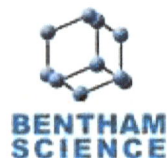

BENTHAM SCIENCE

CONTENTS

Monir Kabiri Sacramento, Javier Alcázar Esteras, Patricia Alfaro de la Torre, Sergi Boada Pie and *Miriam Sánchez Merchante*

Patricia Alfaro de la Torre, Monir Kabiri Sacramento, Irene Riquelme Osado and *Rosa Fernández García*

Míriam Sánchez Merchante and Eugenio D. Martinez Hurtado

PREFACE

Obstetric anesthesia encompasses the anesthetic and analgesic procedures performed during all the stages of labor for vaginal delivery as well as cesarean section. Anesthesiologists have cared for the security of pregnant women since 1847 when James Young Simpson performed the first analgesia for labor. Since then, and even more in the last decades, obstetric anesthesia has become an important aspect of routine anesthetic practice, as women demand to be able to enjoy painless childbirth.

Obstetric anesthesia is a challenge for all of us, because it involves two patients in the same procedure, with different physiologic characteristics, and with different needs. For this reason, our primary target should be to promote a painless and safe delivery, without disturbing uterine contractions or fetoplacental circulation.

Obstetric anesthesia requires a comprehensive approach, not only limiting us to pain relief during labor, but also including the appropriate management of cesarean section and of any potential complications derived of both labor and surgery, while avoiding any fetal compromise.

The Editors of this handbook consider it essential that anesthesiologists understand the importance of obstetric anesthesia in our daily practice. In this handbook, we intend to compile all updated, didactic, and exhaustive information, and we deem every professional should know to face the act of anesthetizing a pregnant patient.

Finally, we would like to thank the co-authors' collaboration for the achievement of this handbook. As we are all professionals from different institutions, we are able to compare different scenarios and ways to conduct anesthesia, which enriches the text content. Lastly, we would like to acknowledge the readers of this handbook, who are responsible for modern, high-quality and safe anesthesia. These last words are dedicated to the new generation of anesthesiologists; we hope that with this handbook they acquire new knowledge and benefit from our experience.

Eugenio Daniel Martínez Hurtado
Department of Anesthesiology and Intensive Care
University Hospital Infanta Leonor
Madrid, Spain

Monica San Juan Álvarez
Department of Anesthesiology and Intensive Care
University Hospital Severo Ochoa
Madrid, Spain

Marta Chacón Castillo
Department of Anesthesiology and Intensive Care
University Hospital Severo Ochoa
Madrid, Spain

List of Contributors

Adriana Carolina Orozco Vinasco	Department of Anesthesiology and Critical Care, University Hospital Severo Ochoa, Leganes, Madrid, Spain
Aleix Clusella Moya	Department of Anesthesiology, Hospital Sant Joan de Déu Esplugues, Barcelona, Spain
Alicia Ruiz Escobar	Department of Anaesthesiology and Intensive Care, Hospital Universitario Infanta Leonor, Madrid, Spain
Ana Plaza Moral	Hospital Clinic, University of Barcelona, Barcelona, Spain
Andrea Alejandra Rodriguez Esteve	Department of Anaesthesiology, Hospital Universitario Fundacion Alcorcon, Madrid, Spain
Andrea Alejandra Rodriguez Esteve	Department of Anaesthesiology, Hospital Universitario Fundacion Alcorcon, Madrid, Spain
Aniza S. González Lumbreras	Hospital Angeles Lomas, 52763 Méx., Mexico
Anna Conesa Marieges	Hospital Universitario Vall d'Hebron, Barcelona, Spain
Antonio López Hernández	Hospital Clinic, University of Barcelona, Barcelona, Spain
Blanca Gómez del Pulgar Vázquez	Department of Anesthesiology and Critical Care, University Hospital Severo Ochoa, Leganes, Madrid, Spain
Carlos Hugo Salazar Zamorano	Department of Anesthesiology and Critical Care, Hospital Universitario 12 de Octubre, Madrid, Spain
Carmen Gomar Sancho	University of Barcelona and University Vic-Central de Catalonia, Barcelona, Spain
Carreño Anna Pascual	Department of Anesthesiology, Hospital Sant Joan de Déu, Esplugues, Barcelona, Spain
Carolina Forero Cortés	Maternal and Child Anesthesiology. Sant Joan de Dèu Hospital, Barcelona, Spain
Clara Hernández Cera	Maternal and Child Anesthesiology. Sant Joan de Dèu Hospital, Barcelona, Spain
Clara Isabel Fernandez Sánchez	Department of Anesthesiology and Critical Care, University Hospital Severo Ochoa, Leganes, Madrid, Spain
Daniel Vieyra Cortés	Genesis Reproductive Medicine, Hospital Ángeles del Pedregal, 10700 Ciudad de México, CDMX, México Universidad Nacional Autónoma de México, 04510 Ciudad de México, CDMX, México
David Orozco Vinasco	Department of Anesthesiology and Critical Care, Clínica Calle 100, Bogotá, Colombia
Elena Sánchez Royo	Hospital Universitario Vall d'Hebron, Barcelona, Spain
Elena Suárez Edo	Hospital Universitario Vall d'Hebron, Barcelona, Spain
Enrique Alonso Rodríguez	Department of Anesthesiology and Critical Care, University Hospital Severo Ochoa, Leganes, Madrid, Spain

Esperanza Martin Mateos	Department of Anesthesiology, Hospital Sant Joan de Déu, Esplugues Barcelona, Spain
Eugenio D. Martinez Hurtado	Department of Anaesthesiology and Intensive Care, Hospital Universitario Infanta Leonor, Madrid, Spain
Eva Maria Blazquez Gomez	Department of Anesthesiology, Hospital Sant Joan de Déu, Esplugues, Barcelona, Spain
Inés Almagro Vidal	Department of Anesthesiology and Intensive Care, Hospital Central de la Defensa - Gómez Ulla, Madrid, Spain
Irene González del Pozo	Department of Anesthesiology and Intensive Care, Hospital Central de la Defensa - Gómez Ulla, Madrid, Spain
Irene León Carsí	Hospital Clinic, University of Barcelona, Barcelona, Spain
Irene Riquelme Osado	Department of Anesthesia, Acute Pain and Chronic Pain, Hospital Sanitas La Moraleja, Madrid, Spain
Javier Alcázar Esteras	Department of Anesthesia, Acute Pain and Chronic Pain, Hospital Universitario de Torrejón de Ardoz, Madrid, Spain
Juan José Correa Barrera	Department of Anesthesiology and Critical Care, University Hospital Severo Ochoa, Leganes, Madrid, Spain
Laura Fernandez Tellez	Department of Anaesthesiology, Hospital Universitario Fundacion Alcorcon, Madrid, Spain
Laura Reviriego Agudo	Department of Anesthesiology and Intensive Care, Hospital Clínico Universitario, Valencia, Spain
Ligia María Pérez Cubías	Maternal and Child Anesthesiology, Sant Joan de Dèu Hospital, Barcelona, Spain
Luis Humberto García Lorant	Hospital Angeles Lomas, 52763 Méx., Mexico
María de la Flor Robledo	Department of Anesthesiology and Critical Care, University Hospital Severo Ochoa, Leganes, Madrid, Spain
María Gómez Rojo	Department of Anesthesiology and Intensive Care, Hospital Ramon y Cajal, Madrid, Spain
Maria Luz Serrano Rodriguez	Department of Anaesthesiology, Hospital Universitario Fundacion Alcorcon, Madrid, Spain
María Mercedes García Domínguez	Department of Anesthesiology and Critical Care Hospital, Universitario Infanta Leonor, Madrid, Spain
Marina Vendrell Jordà	Hospital Clinic, University of Barcelona, Barcelona, Spain
Marta Chacón Castillo	Department of Anesthesiology and Critical Care, University Hospital Severo Ochoa, Leganes, Madrid, Spain
Marta López Doueil	Department of Anesthesiology, Hospital Virtual Valdecilla, Santander, Spain
Marta María Galnares Gómez	Midwifery Unit, Hospital Virtual Valdecilla, Santander, Spain
Miguel Ángel Fernández Vaquero	Department of Anesthesiology and Critical Care, Clínica Universidad de Navarra, Madrid, Spain

Mireia Pozo Albiol	Department of Anesthesiology, Hospital Sant Joan de Déu, Esplugues, Barcelona, Spain
Miriam Sánchez Merchante	Department of Anesthesiology and Critical Care, Hospital Universitario Fundación Alcorcón, Madrid, Spain
Mónica San Juan Álvarez	Department of Anesthesiology and Critical Care, University Hospital Severo Ochoa, Leganes, Madrid, Spain
Monir Kabiri Sacramento	Department of Anesthesiology and Critical Care, Grupo Hospitalario Universitario, Hospital Universitario HM, Madrid, Spain
Montserrat Franco Cabrera	Hospital Angeles Lomas, 52763 Méx., México Hospital Ángeles Pedregal, 05370 Ciudad de México, CDMX, México Hospital Español de México, 11520 Ciudad de México, CDMX, México The American British Cowdray Medical Center (ABC), 05370 Ciudad de México, CDMX, México
Natalia Martos Gisbert	Department of Anesthesiology and Critical Care, University Hospital Severo Ochoa, Leganés, Madrid, Spain
Pablo Solís Muñoz	Department of Anesthesiology and Critical Care, University Hospital Severo Ochoa Leganes, Madrid, Spain
Patricia Alfaro de la Torre	Department of Anesthesia, Acute Pain and Chronic Pain, Hospital Joan XXIII, Tarragona, Spain
Paula Agostina Vullo	Department of Anesthesiology and Intensive Care, Hospital Central de la Defensa - Gómez Ulla, Madrid, Spain
Pedro Charco Mora	Department of Anesthesiology and Intensive Care, Hospital Universitario y Politécnico La Fe, Valencia, Spain
Pilar Hernández Pinto	Department of Anesthesiology, Hospital Virtual Valdecilla, Santander, Spain
Rodrigo Sancho Carrancho	Department of Anesthesiology, Hospital Virtual Valdecilla, Santander, Spain
Rosa Fernández García	Department of Anesthesia Acute Pain and Chronic Pain, Hospital Universitario Príncipe de Asturias, Madrid, Spain
Sara Hervilla Ezquerra	Department of Anaesthesiology, Hospital Universitario Fundacion Alcorcon, Madrid, Spain
Serafín Alonso Vila	Hospital Universitario Vall d'Hebron, Barcelona, Spain
Sergi Boada Pie	Department of Anesthesia, Acute Pain and Chronic Pain, Hospital Joan XXIII, Tarragonay, Spain
Susana Manrique Muñoz	Hospital Universitario Vall d'Hebron, Barcelona, Spain
Yobanys Rodríguez Téllez	Maternal and Child Anesthesiology, Sant Joan de Dèu Hospital, Barcelona, Spain

CHAPTER 1

Fetomaternal Physiology: Physiological Changes during Pregnancy

Adriana Carolina Orozco Vinasco[1,*], **Mónica San Juan Álvarez**[2] **and David Orozco Vinasco**[2]

[1] *Department of Anesthesiology and Critical Care, University Hospital Severo Ochoa, Leganes, Madrid, Spain*

[2] *Department of Anesthesiology and Critical Care, Clínica Calle 100, Bogotá, Colombia*

Abstract: Anesthesia during pregnancy is challenging due to the extreme physiological and anatomical changes that occur. Deep knowledge of these changes and how they influence anesthesia is critical in order to offer safe anesthetic care to both, mother and the child. In this chapter, we will review the main features that occur in the respiratory, cardiovascular, central nervous, renal, and gastrointestinal systems, among others, and how it affects pharmacodynamics, pharmacokinetics, airway management and conduct of anesthesia. Fetomaternal circulation and fetal physiology focused on anesthesia will also be discussed.

Keywords: Anesthesia, Fetoplacental circulation, Fetal-maternal exchange, Placenta, Pregnancy.

INTRODUCTION

Changes during pregnancy are meant to serve a double objective: providing fetal well being, guaranteeing oxygen, nutrients supply, carbon dioxide and waste products removal, and preparing the maternal body for labor, delivery and lactation.

These changes can persist weeks after delivery and some may be long lasting [1, 2]. Maternal changes during pregnancy changes are summarized in Table **1**.

Respiratory System

Changes begin in the first trimester. Higher basal metabolism causes oxygen consumption to augment by about 60%; subsequently, a larger amount of carbon

---
[*] **Corresponding author Adriana Carolina Orozco Vinasco:** Department of Anesthesiology and Critical Care, University Hospital Severo Ochoa, Leganes, Madrid, Spain; E-mail: aorozcovi@yahoo.es

Eugenio Daniel Martinez-Hurtado, Monica Sanjuan-Alvarez & Marta Chacon-Castillo (Eds.)
All rights reserved-© 2022 Bentham Science Publishers

dioxide is produced. Greater minute ventilation is required to cope with this demand. Progesterone has stimulating effects on respiration, by raising sensitivity to carbon dioxide in the central nervous system (*CNS*). The net result is an increase of 50% in minute ventilation due, mostly, to higher tidal volume, causing physiological hypocapnia of around 30 mmHg. Renal compensation occurs so pH remains near 7.44. Despite this the hemoglobin dissociation curve shifts to the right due to an increase in 2,3-bisphosphoglycerate raising maternal P50 (partial pressure at which hemoglobin is 50% saturated), easing the offload of oxygen across the placenta [1 - 3]. Residual volume (*RV*) and residual functional capacity (*RFC*) are diminished (15% and 20%, respectively), the latter sometimes exceeded by closing capacity (*CC*). Owing to raised oxygen consumption and changes in RV and RFC, pregnant women desaturate more rapidly than their non-pregnant counterparts [3 - 5]. Inhalational anesthetics are up taken and eliminated more rapidly due to the greater minute ventilation and cardiac output [5, 6].

Table 1. Main physiological and anatomical changes during pregnancy.

Respiratory Changes	
Oxygen consumption	+ 60%
Minute ventilation	+ 50%
PCO_2	Decrease to 30 mmHg
Residual volume	- 15%
Functional residual capacity	- 20%
Airway capillaries	Engorgement
Diaphragm	Displaced cephalad
Ribs	Flaring
Cardiovascular	
Left ventricle mass	+ 50%
Cardiac output	+ 40-50%
Heart rate	+ 25%
Stroke volume	+ 25%
Systemic/Pulmonary vascular resistance	- 20%/-34%
Systolic blood pressure	- 6-8%
Diastolic blood pressure	- 20-25%
Hematological and Fluid Changes	
Red blood cells mass	+ 25%
Hemoglobin and hematocrit	-15%

(Table 1) cont.....

White blood cells during labor	Raise 9-11 x 10^9/L Up to 15 x10^9/L
Total plasma protein	- 18%
Plasmatic cholinesterase	- 20-25%
Colloid osmotic pressure	-18%
Plasma volume	+ 50%
Extravascular volume If edema	+ 1.7 L + 5 L
Platelets	=/-10%
Prothrombin time/Activated partial thromboplastin time	- 20%
Antithrombin III	- 10%
Protein S	Decrease
Protein C	No change
Fibrinolysis	Raise
I, VII, IX, VIII factors	+ 100- 150%
X, XII factors	+ 30%
II, V factors	=
XI, XIII factors	- 40-50%
Renal Changes	
Renal blood flow, Glomerular filtration rate	+ 50%
Na^+, H^2O and Cl^- reabsorption	+ 50%
Creatinine clearance	Raise
Serum creatinine	Decrease (~0.5-0.6 mg/dL)
Glucose, amino acids and uric acid reabsorption	Decrease
Urinary tract smooth muscle	Relaxation
HCO_3^- excretion	Raise
Gastrointestinal and Hepatobiliary Changes	
Esophagus	Displaced cephalad
Lower esophageal sphincter pressure	Decrease
Barrier pressure	- 45-50%
Alkaline phosphatase	Raise up to 4 times
Bilirubin, lactic deshydrogenase and transaminases	No change or raise
Cholecystokinin	Decrease
Neurological Changes	
Minimum alveolar concentration	- 40%
Pain threshold	Raise

(Table 1) cont.....

Epidural space size	Decrease
Local anesthetic requirements	- 40%
Cerebral spinal fluid volume	Decrease
Sympathetic tone	Raise
Metabolic and Endocrine Changes	
Metabolic basal rate	+ 15%
Cortisol level and half life	Increase
Insulin	Resistance
Immunological Changes	
T-cell activity	Decrease
Cell immunity	Decrease
Immunoglobulin G	Decrease
Immunoglobulin E	Raise
Neutrophils	Raise
Neutrophil chemotaxis and adherence	Decrease

Regarding anatomical changes, capillaries in the upper airway are engorged, causing edema and friability. Facemask ventilation and intubation may be hindered. Thoracic cage diameter is increased by 5-7 cm due to flaring of the ribs, and thus restricting movement. Changes in the subcostal angle persist after delivery. The diaphragm is displaced cephalad by the growing uterus [2, 4, 5].

Compared to pre-gestation values, during labor, minute ventilation may reach as high as 200% and oxygen consumption rises up to 75%. FRC returns to the pre-pregnancy values after two weeks. After birth, minute ventilation, PCO_2 and oxygen consumption gradually return to pre-gestational values during the next 6 to 8 weeks [2].

Cardiovascular Changes

The gravid uterus causes the heart to move anteriorly and to the left, so a left axis can be seen in ECG. Other electrocardiographic changes include T flattening and ST depression. Left ventricular hypertrophy is also common. A raise in cardiac output (*CO*) of 40-50% is seen at term due to greater heart rate (+25%) and stroke volume (+25%) [2 - 4]. The increase in cardiac output may cause a reduction in the latency of drugs acting peripherally [6]. Blood flow is diverted to the uterus, but is also increased in the kidneys and skin, when compared to non-pregnant women. A supplementary CO increase occurs during labor (40-60%, depending on contractions) and immediately after labor, where it can meet 80-100% when compared to values before labor. This occurs because of placental transfusion and aortocaval decompression [1, 2, 4]. Systemic vascular resistance (*SVR*) decreases by 20% due to both, vasodilatory mediators (estrogens, prostacyclin, progesterone) and low resistance bed (uteroplacental). Diastolic pressure is more affected than systolic (decrease of 25% and 8%, respectively). Pulmonary vascular resistance declines by 34%. Hypotension can occur in the supine position due to the compression of the inferior vena cava and aorta, which leads to a drop in CO. This effect is more pronounced when sympathetic activity, one of the compensatory mechanisms, is attenuated (*e.g.* spinal anesthesia). The aortocaval compression causes right heart filling pressures to diminish and lower limbs venous hypertension. Lateral positioning may partially relieve hypotension [2 - 4]. After delivery, CO returns to pregnancy levels after 24 hours, and to pre-pregnancy values after up to 24 weeks; the heart rate becomes normal after two weeks [2, 3].

Hematological and Fluid Status Changes

At term, despite a 25% raise in red blood cell mass, physiological anemia (hemoglobin and hematocrit decrease by 15%) takes place on a dilutional basis, due to a 50% increase in plasma volume. The latter is the consequence of changes in the release of renin and aldosterone, as well as other hormones. These mechanisms compensate the blood loss during delivery. After which, placental autotransfusion should outweigh the physiological blood loss. Extravascular volume is as well increased by 1.7 L in the absence of edema; in case it is present, the raise may be as much as 5L [3, 4]. Plasma protein concentration is reduced and consequently is colloid osmotic pressure. Plasma cholinesterase is reduced up to 25% and thus the effects of succinylcholine may be longer lasting, but not clinically relevant. Infection unrelated leukocytosis develops throughout gestation, reaching 15×10^9/L during labor. Nevertheless, polymorphonuclear cells function is diminished accounting for reduced neutrophil chemotaxis and adherence [2, 3].

During pregnancy, the concentration of most coagulation factors is augmented, noticeably of factors I, VII, VII and IX; and mildly of X and XII. Factors II and V hover pre-pregnancy values, whereas factors XI and XII are decreased. Regarding anticoagulation factors, protein C remains unchanged and antithrombin III and protein S are diminished. Blood viscosity is augmented. All these changes result in hypercoagulability. There is increased platelet consumption and turnover that, along with dilution, may lead to a decrease of up to 10% [1, 3]. Fibrinolysis is enhanced leading to a 100% rise in fibrin degradation products [3]. Coagulation and anticoagulation factors return to basal values after two weeks. The rest of the hematological and fluid changes reverse after 8 weeks [2].

Renal Changes

Renal blood flow and glomerular filtration rate increase by 50% because of vasodilation, and thus is creatinine clearance. Therefore, a decrease in serum creatinine is observed. Sodium, water and chloride reabsorption are enhanced up to 50% as a result of hormones with a mineralocorticoid effect such as cortisol, renin, aldosterone and progesterone. However, glucose, amino acids, and uric acid reabsorption decline, hence, proteinuria is considered above 300 mg per day. Bicarbonate excretion is raised to counteract the increase in minute ventilation [2, 3]. Renal changes cause unaltered drug elimination to increase, *e.g.* cephalosporins [6].

Progesterone has a potassium-sparing effect and can also lead to urinary stasis due to smooth muscle relaxation in the urinary tract. Hydronephrosis incidence is 80% in the second trimester. Therefore, during pregnancy, there might be more urinary tract infections [3].

Gastrointestinal and Hepatobiliary Changes

Bioavailability after oral absorption remains unchanged [6]. From mid-pregnancy onwards, women are at higher risk of regurgitation and aspiration, so they should be considered full stomach [4, 5]. The gravid uterus raises intrabdominal pressure and displaces the esophagus cephalad, lowering the inferior esophageal sphincter pressure. Estrogens and progesterone further reduce this pressure owing to muscle-relaxing effects. Gastrin production by the placenta may increase gastric acid production [3]. These factors contribute to the development of gastroesophageal reflux. Gastric emptying is not delayed, except for labor and delivery, followed by return to the basal status within 18 hours after delivery [2, 5].

Hepatic blood flow remains at pre-pregnancy values, but minor increases in hepatic markers, such as bilirubin, lactic dehydrogenase and transaminases, may occur [2 - 4]. However, the activity of most P450 cytochrome enzymes is increased, affecting the metabolism of phenytoin, midazolam and morphine [2].

There is a supplementary production of alkaline phosphatase by the placenta; hence its value is raised up to four times. Cholecystokinin release is diminished and thus is gallbladder contraction. Therefore, pregnant patients are prone to gallstone formation [2, 4].

Neurological Changes

By eight to twelve weeks of gestation, a 40% reduction in the minimum alveolar concentration (*MAC*) for inhaled anesthetic agents takes place. The underlying mechanism is unclear, but is probably a consequence of the rise in progesterone, β- endorphin and other endocrine factors [2 - 5]. There is also a rise in pain threshold, due, apparently, to the actions of estrogens and progesterone in spinal opioid receptors and in descending noradrenergic pathways [2].

During pregnancy, epidural venous plexus is engorged, thus conditioning a decrease in the size of the epidural space and in the cerebral spinal fluid (*CSF*) volume in the subarachnoid space [3]. There may be an increase in epidural fat, further shrinking the epidural space. At term, local anesthetic requirements in neuroaxial techniques are diminished by 40% approximately. Nevertheless, these changes begin in the first trimester (before aortocaval compression and the other changes occur), suggesting other mechanisms [2 - 4, 6].

An increase in the sympathetic tone takes place to neutralize the effects of aortocaval compression. As said before, the sympathetic block can result in profound hypotension [3].

Metabolic and Endocrine Changes

Several factors contribute to a 15% augmentation in metabolic basal rate, especially after mid pregnancy [1, 3, 5]. Thyroid gland size and function are increased, but free plasma thyroid hormones do not change due to a two-fold increase in Thyroid-binding globulin level. Cortisol plasma level is increased, and the half life is lengthened. Pituitary gland increases in size thus becoming vulnerable to ischemia and hemorrhage as its perfusion occurs at venous pressure [3].

Despite a rise in the number of ß cells in the pancreas and of the insulin receptor sites, a resistance to insulin occurs. This is probably the result of cortisol, prolactin, human placental lactogen and other hormones. Pregnant women are prone to hyperglycemia and ketosis; reversion of this phenomenon occurs 24 hours after delivery [2, 3].

Melanocyte stimulating hormone is increased, and causes hyperpigmentation [3].

Immunological Changes

The maternal immunological system is modified to offer "*tolerance*" to the fetus, as it expresses foreign (paternal) antigens. The main changes are summarized in Table **1**.

Other Changes

Fetus, placenta, amniotic fluid and increase in maternal water and fat, cause pregnant women to gain 10-12 kg (17%) in average. This conditions a greater distribution volume of both, lipo- and hydrophilic drugs. Nevertheless, the reduction in plasma proteins causes an increase in plasma-free drug, due to reduced binding, and toxicity is more likely [3, 4, 6].

Breasts are enlarged and may interfere with ventilation and intubation [2 - 4]. Blood flow to mucosa and skin is increased; if drugs are administered to these areas, absorption may be enhanced [6].

The placenta produces relaxin, which causes generalized relaxation in ligaments. Lumbar lordosis is increased and it may alter neuroaxial distribution of anesthetics [2, 3].

PLACENTAL PHYSIOLOGY

The placenta is a large area of exchange between the mother and the fetus; it supplies blood and nutrients, and removes waste products. The placenta contains maternal tissue (intervillous space) and fetal tissues (chorionic villi). Its greatest growth occurs in the third trimester, when it usually reaches a weight of about 500 g [3, 4]. The placenta has also endocrine and immunological functions and is metabolically active by producing enzymes involved in biotransformation [2] (Table **2**).

Table 2. Other functions of the placenta.

- Endocrine
- Human placental lactogen
- Human chorionic gonadotrophin
- Relaxin
- Estrogens and/or Progesterone
- Thyroid- stimulating hormone
- Prostaglandins
- Immunological
- Barrier to some infections

Blood Supply

The uterine arteries provide blood to the placenta through the spiral arteries, which penetrate the intervillous space, where the exchange takes place. In the nongravid uterus, blood flow is about 100 ml/min, but it may be as high as 800 ml/min (500-800 ml/min) by term. Only 20% blood flow is distributed in the myometrium. Placental blood flow is dependent on maternal CO, as it lacks autoregulation. So if hypotension occurs (*e.g.* hypovolemia, sympathetic block, aortocaval compression) uterine blood flow can be severely impaired. Normally, uterine arteries remain dilated due to several humoral factors such as estrogens, prostacyclin and nitric oxide. Nevertheless, endogenous and exogenous vasoconstrictors, as well as preeclampsia/eclampsia, can alter vascular resistance thus decreasing uterine blood flow. Another situation, where uterine blood flow can decrease, is when there is a raise in venous pressure, for example during contractions, aortocaval compression and during the second stage of labor. Normal placental circulation is a low resistance system [3, 4].

Transfer Across the Placenta

Oxygen and Carbon Dioxide

Oxygen and carbon dioxide cross the placenta by simple diffusion. The placenta is about 20 times more permeable to carbon dioxide than oxygen; only dissolved carbon dioxide crosses.

The main determinant of oxygen transfer is the gradient between maternal and fetal PO_2, but fetal hemoglobin concentration is also important. Maternal hemoglobin dissociation curve is shifted to the right so it has less affinity for oxygen, and conversely fetal hemoglobin is left shifted, so its affinity for oxygen is higher. Furthermore, fetal pH increases during exchange (increasing affinity for oxygen by further shifting the dissociation curve to the left), because CO_2 is transferred to the mother, whose blood pH in turn decreases thus enhancing oxygen offload. This phenomenon is known as the double Bohr effect and 2-8% of oxygen is transferred by this mechanism [1, 2].

A similar effect, the double Haldane effect occurs, regarding carbon dioxide transport. As maternal blood becomes more deoxygenated, its affinity for carbon dioxide increases, while as fetal blood becomes more oxygenated, carbon dioxide offload is enhanced. This phenomenon is responsible for up to 46% of carbon dioxide transport across the placenta. There is also a favorable carbon dioxide concentration gradient between the fetus and the mother [1, 2].

Nutrients (summarized in Table **3**).

Table 3. Placental transfer mechanism of nutrients.

Nutrient	Transport Mechanism
- Sodium - Water - Potassium - Fatty acids	- Simple diffusion
- Glucose	- Facilitated diffusion
- Calcium - Iron - Iodine - Phosphate	- Active transport
- Amino acids	- Secondary active transport (linked to sodium)
- Proteins (immunoglobulin G)	- Pinocytosis
Adapted from: Mushambi, M. Physiology of pregnancy. In: Lin, T, *et al.*, Eds. *Fundamentals of anaesthesia*. 4th ed. Cambridge: Cambridge University Press, 2016; pp. 512-30.	

Drug Transfer

Most drugs, except for muscle relaxants, cross the placenta. Several factors are involved in drug transfer degrees.

- **High Lipid Solubility**: Volatile and intravenous induction drugs are highly lipophilic and cross the placenta, for example, halothane, nitrous oxide, sodium thiopental, ketamine, and propofol. The latter is greatly protein bound, so its transfer is increased when maternal proteins are lowered (*e.g.* preeclampsia). There is a hazard of diffusion hypoxia in the newborn, in case nitrous oxide is used. Benzodiazepines also cross, as they are lipophilic and non-ionized.
- **Molecular weight**: Substances weighing <500-600 daltons, such as most drugs, cross the placenta readily. Succinylcholine has a low molecular weight, but is highly ionizated, so crossing is hindered [2, 3].
- **Ionization**: Only non-ionized fraction of the drug crosses the placenta. Most drugs used in the anesthetic field have high non-ionized fraction. Muscle relaxants are an exception; they do not cross the placenta as they are poorly ionizated and are not very lipophilic [3, 4].
- **pH**: It can alter ionization, especially if the pKa of the drug is near physiological pH, whereas even small pH changes can cause great changes in ionization. Furthermore, fetal pH is always lower, so once some un-ionized drugs cross the placenta, they became ionized in fetal blood, hindering a reverse diffusion. This

can cause accumulation and happens with weak bases such as opioids and local anesthetics. This phenomenon is known as "ion trapping" and occurs especially when the fetal pH decreases, *e.g.* fetal distress [2 - 4].

- *Protein binding*: During pregnancy, proteins decline globally and it can result in a major free drug fraction that diffuses across the placenta. Situations where binding is further decreased include acidosis and preeclampsia [3, 4].
- *Fetomaternal gradient*: when the underlying transfer mechanism is simple diffusion [3].
- *Uterine blood flow*: It affects drugs that readily cross the placenta. At a higher blood flow, a greater transfer occurs [3].

Fetal Circulation

At term, the fetus will have a blood volume between 120-160 ml/kg [4]. Before birth, the lungs and the liver are poorly functional, so only a small blood fraction will cross these organs. Blood enters the fetus *via* one umbilical vein, then it flow diverts, with the majority passing trough the *ductus venosus* directly to the inferior vena cava (*IVC*) and thus bypassing the liver. Most of the well-oxygenated blood entering the right atrium passes across the *foramen ovale* to the left atrium, then to the left atrium and aorta, from where it is distributed among arteries to the head and limbs. Deoxygenated blood entering the right atrium trough the superior vena cava (*SVC*) passes though the tricuspid valve to the rigth ventricle and then to the pulmonary artery. Most of this blood crosses the *ductus arteriosus* to the descending aorta, only a small fraction reaches the lungs. The blood returns to the placenta by two umbilical arteries (Fig. **1**) [1, 4, 7].

CONCLUSION

Changes during pregnancy are meant to serve a double objective: providing fetal well being and preparing the maternal body for labor, delivery and lactation.

Owing raised oxygen consumption and changes in RV and RFC, pregnant women desaturate more rapidly, than their non-pregnant counterparts.

Supine Hypotension can occur due to the compression of inferior vena cava and aorta, which leads to a drop in CO, being more pronounced when sympathetic activity is attenuated. Dilutional anemia and hypercoagulability are typical during pregancy.

At term, the requirements of both local anesthetics in neuroaxial tecniques and MAC, lessen by 40%. Most drugs, except for muscle relaxants, cross the placenta.

Deep knowledge of the physiological and anatomical changes during pregnancy and how they influence anesthesia is critical in order to offer a safe anesthetic care to both, mother and child.

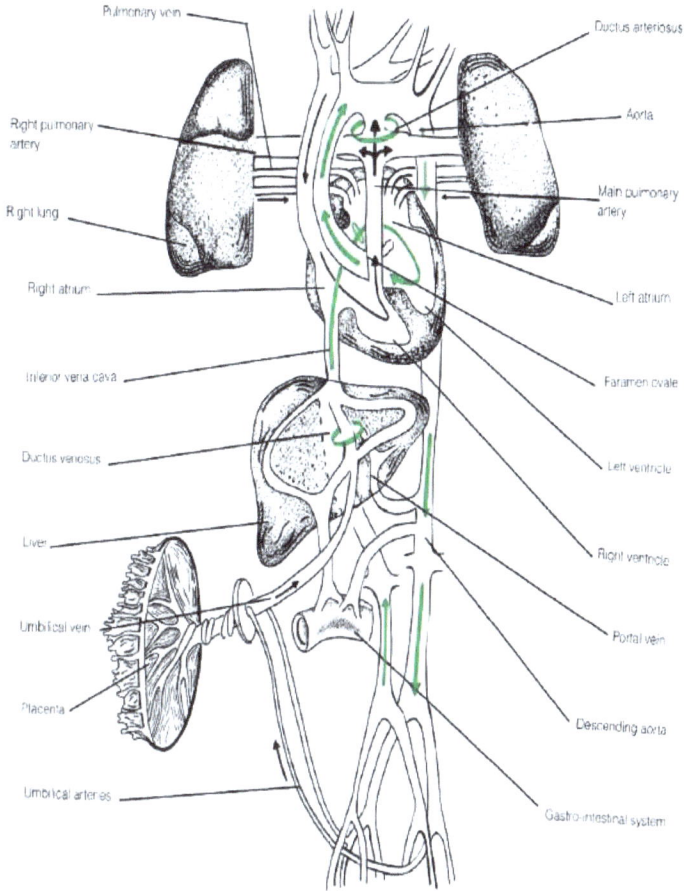

Fig. (1). Fetal circulation.

CONSENT FOR PUBLICATION

Not applicable.

CONFLICT OF INTEREST

The authors declare no conflict of interest, financial or otherwise.

ACKNOWLEDGEMENT

Declared none.

REFERENCES

[1]   Hall JE. HME Guyton and Hall Textbook of Medical Physiology International Edition. 2020; 1045-59.

[2]   Kacmar RMGR. Physiologic Changes of Pregnancy. In: Chestnut DH, Ed. Chestnut's obstetric anesthesia: principles and practice 6th ed. 2019; 13-37.

[3]   Lin T, Ed. M. M. Physiology of pregnancy. Fundamentals of anaesthesia 4th ed. 2016; 512-30.

[4]   Flood PR. Anestesia en Obstetricia. In: Miller RD, Ed. Anestesia 8th ed. 2015; 2328-58.

[5]   Braveman F, Scavone BM, Blessing ML, *et al.* Obstetric Anesthesia. In: Barash PG, Ed. Clinical Anesthesia 8th ed. 2017; 2841-925.

[6]   Chestnut DH, Ed. T. G. Pharmacology during pregnancy and lactation. Chestnut's obstetric anesthesia: principles and practice 6th ed. 2019; 313-35.

[7]   Lin T, Ed. A. W. Fetal and newborn physiology. Fundamentals of anaesthesia. 4th ed. 2016; 531-6.

CHAPTER 2

Safety in the Obstetric Patient: Simulation Training for Anesthesiologists in the Obstetrics Field

Pilar Hernández Pinto[1,*], **Marta López Doueil**[1], **Rodrigo Sancho Carrancho**[1] and **Marta María Galnares Gómez**[2]

[1] *Department of Anesthesiology, Hospital Virtual Valdecilla, Santander, Spain*

[2] *Midwifery Unit, Hospital Virtual Valdecilla, Santander, Spain*

Abstract: The principal goal of health systems is to provide safe and quality healthcare for the patient. Deficiencies in the environment in which obstetric care is provided, inadequate teamwork and communication, and poor individual performance during emergencies have been identified as preventable causes of harm to obstetric patients. There is growing evidence about training in Emergency Obstetric Care (*EmOC*) that reduces the risk of maternal and newborn mortality and morbidity. The Institute of Medicine identifies team-based training and simulation as methods to improve patients' safety, especially in the obstetrics field, these may add value to it. Recent research works review the effectiveness of training in EmOC and the use of simulation in improved health outcomes. It remains unclear whether this translates into improved patient outcomes.

Keywords: Communication, Competency-Based Medical Education, Emergency Obstetric Care, Maternal Mortality, Multidisciplinary Care, Nontechnical and Technical Skills, Obstetric Anaesthesia, Patient Safety, Simulation, Teamwork, Team Training.

INTRODUCTION

Safety and Quality in Obstetrics

The Institute of Medicine (*IOM*) recognizes patient safety as indistinguishable from the provision of quality healthcare. Safety and quality are closely intertwined. Safety methodologies try to avoid preventable adverse events (*pAEs*) while quality projects aspire to achieve the best possible results as health outcomes, patient satisfaction, access, and equity [1, 2].

---

* **Corresponding author Pilar Hernández Pinto:** Department of Anesthesiology, Hospital Virtual Valdecilla, Santander, Spain; E-mail: pilar.hernandezp@scsalud.es

Eugenio Daniel Martinez-Hurtado, Monica Sanjuan-Alvarez & Marta Chacon-Castillo (Eds.)
All rights reserved-© 2022 Bentham Science Publishers

Patient safety and quality improvement in obstetrics is an important issue having three factors: obstetric admissions are one of the main reasons for hospitalization; secondly, family's expectations for a healthy and happy outcome, and lastly the increase in medical litigation claims and trials with costs associated [3]. At a global level, the goal is to achieve safe and quality care in obstetrics and labor settings with a reduction of maternal and neonatal morbidity and mortality.

Maternal survival has significantly enhanced since the incorporation of the United Nations Millennium Development Goal (*MDGs*), the maternal mortality ratio (*MMR*) has decreased in 43.9% of the countries from 1990 to 2015 [4]. However, MMR remains high in many parts of the world, especially in low-income and middle-income countries (*LMICs*). Nearly 50% of these direct maternal deaths are caused by hemorrhage and hypertensive disorders of pregnancy. In high-income countries (*HICs*), indirect maternal deaths (underlying cardiac and embolic diseases and associated conditions like obesity, multiple gestations, and assisted reproductive technologies) outnumber direct deaths. The United Nations Sustainable Development Goal (*SDG*) aspires to reduce the global MMR to less than 70 per 100.000 live births by the year 2030. Evidence suggests that the majority of these and other potentially life-threatening complications such as sepsis, complications from delivery, and unsafe abortion could be prevented by timely and effective emergency obstetric care [5, 6]. However, it has been shown that more than half of all women with obstetric complications lack access to this life-saving intervention [7].

Strategies to Improve Quality in Obstetrics

The minimum care package required during pregnancy and childbirth addresses the main causes of maternal death, stillbirth and early neonatal death referred to as emergency obstetric care (*EmOC*) [8]. The basic components include antibiotics, oxytocic drugs, anticonvulsants, manual removal of placenta, removal of retained products of conception, assisted vaginal delivery and resuscitation of the newborn baby using a bag and mask. It has been argued that a more comprehensive set of signal functions includes caesarean section, blood transfusion and care for small and sick newborns [9]. In many cases, the required infrastructure (as equipment and consumables) is available, but staff may lack the competency to provide all EmOC signal functions. EmOC relies on the presence of suitably trained and competent healthcare providers. Short competency-based training in EmOC results in significant improvements in healthcare provider knowledge/skills and change in clinical practice [9]. Regular training is recommended and, in some cases, mandatory, to ensure the continued accreditation of healthcare providers. In the early 1990s, EmOC training courses such as the Advanced Life Support in obstetrics (*ALSO*) and Managing Obstetric Emergencies and Trauma (*MOET*) were developed to meet this need in high-income settings. However, in the era of the SDGs, competition for limited resources is high, and the cost-effectiveness of training packages is important to aid decision-makers in the most efficient use of resources and assess value-for-money. Very little is published about the costs and cost-effectiveness of training [10]. The wider health, social and economic benefits resulting from relatively small investments in training can be substantial, suggesting that these investments are likely to be of good value for money [11].

Guidelines and protocols endorsed by maternal safety organizations have been developed. They emphasize early and aggressive management of obstetric hemorrhage starting with risk factor identification, rapid diagnosis, timely management and multidisciplinary review. Systems to accelerate the initial response include an obstetric emergency response team, a postpartum hemorrhage cart ("*PPH cart*") and emergency hemorrhage medication packs.

Guidelines and protocols for acute management of hypertension focus on early diagnosis, prompt antihypertensive therapy, and seizure prophylaxis with magnesium sulfate [12].

How About Safety in the Obstetric Field?

The combination of gradually more complex systems controlled by "*imperfect*" humans is the basis of the patient safety problem in current medicine.

The World Health Organization (*WHO*) defines patient safety as the "*absence of preventable harm to a patient during the process of health care and reduction of risk of unnecessary harm associated with health care to an acceptable minimum*".

The Institute of Medicine observed that the root cause of 70% of errors in general and up to 80% of obstetric sentinel events can be traced to the process of team skills [13]. As many as 9% of pregnant patients will experience an adverse event during their delivery and up to 87% of adverse events in the obstetric population are deemed preventable [14]. In 2004, Joint Commission Sentinel Event Alert studied 47 perinatal deaths and identified non-medical factors topped the list of identified root causes, particularly communication and organizational culture, which contributed significantly to deficient perinatal outcomes [15]. This sentinel event alert was essential for clarifying obstetric safety threats and for risk reduction strategies that any unit starting a patient safety program should focus on.

Taking into account the five root causes of adverse perinatal events from the Joint Commission Sentinel Event Alert, possible safety interventions would focus on communication, organizational culture, staff competence, orientation, and training, and fetal monitoring.

- *Communication*: Staff resource management is a method to improve communication and coordination between members of a healthcare team. Topics covered in staff resources management programs such as Team STEPPS (Team Strategies and Tools to Enhance Performance and Patient Safety) and Med Teams address four main skills: leadership, situation monitoring, mutual support and communication. Team STEPPS identified communication tools such as *check-back* (or closed loop communication) to ensure the recipient has understood the sender´s information correctly, *SBAR* (an acronym standing for situation, background, assessment and recommendation) which can be used when requesting help in emergency situations, *call-out*, which is used to convey critical information to a larger group of people efficiently and *checklist* for handovers, have improved both teamwork and relevant outcomes [16].
- *Organizational Culture*: It integrates safety thinking and practices into clinical activities, changing from the traditional culture of hierarchy and blames a just culture for uncovering the systems that lead to risky activities or adverse outcomes. Safety Attitudes Questionnaire is the only safety climate survey that demonstrated a relationship between improvements in safety culture and patient outcomes, both in general medicine and obstetrics.
- *Staff Competence*: Competence is the ability to do something successfully and competently. One way to achieve this is by developing protocols, guidelines and checklists from a multidisciplinary process. This allows for the application of evidence-based standards and the creation of a shared mental model of how care should be provided in certain conditions and situations.
- *Orientation and Training*: To improve practical and communication skills and to train for unusual events.
- *Fetal Monitoring*: There is very little evidence of the effect of accreditation in fetal monitoring on outcomes.

Strategies to Improve Safety in Obstetrics

Most safety strategies need multidimensional solutions, including health provider education and training, work to improve team coordination and communication, and organization of administrative and structural processes. The growing effort of healthcare institutions to implementing training programs to address these issues has raised new questions about how to best train for effective performance in such systems.

Simulation in obstetrics has been rapidly expanding and the amount of published research in this area has increased in recent years. In 2011, Riley *et al.* [17]

showed that establishing multidisciplinary training programs and simulation exercises improved perinatal outcomes. The introduction of shoulder dystocia training for all maternity staff was associated with improved management and neonatal outcomes of births complicated by shoulder dystocia [18]. Simulation has been tested as an educational tool and as an intervention to improve outcomes in specific drills scenarios such as surgical delivery, eclampsia, postpartum hemorrhage and shoulder dystocia. Clinical topics in which simulation training is associated with improved clinical outcomes are: shoulder dystocia management, forceps delivery, emergency unplanned Cesarean delivery, postpartum hemorrhage, and neonatal resuscitation [19].

The management of obstetric emergencies, not only requires technical ability but also requires a range of non-technical skills such as communication, leadership and situational awareness. Simulation has been used to train technical and nontechnical skills, to review the environmental design of an existing or new obstetric unit, and is effective in assisting in the implementation of new technology or in the optimization of a plan [20].

Obstetric emergencies and team-based drills are common in obstetric simulation curricula. Simulation-Based Team Training (*SBTT*) and Multidisciplinar Simulation-Based Team Training (*MD-SBTT*) programmes have been developed and implemented across the globe [21]. The most popular are MOSES (Multidisciplinary obstetric simulated emergency scenarios), ESMOE (essential steps in managing obstetric emergencies), PROMPT (Practical Obstetric Multi-professional training), ASLO (Advanced Life Support in Obstetrics) or the MOET (Managing Obstetrics Emergencies and Trauma) where obstetrics, midwives and anesthesiologists can train together in emergency obstetric and newborn care. Simulation-based communication-training programs have been aimed to help obstetrics and gynecology trainees to develop communication skills [22].

Lately, there is a need for a robust evaluation of the effectiveness of training to improve training programmes and to provide information on how these can be developed and delivered to have the desired effect [23]. Data on the retention of knowledge and skills over time are useful to determine how frequently healthcare providers should be *"re-trained"* to maintain competency in EmOC. There is limited data to suggest the optimum length of a training EmOC. Longer training programmes were associated with greater improvement in skills compared with shorter programmes. Ameh *et al.* [9] conducted a systematic review of studies that evaluated the effectiveness of training in EmOC assessing four levels: participant reaction, knowledge, and skills, change in behaviour and clinical practice and availability of EmOC and health outcomes. They found strong evidence for improved clinical practice (adherence to protocols, resuscitation technique, communication and teamwork) and improved neonatal outcomes reduced trauma after shoulder dystocia, reduced the number of babies with hypothermia and hypoxia). Less strong evidence was found for the reduction in the number of cases of postpartum haemorrhage, case fatality rates, stillbirths and institutional maternal mortality. Knowledge and skills can be retained for up to 1-year post training and healthcare providers report being confident to provide EmOC for up to 1-year post-training. Skills decline at a faster pace than knowledge. No studies assessing knowledge and skills retention > 12 months because there will be several confounding factors to account for. Some obstetric complications are not common and to retain the ability to correctly manage such complications, health care workers should have the opportunity to have "*booster*" training at regular intervals [24].

Furthermore, means of assessing the communication, behavioral and nontechnical skills (*NTS*) of a team are necessary because these are important factors in team interactions. Recently, Onwochei *et al.* [25] reviewed the tools available to assess team effectiveness in obstetric emergencies. They found the most reliable tools identified were the Clinical Teamwork Scale, The Global Assessment of Obstetric Team Performance and the Global Rating Scale of performance. However, they were still lacking in terms of quality and validity. Further studies are required to assess how outcomes, such as performance and patient safety are influenced when using teamwork assessment tools.

In the obstetrics area, patients and families should play a central role in their own safety. Communication with expectant mothers/patients and their partners, close relatives or friends providing social support should be improved to ensure patient safety, including the avoidance of pAEs. Thus, applications (*app*) are even being developed to offer an effective and inexpensive way to promote effective communication between staff, patients, and their social support providers. Improving communication is expected to reduce pAEs and increase both work and patient satisfaction [26].

Not all women benefit from robust support. Race, ethnicity, primary spoken language, poverty, social capital, literacy, numeracy, and racism at the interpersonal and system level all contribute to a woman´s capacity to safely navigate the healthcare system. Women from vulnerable backgrounds are least able to engage in effective partnerships with their clinical care teams, and the resulting disconnects can increase the risk for serious patient harm. A culture of equity can support and advance a culture of safety by converging both clinical attention and system innovations on those individuals and groups who are most likely to benefit [12].

At hospitals, the risks associated with patient care can never be completely eliminated. Incident reporting systems make it possible to report incidents related to health care and obtain useful information on the sequence of events that led to their production, facilitating learning opportunities to avoid their repetition. Incident reporting systems are explicitly recommended by the WHO and by the Council of the European Union. They are a useful learning tool that favors the dissemination of the culture of patient safety, as long as professionals are adequately and promptly informed about the problems identified and improvement measures taken.

The Role of Anesthesiologist in the Safety of the Obstetric Patient

The role of anesthesiologists in obstetrics units and labor suites, considered high-risk areas in the hospital setting, is crucial. The anesthesiologist is a member of the delivery unit team which involves many different clinicians, patients and their relatives. The Anesthesia Patient Safety Foundation articulated the vision that "*no patient shall be harmed by anesthesia*", leading the movement toward a safer future [27]. A reduction in maternal morbidity and mortality should be the number one concern for obstetric anesthesiologists who have the role of a perioperative/peripartum physician.

Anesthesia-related maternal deaths are extremely rare. Airway disasters account for most deaths from general anesthesia. Technological advances, including pulse oximetry, capnography, airway management aids, along with improvements in drugs markedly reduced the risk associated with general anesthesia. Neuraxial anesthesia is considered a safe technique. The most frequent causes of serious complications (1:3000 obstetric anesthetics) of neuraxial anesthesia are high neuraxial block (1:4.336), peripartum respiratory arrest (1:10.042) and unrecognized spinal catheter (1:15.435) [12]. Sobhy *et al.* [28] estimated that in low-and middle-income countries, the risk of death from anesthesia is 1,2 per 1000. Anesthesia contributed to 3.5% of all direct maternal deaths and 13.8% of deaths after cesarean delivery. These complications (failed tracheal intubation, pulmonary aspiration and high spinal block) could be significantly reduced by safety improvements in practice. Safe induction of general anesthesia and airway management algorithms have been suggested.

There are a lot of individual improvements that have produced the safe practice that is provided by obstetric anesthesiologists today. Birnbach and Bateman [29] highlight innovations as:

- Safer and more effective labor analgesia (supporting the use of neuraxial blocks rather than the use of general anesthesia for cesarean delivery, improving safety).
- Safer treatments for hypotension associated with neuraxial blockade using ephedrine and phenylephrine.
- Advances in spinal and epidural techniques for operative deliveries with the development of new drugs, use of test doses (to identify catheters inadvertently threaded into blood vessels or the intrathecal space) availability of intralipid antidote to local anesthetic toxicity among others.
- Lower incidence of postdural puncture headache through improved technology with new spinal needles commonly termed "*pencil point*".
- Safer parental agents for labor analgesia. Fentanyl and remifentanil offer safer and more effective alternatives although still requiring close patient monitoring.
- Improved safety of general anesthesia in obstetrics with better monitoring, better laryngoscopes, airway adjuncts and better training,in addition to the development of difficult intubation algorithms.
- Improved education and the use of simulation including team training. Anesthesiologists play a key role in cases of severe preeclampsia, eclampsia, hemorrhage or critically ill patients.
- Reductions in operating room (*OR*) related infections with hand hygiene.

There is a growing movement toward the effective use of crisis checklists, emergency manuals, and other cognitive aids in the OR. There is little evidence that their use has been routinely implemented in labor and delivery suites. Anesthesiologists can play a key role in not only embracing checklists, but also in championing their use in labor and delivery suites,for example, keeping local anesthesia systemic toxicity checklists available in all areas where local anesthetics are used.

SIMULATION TRAINING FOR ANESTHESIOLOGISTS IN THE OBSTETRICS FIELD

Simulation has been a part of anesthesia for decades. Although it was not until the 1980s that popularity increased by combining task training with the concept of Crisis Resource Management [30].

For decades the procedures and techniques in anesthesia have been learned by direct contact with the patient, through the maxim "see one, do one, teach one" which increases the risk and discomfort of the patient, which is inadmissible for today. This has led to a change in medical education thanks to the use of clinical simulation. Simulation is the piece that allows us to go from the theoretical knowledge acquired through books, papers or essays to its application in a real patient, because it allows us to apply what has been learned without putting the patient's safety at risk. It also allows the repetition of skills as many times as necessary to obtain the necessary skill.

Simulation comes from Latin and means to imitate or copy and offers the opportunity to learn and practice both individually and in groups in a safe environment without risk of injury to the patient. Dr. Gaba, simulation is an instrument that replaces real encounters with patients. The objective is to replicate real, predictable, standardized and reproducible scenarios and environments in order to give feedback and evaluate the participant's performance. The simulation can be verbal, with standardized patients (actors), task trainers, simulated patients (mannequins) or virtual reality.

Simulation can play a very important role in medical situations with low opportunity to experience and high urgency for medical intervention such as obstetrics emergencies. Obstetric units expose the anesthesiologist to a completely different setting and environment than usual, with two potential patients (mother and child) simultaneously, involving many different clinicians.

Competency-Based Curriculum in Anesthesia

Due to the complex reality that occurs in delivery rooms, anesthesiologists with high professional experience are required, capable of handling stressful situations with communication skills, not only with the woman in labor and family members but with the entire multidisciplinary obstetric team.

Training residents in these practices is complex, as is maintaining the degree of professionalism of the anesthesia attending physician. Simulation has become a very important and well-accepted method in education and training of health providers practitioners making learning more effective. For this reason, in different countries and Anesthesia Societies, simulation is part of the residents' training program, allowing students to acquire and maintain capacities, competencies and technical skills that allow progressive development while making performance evaluation possible [31, 32] It is the competency-based medical education (*CBME*), which can be defined as an approach to prepare anesthesiologists for their professional practice that is fundamentally oriented to the outcome skills of graduates and organized around competencies derived from an analysis of social and patient needs. It is time-based, flexible, learner-centered and cost-effective learning. It allows the student to focus efforts on developing aspects of their performance that need improvement (deliberate practice), all in a safe environment, without risk to the patient. It also requires an evaluation of the program to receive feedback from the learners and check their progress. Learning is defined by objectives achieved, not by the number of procedures performed.

The CMBE uses a methodology that assesses technical and non-technical skills in simulation or in clinical practice, unlike traditional assessment methods through subjective questions or summaries by a supervisor. Through the CMBE the competencies are progressively achieved and each one is based on the basis of the one that precedes it. It can be represented as a pyramid (Fig. **1**).

Simulation education improves the performance of participants, patient care, patient outcomes, and promotes retention and saves costs. This has been demonstrated in programs such as central line placement [33], the use of the bronchofibroscope for difficult intubation [34], lumbar puncture technique [35] or thoracentesis [36], and cardiopulmonary resuscitation technique [37].

In obstetric anesthesia, there are four broad uses of simulation: Improvement of technical skills, nontechnical or teamwork skills, individual clinical competence and the safety of the clinical environment [38] (Fig **1**).

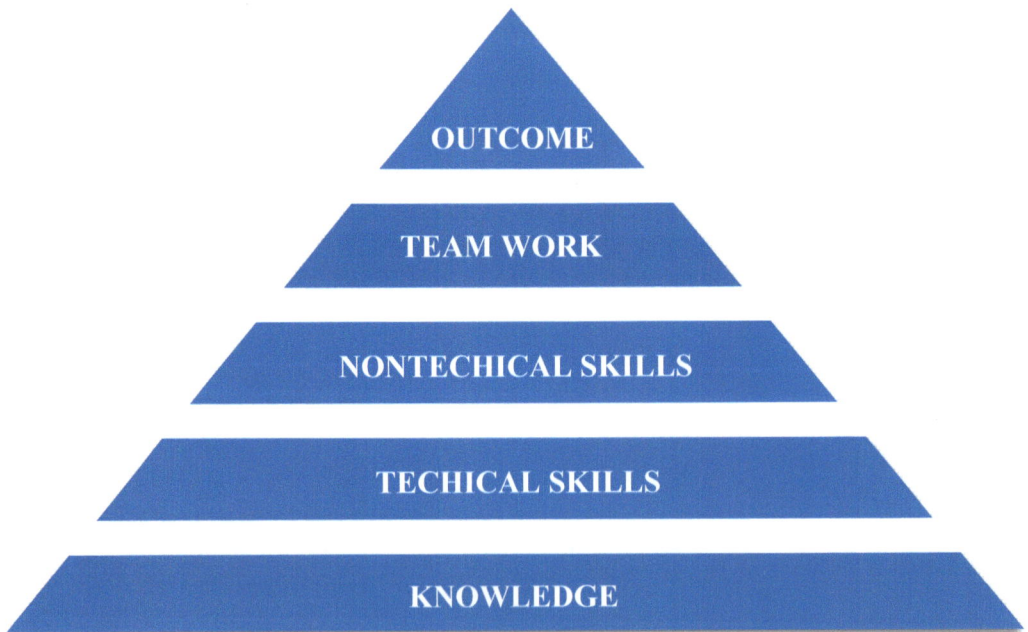

Fig. (1). Based on Vasco´s Pyramid of clinical competence. Modified by Vasco from the Bloom and Miller Pyramids. From: M. Vasco Ramírez. Training future anesthesiologists in obstetric care. Curr Opin Anesthesiol 2017, 30:313–318.

Improvement Technical Skills

Technical skills can be easily trained in lower-risk areas without exposition to time pressure, observation by other colleagues or relatives or the difficulties of an unfamiliar environment. Simulation in this field has focused on airway management and general anesthesia for emergent cesarean delivery, training epidural and intrathecal access and estimating the volume of blood loss [31].

The management of the airway in the obstetric patient is usually more difficult due to changes in the maternal airway during pregnancy and labor. In addition, the predominant use of neuraxial techniques in obstetric anesthesia makes the management of the airway in the parturient infrequent, being limited to emergent cesarean delivery, which reduces provider familiarity and increases the risk of airway mismanagement in emergent situations. For these reasons, simulating with airway management is a logical intervention. In fact, there are several studies that show that airway training increases airway management performance. There are also a couple of studies that show a high rate of skill retention for a few weeks, using a previously validated scoring system. A long-term retention has not been reported [39].

Neuraxial techniques are a fundamental part of current obstetric anesthesia practice. Simulators provide a training ground for both epidural and intrathecal access, enhancing the teaching of these skills. There are commercial simulators of the spinal column, but some studies suggest that cheap self-made low fidelity simulators or *"task trainers"*, using common materials, such as globes, polyethylene foam or different fruits, provide similar experience to that other more expensive [40, 41]. These simulators provide the possibility of becoming familiar with the steps of the procedure and the function of the equipment components, practice of the skills with feedback, easy access to repeated practice and improve the degree of self-efficacy [41].

Simulation can also be used to assess technical skills. The gold standard for evaluation of these skills in anesthesia consists of a combination of global rating scales and previously validated checklist, used after the execution of the procedure, in a real or simulated patient, by a trained observer. There are different methods to evaluate technical skills, but the Cumulative sum (*Cusum*) analysis has appeared as an important objective method, a statistical and graphical instrument that can objectify the success and failure at technical skill and analyze learning trends over time. This tool can be used to define learning curves for specific technical skills to detect deviations from the practice norms and to provide an estimated number of cases that are necessary to achieve competency in a particular skill [42]. Anesthesia residents will achieve a 90% success rate for epidural technique after carrying out around 75 procedures [43]. Practice using a simulator might be used to reduce the number of procedures required for success by a resident in clinical situations and reduce the time to surgical incision in emergency cesarean delivery under either general or regional anesthesia.However, to date, although it is suspected, there is no evidence that these practices translate into better patient outcomes.

As a novel concept to improve technical skills, it is worth highlighting the so-called *"virtual warm-ups"*. It is about preparing and refreshing a complex procedure immediately before carrying it out in a real setting [39]. Fiberoptic intubation (*FOI*) is a good example: technique in which it has been demonstrated that the simulated FOI just before the real one reduces intubation time by approximately 30% [44].

Another interesting innovative concept is three-dimensional printing. In medicine, some specialities are using 3D printing mostly in surgery. In anaesthesia, the use has been more limited to date. But it has been used for modelling airways or producing ultrasound *"phantoms"* for spinal injections. In the field of obstetric anesthesia it has not yet been fully explored [42].

Improvement Non-Technical Skills

Non-technical skills (*NTS*) are behaviours within the perioperative environment, not directly related to the use of drugs, equipment, or the experience of the anesthesiologist. Human behavior is responsible for 50 to 80% of errors in medicine and is the largest contributor to adverse effects in obstetrics.

In obstetric emergencies, as mentioned throughout the chapter, non-technical skills are of vital importance. We are going to find ourselves in chaotic situations, due to the unexpected nature of the emergency, having to communicate with many professionals, work as a team and where leadership is essential. These types of essential emergency skills are non-technical skills and they can be practiced, trained and evaluated through simulation [45]. The principles of *"Crisis Resource Management"* have been used effectively to guide this learning of non-technical skills [46].

David Gaba [47] identified gaps in the curriculum of anesthesia residents due to the lack of programs based on social skills such as communication, decision-making or leadership. The training of these non-technical skills is beneficial even without the use of simulation. If this training also involves simulation, the benefits will be greater. He also advocates a multidisciplinary simulation, as it reflects much better reality and the environment in the obstetric area. In this way, not only teamwork is improved, but it specifically contributes to improving mutual understanding between the different specialties that work together in the delivery room.

The European Society of Anesthesiology published the Helsinki Patient Safety Declaration in 2010. The declaration demanded that Team training should be part of the curricula to enhance communication and teamwork. However, implementation of these demands is usually based on local "bottom-up" efforts rather than nation-wide "*top-down*" approaches. Anesthesia and healthcare in general would benefit from regulations like in aviation [48].

To improve teamwork skills, healthcare organizations should encourage participation in simulation education programs and create a culture of learning and teaming. These activities should be designed taking into account the principles of "*Crisis Resource Management*". These programs should provide learning opportunities that allow for constructive reflection and debriefing.

Non-technical skills should not be assessed in isolation, but together with the rest of the skills. Thus, simulation scenarios designed to train individual skills can be used to evaluate group skills such as communication skills, workload distribution skills, or problem-solving skills.

There is no need for expensive models for non-technical skills training or assessment and low-cost simulation models have been described during a cesarean section with good psychological fidelity, which are very useful for non-technical skills training.

The use of checklists in obstetrics is of great help in a crisis situation but by itself does not change the outcome. Their use must be accompanied by the dissemination of their existence and training in simulation scenarios. They help guide decision making and prevent errors caused by forgetfulness. They also have a positive impact on communication and encourage leadership and effective communication. The check list has been used in simulation during pediatric emergencies, obstetric hemorrhage or surgical crises, managing to reduce maternal mortality [49]. Simulation has also been used to train checklists, emergency manuals, or other cognitive aids. During an emergent cesarean delivery, it has been seen that the monitoring of these cognitive aids decreases, simulation has been shown to improve adherence to the checklist. Therefore, the potential effectiveness of improvement with the use of simulation is confirmed.

A high level of fidelity of the simulated scenarios is not necessarily associated with a high level of perception. Learning according to Kolb [50] is directly proportional to the experience lived by the participant. It is important to remember that simulators do not teach, they are only effective tools for learning, but they need wise and competent educators, with debriefing skills. Furthermore, exposing participants to a simulation scenario without feedback has a little effect on the students, while a good debriefing with good judgment, supported by video assistance, will have a greater impact [51]. It is not necessary to invest in simulators, but in training and maintaining educators capable of guiding good learning.

Improvement Individual Clinical Competence

Although the literature is in favor of the use of simulation as a method of continuous training, it represents an important cultural change. But it should be considered to create a certification process by the different anesthesia societies. Our situation should not be different from the aviation industry, where airlines legally require their pilots to perform annual simulation evaluations in order to certify their level of professionalism. To do this, the curriculum of residents and attending physicians should be redesigned.

For Epstein [52] professional competence is not an achievement but a lifelong learning habit, so that level of competence is important to maintain throughout life. The level of competence should be achieved at all 3 levels of knowledge: cognitive, technical skills, and team skills.

Improvement Safety of the Clinical Environment

Last, but probably the most important use of the simulation, is to assess the work environment. Using a simulation approach similar to team training, the work system as a whole is analyzed, trying to identify weaknesses of the system, whether they are clinical or organizational [53, 54].

It is well known from other high-risk industries, that these work environment simulations are the most effective ones, because problems of the system are more significant and better solvable than individual deficiencies.

The simulation of these scenarios is more complex, more expensive and means an additional overload of the system, but it identifies latent insecure conditions of the system that can often be resolved. There is little data about the prevalence of these in situ drills simulation. For example, in England almost half of the obstetric units carry out drills once per month [40].

For the obstetric environment, some simulation scenarios have been implemented; cardiac arrest, massive hemorrhage, eclampsia, fire in the operating room and failed intubation.

Several studies developed in the most frequent scenarios, such as hemorrhage and eclampsia, have revealed latent errors or problems in the system, which are solved afterwards as a consequence of the simulation, without putting patients at risk and offering the possibility of improving care in the future [55]. These failures become more apparent as the urgency of the situation increases. One of the errors detected was the amount of time that was lost looking for the necessary elements for the treatment of seizures, which was solved by creating an *"Eclampsia box"*, destined to contain all the medication and material necessary to manage the situation [40].

Although the bibliography shows that in situ and offsites simulation have a similar effectiveness when learning technical and non-technical skills, in particular the detection of system weakness is easier if the simulation is conducted in situ [39].

CONCLUSION

A system with a strong culture of patient safety works to avoid errors and harm, learns of errors that do happen, is based on a culture that prioritizes safety, using strategies to improve it and encompasses the entire healthcare team [3].

Health Care systems are complex and patient safety systems, teamwork strategies, and medical simulation can improve outcomes and are recommended as part of comprehensive patient safety programs in obstetrics.

Safety is a never-ending process. Hospitals can build their integrated patient safety system - in which staff and leaders work together to eliminate complacency, promote collective mindfulness, treat each other with respect and compassion, and learn from patient safety events.

Simulation training for anesthesia in obstetrics is an important tool which can improve both individual technical and team performance. Multidisciplinary simulation training is of great importance for an optimal cooperation during obstetric emergencies.

CONSENT FOR PUBLICATION

Not applicable.

CONFLICT OF INTEREST

The authors declare no conflict of interest, financial or otherwise.

ACKNOWLEDGEMENT

Thanks to Dr. Jose Maria Maestre, Education Director at Valdecilla virtual Hospital, for his collaboration in the critical reading and his contributions to this manuscript.

REFERENCES

[1]   Smith A, Siassakos D, Crofts J, Draycott T. Simulation: Improving patient outcomes. Semin Perinatol 2013; 37(3): 151-6.
[http://dx.doi.org/10.1053/j.semperi.2013.02.005] [PMID: 23721770]

[2]   Institute of Medicine (US) Committee on Quality of Health Care in America. To Err is Human: Building a Safer Health System. Kohn L, Corrigan J, Donaldson M, editors. Washington, DC: National Academies Press 2000.

[3]   Pettker CM, Grobman WA. Obstetric Safety and Quality. Obstet Gynecol 2015; 126(1): 196-206.
[http://dx.doi.org/10.1097/AOG.0000000000000918] [PMID: 26241273]

[4]   Alkema L, Chou D, Hogan D, *et al.* Global, regional, and national levels and trends in maternal mortality between 1990 and 2015, with scenario-based projections to 2030: a systematic analysis by the UN Maternal Mortality Estimation Inter-Agency Group. Lancet 2016; 387(10017): 462-74.
[http://dx.doi.org/10.1016/S0140-6736(15)00838-7] [PMID: 26584737]

[5]   Paxton A, Maine D, Freedman L, Fry D, Lobis S. The evidence for emergency obstetric care. Int J Gynaecol Obstet 2005; 88(2): 181-93.
[http://dx.doi.org/10.1016/j.ijgo.2004.11.026] [PMID: 15694106]

[6]   Adegoke AA, van den Broek N. Skilled birth attendance-lessons learnt. BJOG 2009; 116 (Suppl. 1): 33-40.
[http://dx.doi.org/10.1111/j.1471-0528.2009.02336.x] [PMID: 19740170]

[7]   Holmer H, Oyerinde K, Meara JG, Gillies R, Liljestrand J, Hagander L. The global met need for emergency obstetric care: a systematic review. BJOG 2015; 122(2): 183-9.
[http://dx.doi.org/10.1111/1471-0528.13230] [PMID: 25546039]

[8]   World Health Organization, UNFPA, UNICEF, AMDD. Monitoring Emergency Obstetric Care: A Handbook. Geneva:World Health Organization 2009.

[9]   Ameh CA, Mdegela M, White S, van den Broek N. The effectiveness of training in emergency obstetric care: a systematic literature review. Health Policy Plan 2019; 34(4): 257-70.
[http://dx.doi.org/10.1093/heapol/czz028] [PMID: 31056670]

[10]   Banke-Thomas A, Wilson-Jones M, Madaj B, van den Broek N. Economic evaluation of emergency obstetric care training: a systematic review. BMC Pregnancy Childbirth 2017; 17(1): 403.
[http://dx.doi.org/10.1186/s12884-017-1586-z] [PMID: 29202731]

[11]   Collins KJ, Draycott TJ. Skills and drills: are they worth the effort? Obstetrics, Gynaecol Reprod Med 2015; 25(12): 372-4.
[http://dx.doi.org/10.1016/j.ogrm.2015.09.003]

[12]   Abir G, Mhyre J. Maternal mortality and the role of the obstetric anesthesiologist. Baillieres Best Pract Res Clin Anaesthesiol 2017; 31(1): 91-105.
[http://dx.doi.org/10.1016/j.bpa.2017.01.005] [PMID: 28625309]

[13]   Institute of Medicine. Crossing the Quality Chasm: A New Health System for the 21st Century. Washington DC: National Academy Press 2001.

[14]   Forster AJ, Fung I, Caughey S, *et al.* Adverse events detected by clinical surveillance on an obstetric service. Obstet Gynecol 2006; 108(5): 1073-83.
[http://dx.doi.org/10.1097/01.AOG.0000242565.28432.7c] [PMID: 17077227]

[15]   The Joint Commission. 2004.http://www.jointcommisssion.org/sentinel_event_alert_issue_30_preventing_infant_death_and_injury_during_delivery

[16]   https://www.ahrq.gov/teamstepps/longtermcare/index.html

[17]   Riley W, Davis S, Miller K, Hansen H, Sainfort F, Sweet R. Didactic and simulation nontechnical skills team training to improve perinatal patient outcomes in a community hospital. Jt Comm J Qual Patient Saf 2011; 37(8): 357-64.

[http://dx.doi.org/10.1016/S1553-7250(11)37046-8] [PMID: 21874971]

[18]   Draycott TJ, Crofts JF, Ash JP, *et al.* Improving neonatal outcome through practical shoulder dystocia training. Obstet Gynecol 2008; 112(1): 14-20.
[http://dx.doi.org/10.1097/AOG.0b013e31817bbc61] [PMID: 18591302]

[19]   Satin AJ. Simulation in Obstetrics. Obstet Gynecol 2018; 132(1): 199-209.
[http://dx.doi.org/10.1097/AOG.0000000000002682] [PMID: 29889745]

[20]   Martíinez-Pérez O, Cueto-Hernández I, Hernández-Pinto P, Odriozola-Feu J. Entrenamiento en Emergencias Obstétricas basado en Simulación. In: Martínez-Pérez OGAECHI, Ed. Manual Práctico de Emergencias Obstétricas 2015; 49-67.

[21]   Hernández Pinto P, Odriozola Feu JM, Maestre Alonso JM, López Sánchez M, Del Moral Vicente Mazariegos I, De Miguel Sesmero JR. Entrenamiento de equipos interdisciplinares en urgencias obstétricas mediante simulación clínica. Progresos de Obstetricia y Ginecología 2011; 54(12): 618-24.
[http://dx.doi.org/10.1016/j.pog.2011.05.009]

[22]   Nguyen N, Watson WD, Dominguez E. simulation-based communication training for general surgery and obstetrics and gynecology residents. J Surg Educ 2019; 76(3): 856-63.
[http://dx.doi.org/10.1016/j.jsurg.2018.10.014] [PMID: 30826262]

[23]   Kirkpatrick DL, Kirkpatrick JD. Implementing the Four Levels a Practical Guide for Effective Evaluation of Training Programs San Francisco: Berrett-Kochler Publishers 2007.

[24]   Ameh CA, White S, Dickinson F, Mdegela M, Madaj B, van den Broek N. Retention of knowledge and skills after Emergency Obstetric Care training: A multi-country longitudinal study. PLoS One 2018; 13(10): e0203606.
[http://dx.doi.org/10.1371/journal.pone.0203606] [PMID: 30286129]

[25]   Onwochei DN, Halpern S, Balki M. Teamwork Assessment Tools in Obstetric Emergencies. Simul Healthc 2017; 12(3): 165-76.
[http://dx.doi.org/10.1097/SIH.0000000000000210] [PMID: 28009653]

[26]   Lippke S, Wienert J, Keller FM, *et al.* Communication and patient safety in gynecology and obstetrics - study protocol of an intervention study. BMC Health Serv Res 2019; 19(1): 908.
[http://dx.doi.org/10.1186/s12913-019-4579-y] [PMID: 31779620]

[27]   Eichhorn JH. The Anesthesia Patient Safety Foundation at 25: a pioneering success in safety, 25th anniversary provokes reflection, anticipation. Anesth Analg 2012; 114(4): 791-800.
[http://dx.doi.org/10.1213/ANE.0b013e3182427536] [PMID: 22253277]

[28]   Sobhy S, Zamora J, Dharmarajah K, *et al.* Anaesthesia-related maternal mortality in low-income and middle-income countries: a systematic review and meta-analysis. Lancet Glob Health 2016; 4(5): e320-7.
[http://dx.doi.org/10.1016/S2214-109X(16)30003-1] [PMID: 27102195]

[29]   Birnbach DJ, Bateman BT. Obstetric Anesthesia. Obstet Gynecol Clin North Am 2019; 46(2): 329-37.
[http://dx.doi.org/10.1016/j.ogc.2019.01.015] [PMID: 31056134]

[30]   Rosen KR. The history of medical simulation. J Crit Care 2008; 23(2): 157-66.
[http://dx.doi.org/10.1016/j.jcrc.2007.12.004] [PMID: 18538206]

[31]   Boker AMA. Toward competency-based curriculum: Application of workplace-based assessment tools in the National Saudi Arabian Anesthesia training program. Saudi J Anaesth 2016; 10(4): 417-22.
[http://dx.doi.org/10.4103/1658-354X.179097] [PMID: 27833485]

[32]   Chiu M, Tarshis J, Antoniou A, *et al.* Simulation-based assessment of anesthesiology residents' competence: development and implementation of the Canadian National Anesthesiology Simulation Curriculum (CanNASC). Can J Anaesth 2016; 63(12): 1357-63.
[http://dx.doi.org/10.1007/s12630-016-0733-8] [PMID: 27638297]

[33]   Hoskote SS, Khouli H, Lanoix R, *et al.* Simulation-based training for emergency medicine residents in

sterile technique during central venous catheterization: impact on performance, policy, and outcomes. Acad Emerg Med 2015; 22(1): 81-7.
[http://dx.doi.org/10.1111/acem.12551] [PMID: 25556399]

[34]   Giglioli S, Boet S, De Gaudio AR, *et al*. Self-directed deliberate practice with virtual fiberoptic intubation improves initial skills for anesthesia residents. Minerva Anestesiol 2012; 78(4): 456-61.
[PMID: 22310190]

[35]   Barsuk JH, Cohen ER, Caprio T, McGaghie WC, Simuni T, Wayne DB. Simulation-based education with mastery learning improves residents' lumbar puncture skills. Neurology 2012; 79(2): 132-7.
[http://dx.doi.org/10.1212/WNL.0b013e31825dd39d] [PMID: 22675080]

[36]   Wayne DB, Barsuk JH, O'Leary KJ, Fudala MJ, McGaghie WC. Mastery learning of thoracentesis skills by internal medicine residents using simulation technology and deliberate practice. J Hosp Med 2008; 3(1): 48-54.
[http://dx.doi.org/10.1002/jhm.268] [PMID: 18257046]

[37]   Wayne DB, Butter J, Siddall VJ, *et al*. Mastery learning of advanced cardiac life support skills by internal medicine residents using simulation technology and deliberate practice. J Gen Intern Med 2006; 21(3): 251-6.
[http://dx.doi.org/10.1111/j.1525-1497.2006.00341.x] [PMID: 16637824]

[38]   Green M, Tariq R, Green P. Improving Patient Safety through Simulation Training in Anesthesiology: Where Are We? Anesthesiol Res Pract 2016; 2016: 1-12.
[http://dx.doi.org/10.1155/2016/4237523] [PMID: 26949389]

[39]   Schormack LA, Baysinger CL, Pian-Smith M. Recent advances of simulation in obstetric anesthesia. Curr Opin Anesthesiol. 2017; 30

[40]   Wenk M, Pöpping DM. Simulation for anesthesia in obstetrics. Baillieres Best Pract Res Clin Anaesthesiol 2015; 29(1): 81-6.
[http://dx.doi.org/10.1016/j.bpa.2015.01.003] [PMID: 25902469]

[41]   Rábago JL, López-Doueil M, Sancho R, *et al*. Evaluación de los resultados de aprendizaje de un curso de introducción a la anestesiología basado en simulación clínica. Rev Esp Anestesiol Reanim 2017; 64(8): 431-40.
[http://dx.doi.org/10.1016/j.redar.2016.12.008] [PMID: 28347552]

[42]   Vasco Ramírez M. Training future anesthesiologists in obstetric care. Curr Opin Anaesthesiol 2017; 30(3): 313-8.
[http://dx.doi.org/10.1097/ACO.0000000000000471] [PMID: 28306682]

[43]   Naik VN, Devito I, Halpern SH. Cusum analysis is a useful tool to assess resident proficiency at insertion of labour epidurals. Can J Anaesth 2003; 50(7): 694-8.
[http://dx.doi.org/10.1007/BF03018712] [PMID: 12944444]

[44]   Samuelson ST, Burnett G, Sim AJ, *et al*. Simulation as a set-up for technical proficiency: can a virtual warm-up improve live fibre-optic intubation? Br J Anaesth 2016; 116(3): 398-404.
[http://dx.doi.org/10.1093/bja/aev436] [PMID: 26821699]

[45]   Sancho R, Maestre JM, Del Moral I. Manejo de las crisis. Papel de la simulación en la seguridad del paciente. Rev Esp Anestesiol Reanim 2012; 59 (Suppl. 2): S53-9.

[46]   Gaba DM, Howard SK, Fish KJ, Smith BE, Sowb YA. Simulation-based training in anesthesia crisis resource management (ACRM): a decade of experience. Simul Gaming 2001; 32(2): 175-93.
[http://dx.doi.org/10.1177/104687810103200206]

[47]   Gaba DM. Human error in anesthetic mishaps. Int Anesthesiol Clin 1989; 27(3): 137-47.
[http://dx.doi.org/10.1097/00004311-198902730-00002] [PMID: 2670768]

[48]   Krage R, Erwteman M. State-of-the-art usage of simulation in anesthesia. Curr Opin Anaesthesiol 2015; 28(6): 727-34.
[http://dx.doi.org/10.1097/ACO.0000000000000257] [PMID: 26485205]

[49]   Shields LE, Wiesner S, Fulton J, Pelletreau B. Comprehensive maternal hemorrhage protocols reduce the use of blood products and improve patient safety. Am J Obstet Gynecol 2015; 212(3): 272-80.
[http://dx.doi.org/10.1016/j.ajog.2014.07.012] [PMID: 25025944]

[50]   Kolb D. Experiential learning: experience as the source of learning and development Englewood Cliffs, New Jersey: Prentice Hall 1984.

[51]   Maestre JM, Rudolph J. Teorías y estilos de debriefing: el método con buen juicio como herramienta de evaluación formativa en salud. [Spanish Edition]. Theories and Styles of Debriefing: the Good Judgment Approach as a Formative Assessment Tool in Healthcare. [English Edition]. Rev Esp Cardiol. 2015.68(4): 282-5.

[52]   Epstein RM. Assessment in medical education. N Engl J Med 2007; 356(4): 387-96.
[http://dx.doi.org/10.1056/NEJMra054784] [PMID: 17251535]

[53]   Marynen F, Van Gerven E, Van de Velde M. Simulation in obstetric anesthesia: an update. Curr Opin Anaesthesiol 2020; 33(3): 272-6.
[http://dx.doi.org/10.1097/ACO.0000000000000874] [PMID: 32371644]

[54]   Maestre JM, Pedraja J, Herrero L, *et al.* Simulación clínica para la mejora de la calidad en la atención a la hemorragia posparto. J Healthc Qual Res 2018; 33(2): 88-95.
[http://dx.doi.org/10.1016/j.jhqr.2018.01.002] [PMID: 31610983]

[55]   Cano M, Suarez C, Agüero B, Odriozola J, Mestre J. Evaluation of the quality improvement process in the care of massive postpartum hemorrhage. Prog Obstet Ginecol 2019; 62(3): 216-20.

CHAPTER 3

Airway Management in Pregnancy

Eugenio D. Martinez Hurtado[1,*], Laura Reviriego Agudo[2], Pedro Charco Mora[3], Miguel Ángel Fernández Vaquero[4] and María Gómez Rojo[5]

[1] *Department of Anaesthesiology and Intensive Care, University Hospital Infanta Leonor, Madrid, Spain*

[2] *Department of Anesthesiology and Intensive Care. Hospital Clínico Universitario, Valencia, Spain*

[3] *Department of Anesthesiology and Intensive Care, Hospital Universitario y Politécnico La Fe, Valencia, Spain*

[4] *Department of Anesthesiology and Critical Care, Clínica Universidad de Navarra, Madrid, Spain*

[5] *Department of Anesthesiology and Intensive Care. Hospital Ramon y Cajal, Madrid, Spain*

Abstract: Airway management in the obstetric patient is a challenge for anaesthesiologists, not only because of the anatomical and physiological changes during pregnancy, but also because of the surgery´s urgency, the location of the procedure, which sometimes takes place even outside the operation theatre, and also due to conflicts emerging between the needs of the mother and fetus. The arising maternal comorbidities such as obesity, contribute to complications in airway management in this population.

Keywords: Airway Management, Apnoeic Times, Cricothyroid Membrane, Difficult Airway, Difficult Intubation, Laryngoscopy, Maternal Death, Neuraxial Anesthetic Blocks, Predictors, Pregnant Patient, Pregnancy, Preeclampsia, Ultrasonography, Video Laryngoscopy.

INTRODUCTION

The rate of failed tracheal intubation in obstetrics has remained unchanged from 1970 to 2015 as demonstrated by reviewing the scientific literature. The incidence of failed tracheal intubation remains at 2.6 per 1,000 general anesthetics during obstetric procedures, and about 2.3 per 1,000 general anesthetics in case of cesarean section [1]. And, in case of tracheal intubation failure, it is usually

* **Corresponding author Eugenio D. Martínez Hurtado:** Department of Anesthesiology and Intensive Care. Hospital Universitario Infanta Leonor, Madrid, Spain; E-mail: emartinez@AnestesiaR.org

Eugenio Daniel Martinez-Hurtado, Monica Sanjuan-Alvarez & Marta Chacon-Castillo (Eds.)
All rights reserved-© 2022 Bentham Science Publishers

preferable to maintain general anesthesia using a rescue device rather than awakening the patient.

Pregnancy implies that a potentially life-threatening event will occur within 9 months, in addition to which the management of pregnant women is different from that of other patients in several respects. The most frequent cause of morbidity and mortality related to obstetric anesthesia is failure or difficulties in airway control after the induction of general anesthesia. Furthermore, the causes of this morbi-mortality are different from those of other surgical patients. Therefore, regional anesthesia is being used more and more frequently [2 - 5].

Although induction of a rapid sequence of general anesthesia and tracheal intubation is a standard of management, regional anesthesia is used in most cesarean sections [6 - 8]. Instead, if there is a primary airway pathology, delaying or modifying the treatment should be considered, in view of the fetal well-being and the evolution of the pregnancy [9].

However, although anesthetic procedures may be very different, technical aspects of airway management in pregnant are similar to that of non-pregnant. Therefore, multidisciplinary teamwork is essential, and should begin in the early stages of pregnancy or when an airway problem becomes apparent [10 - 12] (Fig **1**).

SPECIFIC CONSIDERATIONS OF THE OBSTETRIC AIRWAY

Anesthetic management of the obstetric patient has changed in the last years [13 - 15], but it was not until 2015 that the first specific obstetric difficult airway guidelines were published by the Obstetric Anaesthetists Association (*OAA*) and the Difficult Airway Society (*DAS*) [9].

Pregnant airway management is greatly modified by anatomical and physiological changes during pregnancy, predominantly in the third trimester, and remain up to 2-3 weeks after delivery.

Anatomic modifications include weight increase and enlargement of breasts. Upper airway mucosa becomes edematous and Mallampati score increases, not only along pregnancy, but also during labour and delivery [16]. This mucosa bleeds more easily as the vascularization increases, and makes nasal intubation more complicated. Other factors like preeclampsia, oxytocin therapy and fluid administration can increase swelling.

Among the physiological respiratory changes, it should be noted that the pregnant uterus produces a cephalic displacement of the diaphragm that progressively decreases the expiratory reserve volume, which makes pregnant more susceptible to hypoxemia and hypercapnia, causing shorter apnea times and facilitating earlier desaturation [17 - 22].

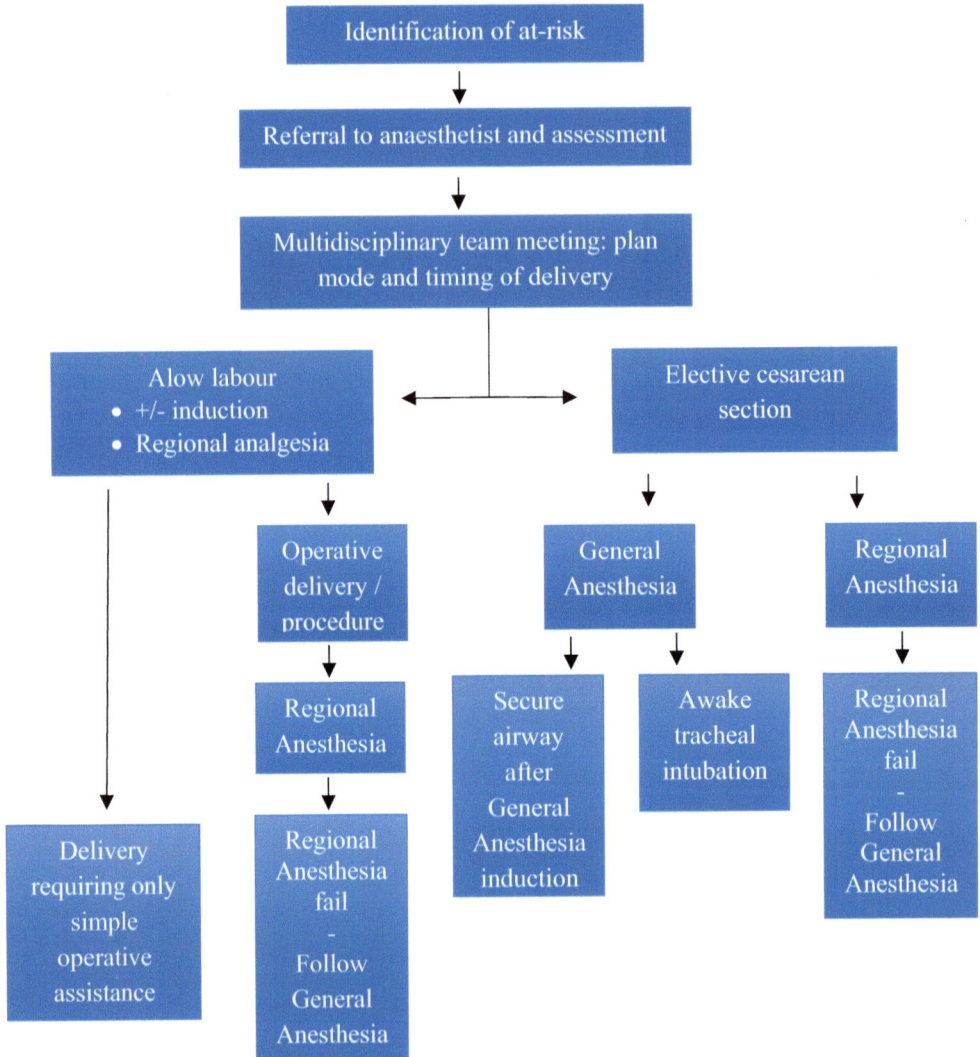

Fig. (1). Management of pregnant women with anticipated difficult airway.

The lower esophageal sphincter is relaxed, and gastric emptying is delayed by the action of progesterone. Increased gastric volume and hydrochloride production are due to placental secretion of gastrin.

Obesity, which is currently a health pandemic, can complicate airway management in pregnant women, as it has been shown that for every 1 kg/m2 increase in BMI, the risk of difficult intubation increases by 7% [23 - 26].

Maternal age and higher BMI are also associated with an increased risk of preeclampsia. This pathology of pregnancy is a specific risk factor for difficult airways due to increased edema and fragility of the oropharyngeal mucosa [27].

There are local and human factors as well, like the isolation of the obstetric ward, frequently located far from the surgical ward, the lack of equipment for management of the difficult airway and insufficient training and familiarity with the available equipment. These factors could be addressed simply by equipping the obstetric unit with its own airway management equipment.

Human factors include communication organization, decision-making process and staff behaviour in a high-stress situation. One of the major contributing factors to disaster in airway management is lack of training. Effective training improves dexterity in airway management [28 - 30].

SAFE GENERAL ANAESTHESIA IN THE OBSTETRIC PATIENT

Problems related to the airway management can be anticipated and minimised once the anatomical and physiological changes are known, and the proper anaesthetic technique has been chosen. To achieve safe management, adequate preparation and planning of the anesthetic strategy is the best practice to achieve adequate oxygenation in these patients.

Table 1. Considerations for the management of pregnant in whom airway management problems are anticipated.

- Appropriate identification of at-risk women by obstetric and midwifery staff when they present to the maternity service; especially cases that are otherwise low risk and who may normally follow a "low-intervention" pathway.
- Appropriate anaesthetic referral pathways for at-risk women who have been identified, to allow adequate time to assess the airway problem.
- Multidisciplinary team management that includes obstetric anaesthetists and obstetricians, and where appropriate, surgeons, physicians and intensivists.
- Consideration of the suitability of allowing labour.
- Consideration of approach to general anaesthesia (Fig 2).

Pre-Operative Evaluation

All pregnant women with a known or suspected difficult airway and with a history of anesthetic problems related to the airway, should be referred prenatally for an in-person anesthetic evaluation (Table 1). History in the medical record that may alert to a possible airway problem includes: head, neck or jaw surgery, mediastinal masses, morbid obesity, obstructive sleep apnoea (*OSA*), juvenile rheumatoid arthritis (*JRA*), and some congenital syndromes [31].

Even though there may be a narrow timeframe for the preoperatory assessment of obstetric patients as a result of urgent situations, the identification of a potentially difficult intubation should always be pursued by a thorough airway assessment [32]. In obstetric patients, preoperatory airway assessment should consider the following Table (**2**):

Table 2. Airway assessment in obstetric patients.

1. History of difficult airway management.
2. Overall face appearance, asymmetry, scars.
3. Mouth opening ability.
4. Length and shape of mandible, prognathism/retrognathia, jaw protrusion ability.
5. Neck movement (flexion / extension) and identification of cricothyroid membrane.

Several studies show that the positive predictive value of these tests is actually low [35]. Recently, in a comprehensive review, the authors concluded than in up to two-thirds of failed tracheal intubation cases in obstetric patients, airway was not supposedly difficult [1]. However, all obstetric patients should be subject to a preanesthetic airway predictors assessment to identify beforehand those cases in which the difficult airway (*DA*) algorithm should be applied.

1. *A history of difficult airway management*: a record of difficult tracheal intubation in prior anesthetic procedures is the most specific difficult airway (*DA*) predictor [9].
2. *Associated conditions such as obesity or preeclampsia/eclampsia syndrome*: Both are considered independent risk factors [33]. The risk for oropharyngeal obstruction is twofold in obese obstetric patients. Moreover, there is an increased risk for difficult face mask ventilation. A recent publication found a higher difficulty for orotracheal intubation in morbidly obese patients (>130 kg) [34].
3. *Anatomical factors associated to difficult or impossible intubation*: in order to properly assess an obstetric patient's airway, she should be sitting, and her airway should be assessed from the front and the side, always in the same order for the sake of completeness. First, from the front, we should apply the Mallampati classification, mouth opening ability (inter-incisor gap) and the upper-lip bite test and then, from her side, assess jaw protrusion, head and neck movement, thyromental distance (*TMD*), sternomental distance (*SMD*) and retrognathia.

Factors associated with intubation difficulty appear to be the same in the general obstetric population as in non-pregnant patients. These include a high Mallampati score, short neck, mandibular retrognathia, protrusion of the maxillary incisors [36], and a large neck circumference [37].

Difficult laryngoscopy and intubation prediction are not the only important questions, but also the evaluation of ventilation with face mask (*FMV*), insertion of supraglottic airway device (*SAD*) and emergency front-of-neck access [30]. They will help in choosing the appropriate device for airway management, formulate the corresponding rescue plan and involve the surgical team when necessary.

Any obstetric patient with anticipated difficult airway should be referred during her pregnancy to an obstetric designated hospital with staff trained in the management of this population's airway.

There are several bedside tests which can be used to assess the airway (Table **3**) such as the Mallampati test, cervical flexion-extension, temporo-mandibular joint function, inter-incisor gap < 3 cm., thyromental distance (*TMD*) < 6 cm., neck circumference and length, micrognathia and maxillofacial abnormalities.

Table 3. Variables and critical values with higher specific values for DL.

- Inter-incisor gap < 3 cm.
- Thyromental distance (*TMD*) < 6 cm.
- Mallampati Samsoon&Young ≥ 3
- Weight >120% ideal weight
- History of difficult airway management
- Neck flexion <80°
- Jaw protrusion impairment
- Failed upper lip bite test (score 3) [38]

Although the Mallampati-Samsoon classification is the most widely used, if used alone it is not an accurate method to identify difficult intubation/laryngoscopy [34]. Since difficult laryngoscopy and intubation have a multifactorial etiology, it seems reasonable to consider that a successful prediction necessarily includes the analysis of different tests, which will have an improved prediction value as a whole than when used alone. The most widely referenced is Adnet's intubation difficulty scale (*IDS*). Other tests with varying sensitivity and specificity are Janssen's and Hastey's classification, Wilson's test, El Ganzouri's test and of late, those by Ebehart and Basaronoglu. The combination of these tests has a higher positive predictive value than when used alone [30].

Higher body mass index (*BMI*), snorers, edentulous patients and age are independent risk factors for difficult face mask ventilation (*DMV*). The combination of two or more factors can significantly increase the risk of MVD or result in the impossibility of mask ventilation. Among obstetric patients, age, BMI and Mallampati score have been identified as independent factors for DMV [23].

It has been proven through Mallampati assessment at 12 and 38 weeks of pregnancy that the classification increases with gestation. Even during delivery, the score can escalate one point in up to 33% of patients and two points in 5% as to pre-delivery values [13]. This escalation can increase the risk for DL, particularly if concomitant with other factors such as a short neck, retrognathia, prominent maxillary incisors, loose dental work or morbid obesity [37]. During delivery we can also find edema of the airway mucosa, due to the existence of hypertensive disease of pregnancy, fluid retention, the antidiuretic effect of oxytocics and the efforts of labour itself. For all these reasons, airway assessment should be performed immediately before the anesthetic procedure in the anticipation of a real deterioration of airway conditions [32].

POINT-OF-CARE ULTRASOUND (POCUS) IN PREGNANCY

Complications during pregnancy are not frequent, but may occur brusquely. Point-of-care ultrasound (*PoCUS*) is an emerging tool which has many obvious benefits (safe, fast, repeatable, transportable, widely accessible and produces dynamic images in real time). It can be realised at the bed-side for patient safety when complications occur.

Ultrasonography is widely used in obstetric practice for fetal monitoring, and also allows for maternal diagnostic and screening procedures, so it is considered an extension of clinical evaluation [39]. Pregnancy is associated with an increased risk of aspiration of gastric contents and difficulty in airway management [30, 40].

Gastric Contents

Pregnant patients at term are considered high-risk for aspiration because of anatomical and physiological changes and the urgency of interventions. In addition, they have a higher chance of a difficult airway, which makes an aspiration event potentially catastrophic.

Rapid sequence induction with tracheal intubation has traditionally been recommended for obstetric general anesthesia because of the risk of regurgitation and pulmonary aspiration in non-fasting ("*full stomach*") pregnant women presenting for emergency surgery, as well as the reduction of lower esophageal sphincter tone during pregnancy. Gastric PoCUS allows the assessment of the stomach contents, both the actual volume and the nature of the stomach. This allows risk decisions to be made and thus aids in decision making [41].

The examination allows a qualitative quantification of the stomach, which will be defined as "*empty*" (flat antrum with juxtaposed anterior and posterior walls in both supine and right lateral decubitus), "*with fluid*" (distended antrum with thin walls and hypoechoic contents) or "*with solid food*" (distended antrum with mixed echogenicity contents). In quantitative analysis, quantification of gastric fluid volume is highlighted using the antrum cross-sectional area (*CSA*). The measurement is performed in the right lateral decubitus (*RLD*), and the area is measured including the entire antral wall thickness. The following mathematical model will be used: gastric volume (ml) = **27.0 + 14.6 x RLD CSA − 1.28 x age**.

This model was validated over a wide range of ages and weights of non-pregnant adults undergoing gastric emptying by endoscopic aspiration, demonstrating a prediction of gastric volume of up to 500 ml. Pregnant women weight at term was used to calculate gastric volumes by weight (mL kg^{-1}). The antrum was classified according to a 3-point grading system (Pearls grade 0e2) based on the presence or absence of clear fluid in the supine and RLD positions (clear fluid was defined as the presence of non-particulate anecogenic content) [42].

Difficult Airway

Recent Association of Obstetric Anesthesiologists/Difficult Airway Society guidelines for the management of difficult and failed tracheal intubation in obstetrics advise that an airway assessment should always be performed before performing induction of general anesthesia. This assessment is intended to predict not only difficult tracheal intubation, but also difficulties in the use of supraglottic devices, face mask ventilation, and surgical access to the frontal airway [9]. Pregnant women are at an increased risk for a difficult airway due to physical changes in the upper airway anatomy.

Airway assessment is the first step in avoiding potential complications, and should always be performed prior to airway management. However, assessment to predict potential intubation difficulties is not reliable. Studies show that ultrasonography may be useful as a predictor of difficult laryngoscopy, as it allows the measurement of anterior neck soft tissue thickness in non-obstetric patients [43]. Therefore, there are ongoing studies that aim to find out whether preoperative ultrasound assessment of neck anatomy can predict difficult airway in pregnant women [44].

Also, the use of ultrasound as an aid in surgical front-of-neck airway access techniques, a rescue technique performed in emergency "*can't intubate, can't oxygenate*" scenarios (1 in 60 failed intubations, approx.), is promising [1].

Identification of the cricothyroid membrane by digital palpation can be complicated, especially in obese non-pregnant and pregnant women [45]. This difficulty in locating it can lead to unsuccessful invasive procedures over the airway, with severe associated morbidity or even risk of death. Ultrasonography of the airway significantly increases the success rate of identification of this membrane compared to manual palpation [46]. In cadavers and mannequins with poorly identifiable airway anatomy, ultrasound has also been shown to improve the identification and performance of cricothyroidotomy.

Finally, we can check endotracheal intubation with airway PoCUS with two methods: directly or indirectly.

Directly at the suprasternal level has been described the TRUE PROTOCOL (Tracheal Rapid Ultrasound Exam). In this technique, the ultrasound probe is placed 1 centimetre above the sternal notch, showing the trachea and allowing the location of the esophagus (the patient can be requested to swallow), Keeping the probe at this level, and while a second operator performs the intubation, it is possible to distinguish sonographically whether an esophageal or tracheal intubation is performed [47]. Although capnography remains the gold standard for confirming orotracheal intubation, this technique would allow us also to assess an adequate intubation in patients before they are ventilated.

Indirectly, anaesthetist can look for bilateral lung sliding to determine that there is no selective intubation and in B and in M mode it can see the "*beach sign*". Although the diaphragmatic variability that occurs when starting ventilation must be taken into account [48].

Fasting and Antacid Prophylaxis

Pregnant women are at high risk of bronchial aspiration secondary to gastroesophageal reflux and delayed gastric emptying, which is why all women undergoing cesarean section are considered at risk of pulmonary aspiration, regardless of the fasting period. This aspiration may occur during intubation or extubation. Indeed, mortality is more likely during extubation rather than during anaesthesia induction [49].

Preparation for caesarean section includes a combination of H_2 antagonists on surgery's eve and two hours prior to surgery, with or without a prokinetic drug. Sodium citrate should be administered before induction. McDonell *et al.* reported high rates of antacid prophylaxis in elective cases, but just 64% in urgent caesarean section [50].

Planning and Preparation

The World Health Organization suggests the application of a checklist before every surgical intervention [51]. The obstetrician should inform the anaesthesiologists of all clinical and surgical details in every case. A second anaesthesiologist should be available for consultation if required. The team must be familiar with the advanced airway trolley and this trolley must be checked regularly. Airway equipment must include different sized laryngeal masks, oropharyngeal cannulas, an alternative laryngoscope with various blades, supraglottic devices, videolaryngoscope and cricothyroidotomy material.

Prior to induction, it is recommended to discuss potential airway problems and to plan airway management, including whether waking up the patient or not if tracheal intubation fails. Final decision depends on mother, foetus, medical team and clinical situation.

Preoxygenation

The reduced functional residual capacity and increased oxygen demand that occur physiologically during pregnancy lead to shorter apnea time and earlier desaturation in pregnant women. The aim of preoxygenation is to provide a sufficient oxygen reserve to the patient, so that apnoea is tolerated without desaturation before the airway can be secured.

Preoxygenation is an effective manoeuvre to extend apnoea time. This manoeuvre is considered successful if an end tidal O_2 above 90% is achieved [52]. Different preoxygenation techniques have been described, including breathing with tidal volume for 3 minutes or until an $ETO_2 > 0.9$ is achieved, or taking 4 to 8 deep breaths for 30 to 60 seconds.

Cricoid Pressure

Sellick first described cricoid pressure in 1961 [53 - 55], and, since then, it has become the routine technique during rapid sequence induction in patients at high risk of bronchoaspiration. It must be applied correctly [56 - 58].

Successful endotracheal intubation must be confirmed by capnography. Cricoid pressure can be terminated as soon as capnography has been detected and the endotracheal cuff inflated.

Face Mask Ventilation during Apnoea

Face mask ventilation in obstetric patients is currently recommended using pressure that does not exceed 20 cm H_2O and applying a correct cricoid pressure [30].

First Intubation Attempt

During the first intubation attempt, the priority is to achieve a high success rate with minimal damage to the airway. Direct laryngoscopy with a low diameter endotracheal tube fitted with a stylet is the gold standard to intubate obstetric patients [4].

The best way to confirm a correct endotracheal intubation is capnography. If intubation fails, face mask ventilation is recommended and a strategy and equipment for the second attempt should be prepared. To achieve this, the anaesthesiologist must have all familiar material available [4].

Second Intubation Attempt

After the first attempt failure, the anaesthesiologist should call for help from a more experienced clinician and should focus on the patient's oxygenation. Face mask ventilation with pressures below 20 cmH $_2O$ must be established. If necessary, an oropharyngeal cannula may be inserted or two-person mask ventilation can be applied. Cricoid pressure may be supressed in case it hinders face mask ventilation.

If face mask ventilation is successful, a second intubation attempt can be made, after optimizing the patient's position or reducing cricoid pressure.

In the presence of a Mallampati grade of IIIb or IV, success rates of blind intubation or intubation with a bougie are low, and airway damage risk is high, especially after multiple attempts.

The videolaryngoscope is gaining grounds in obstetric airway management strategy for this second attempt, and for some authors, its use should be included in the previous step [59 - 62].

FAILED TRACHEAL INTUBATION

Failure to intubate is defined as the impossibility to place an intratracheal tube after two laryngoscopies. If failed intubation happens, asking for help from a more experienced anesthesiologist is one of the priorities. The primary goal is to maintain the patient's oxygenation. Failure to oxygenate in these patients can lead to fetal distress.

Second-generation supraglottic devices are generally recommended in this point, since they allow for gastric aspiration and seal the airway better if positive pressure ventilation is used [63]. The laryngeal mask pressure must not be over 60 cm H2O [64]. It is recommended a maximum of two attempts when placing the supraglottic device to minimize the traumatism to the airway [30]. If the first device used does not seal the airway properly, a different size or a new device must be used.

CAN´T INTUBATE, CAN´T OXYGENATE

Oxigenation failure is a critical situation, which demands an emergent management. The team should call for help and put the patient in cricothyroidotomy position. The equipment needed for a surgical approach should be readily available after the second supraglottic device insertion attempt. Ultrasound is helpful in identifying the cricothyroid membrane, but its use in an emergency situation remains limited [65]. Cricothyroidotomy failure can result in maternal arrest.

AWAKEN PATIENT *VS* CONTINUE SURGERY

If awakening has been chosen, oxygenation should be maintained, while avoiding vomiting and regurgitation.

If the decision is continuing surgery, and thus general anaesthesia, several factors should be considered: proper device election, ventilation and anaesthesia maintenance strategies, cricoid pressure, gastric content aspiration and an intubation plan if necessary.

EXTUBATION

Any extubation must be considered as a potential reintubation, especially if it is a difficult airway case. Airway related problems that appear during extubation and immediate postoperative period are often due to insufficient monitoring and residual neuromuscular blockade [66]. NAP4 study revealed that up to 30% of anesthesia-related adverse events occurred at the end of anesthesia or during patient awakening [67, 68].

To achieve a successful extubation, proper planning and preparation must be done and all necessary equipment and staff must be available in case reintubation is required [69].

UNANTICIPATED DIFFICULT AIRWAY IN OBSTETRIC PATIENTS

The following recommendations refer to the action sequence for an obstetric patient scheduled for elective or emergent cesarean section who, after an appropriate preoperatory assessment, presents no predictors for difficult intubation. If this were the case, regional techniques or awake intubation should be performed [32].

The efficient and secure management of unplanned difficult airway in obstetric patients (most frequently in emergency situations) requires the application of standardized and predetermined algorithms, same as for non-obstetric patients [9, 32, 33]. These should include airway management techniques that have greatly advanced in recent decades, supraglottic airway devices (*SAD*) and, most recently, videolaryngoscopes. Equally important are human factors such as team communication and stress responsiveness.

Decision-making for difficult airway management in obstetric patients rests on the capacity of maternal oxygenation and fetal wellbeing. When fetal extraction is compulsory, surgical discontinuation will not be an option.

The initial intubation plan for obstetric patients must include the usual measures of rapid-sequence induction and intubation (*RSI*) (see Table **4**).

Table 4. Timeframe for rapid sequence induction and intubation.

1. Planning and Preparation (- 10 min).
2. Pre-induction: - Preoxygenation (- 5 min). - Premedication (- 3 min).
4. Apnea (± 1 min): - Induction (Paralysis and simultaneous loss of consciousness): 0 min. - Patient positioning and cricoid pressure +20 seg. - Laryngoscopy: +45-60 seg. - Intubation: <1 min.
5. Intubation confirmation (auscultation and capnography).
6. Post-intubation.

Despite direct laryngoscopy remains the gold-standard for tracheal intubation in obstetric patients, the current development and extensive use of videolaryngoscopy would suggest considering this the initial approach to tracheal intubation, although its use is the obstetric population still is exceptional (DREAMY study <1.9%) [33, 70, 71].

Upon a first failed attempt of intubation, light mask ventilation should be performed while evaluating efficient oxygenation and preparing for the second attempt. The most experienced anesthesiologist should be consulted as soon as a difficult airway is suspected or identified. If oxygenation is adequate, a second intubation attempt may be attempted after performing appropriate optimization manoeuvres (Table **5**).

Table 5. Intubation optimization manoeuvres.

Patient
- Improved positioning. - External manipulation of head, neck and larynx. - Adequate aspiration device. - Muscular tone (deeper neuromuscular blockade).
Technique
- Videolaryngoscopy. - Consider change of device. - Consider change of blade (type or size). - Bougie. - Most experienced anesthesiologist

At this point, if it was not used before, a videolaryngoscope (*VL*) with a difficult intubation blade is preferred [32]. VL improve glottic visualization and ease of intubation in most difficult cases. We should perform this second and last attempt after careful and appropriate optimization. In the scenario of a repeated failed intubation, a CAN'T INTUBATE situation should be openly declared. If facemask ventilation remains easy and there is no fetal compromise, surgery should be terminated, and the patient awakened. Cricoid pressure should be applied during the whole procedure, and it is recommended that the patient be positioned slightly towards her left side. Once conscience is regained, the recommended intubation technique would be awake fibre-optic intubation (*AFOI*) [9, 72, 73].

If there is fetal compromise that requires continuation of the surgical procedure, and the oxygenation is convenient, C-section can be carried out with facemask ventilation or by means of a supraglottic airway device (*SAD*) to set the anesthesiologist's hands free. At this point, the priority will be to ensure appropriate oxygenation and avoid pulmonary aspiration.

We should use a SAD if oxygenation cannot be ensured with a face mask (SO_2 <90%). Classical laryngeal masks are the most widely used device according to several studies [1]. However, currently we should consider their capacity to protect against potential aspiration and to ensure optimal ventilation (with higher sealing pressures), and therefore second-generation SAD are a must, which can also be used for fibre-optic intubation.

If adequate oxygenation cannot be maintained by face mask or SAD, a *"can't intubate, can't oxygenate"* scenario should be clearly communicated. Rescue will then proceed with surgical front-of-neck airway access (cricothyrotomy). Although all front-of neck access techniques are not exempt from risks, this should not delay attempts to re-establish oxygenation since this is the most important complication after the onset of hypoxia [9].

Nevertheless, in the event that oxygenation cannot be adequately restored and cardiac arrest occurs in the pregnant woman of more than 20 weeks' gestation, a perimortem cesarean section will be performed within 5 minutes of cardiac arrest. This allows, on one hand, optimization of advanced life support techniques by improving hemodynamic and respiratory conditions and on the other, independent fetal CPR.

For critical situations in Anesthesiology, such as an unanticipated difficult airway, simulation-based training is becoming increasingly important to learn a coordinated and effective action sequence. The VORTEX model described by N. Chrimes [74 - 76] is a cognitive aid that allows the application of an orderly sequence of actions and devices in order to overcome the difficulty in achieving adequate oxygenation. It counts upon widely used devices such as ordinary facemask ventilation, tracheal intubation, SADs and rescue front-of neck access via cricothyrotomy. It passes from one to another as to employ the most convenient in each situation until the problem is overcome, with a maximum of three attempts per device and optimization manoeuvres (Table **5**). After achieving adequate oxygenation, it is necessary to stop and consider the next step, to better reach the resolution of the crisis situation.

ANTICIPATED DIFFICULT AIRWAY DURING OBSTETRIC GENERAL ANAESTHESIA

In some patients, an elective caesarean section may be indicated because of the possibility of a very difficult airway management in the event that an emergency caesarean section is needed [73, 77, 78].

When planning an elective cesarean section, the contingency that an emergency cesarean section may be required after early onset of labour or because of obstetric complications should also be anticipated. Some units will have facilities to be able to perform awake intubation with fibrobronchoscope after hours (usually considered the safest method for treating the woman with extreme airway difficulties). However, even in skilled hands, the time required is likely to be significantly longer than for rapid sequence induction [79].

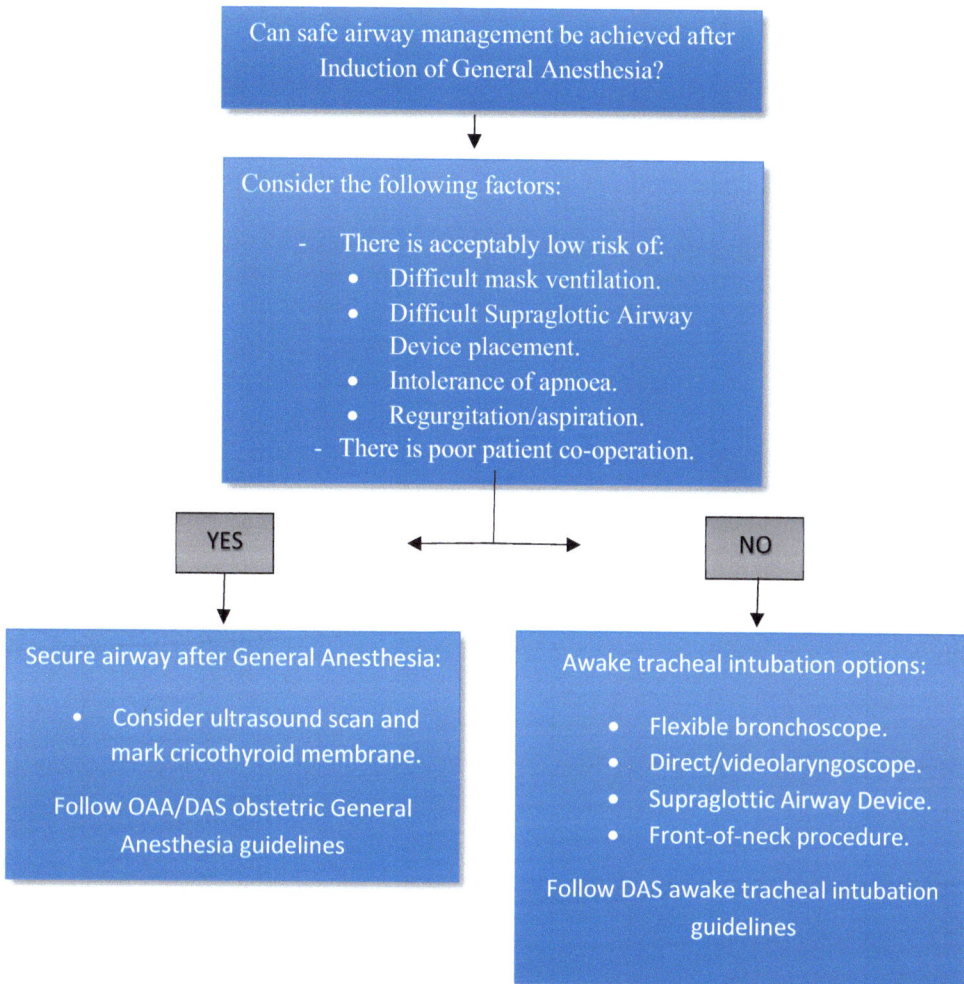

Fig. (2). General anaesthetic approach for pregnant women with anticipated difficult.

In addition, pregnant women with an expected difficult airway may also have anatomic or physiologic features that make regional anesthesia difficult or impossible. Therefore, one must anticipate the potential failure of regional anesthesia, something that could include: ultrasound and marking of cricothyroid membrane, local anaesthetic application, flexible nasendoscopy, awake direct or indirect laryngoscopy. If primary or secondary general anaesthesia is required (*i.e.* after failed regional), the first question will be to decide whether anesthesia will be induced before or after securing the airway (Fig **2**).

Awake fiberoptic intubation (*AFOI*) is probably the safest option for managing the anticipated difficult airway, particularly if difficult or impossible mask ventilation is also anticipated [67].

Preparation and performance of awake tracheal intubation [80] include: procedure preparation, oxygenation, airway topicalization, sedation (if necessary), and performance of an awake tracheal intubation technique. This technique may be modified for special circumstances, such as in the pregnant woman.

AFOI is especially indicated if there is a restricted mouth opening or distorted oropharyngeal passage. However, the disadvantages are the presence of blood or secretions in the airway, or the limited time [69].

Quite possibly video laryngoscopy will end up being the intubation technique of choice after induction of general anesthesia in the woman with an anticipated difficult airway. This will be compounded by the increasing availability of high-flow nasal oxygenation in anesthesia in general, and specifically in the delivery room. Videolaryngoscopes have been repeatedly suggested as a first-line instrument for routine intubation [81], and are gaining popularity as an awake technique for assessing the airway or intubating [82].

Women who are scheduled for airway surgery in addition to cesarean section, or in whom extracorporeal oxygenation methods are planned, may be required to deliver in a different unit, such as a cardiothoracic centre [83 - 86], or an operating room away from the delivery room [87].

CONCLUSION

The different anatomical and physiological changes that occur during pregnancy increase the frequency of difficulties that may arise during airway management. General anesthesia plays an essential role in obstetric surgery when the case is urgent, as well as when regional anesthesia is contraindicated, or it fails. Obstetric airway management is a unique area that requires teamwork between the gynecologist, neonatologist, and the anesthesiologist. We need to get acquainted with the available equipment in our facility, especially with second-generation supraglottic devices. The anesthesiologist must be specifically prepared to manage the event of a difficult airway in these patients. For that, the specialist in anesthesiology needs to verify his equipment and to continue learning about all devices, old and new, that are mentioned in the clinical algorithms.

CONSENT FOR PUBLICATION

Not applicable.

CONFLICT OF INTEREST

The authors declare no conflict of interest, financial or otherwise.

ACKNOWLEDGEMENT

Declared none.

REFERENCES

[1]   Kinsella SM, Winton AL, Mushambi MC, *et al.* Failed tracheal intubation during obstetric general anaesthesia: a literature review. Int J Obstet Anesth 2015; 24(4): 356-74.
        [http://dx.doi.org/10.1016/j.ijoa.2015.06.008] [PMID: 26303751]

[2]   Sumikura H, Niwa H, Sato M, Nakamoto T, Asai T, Hagihira S. Rethinking general anesthesia for cesarean section. J Anesth 2016; 30(2): 268-73.
        [http://dx.doi.org/10.1007/s00540-015-2099-4] [PMID: 26585767]

[3]   Biro P. Difficult intubation in pregnancy. Curr Opin Anaesthesiol 2011; 24(3): 249-54.
        [http://dx.doi.org/10.1097/ACO.0b013e328345ace3] [PMID: 21451403]

[4]   Mhyre JM, Healy D. The unanticipated difficult intubation in obstetrics. Anesth Analg 2011; 112(3): 648-52.
        [http://dx.doi.org/10.1213/ANE.0b013e31820a91a6] [PMID: 21350228]

[5]   Cooper GM, McClure JH. Anaesthesia chapter from Saving Mothers' Lives; reviewing maternal deaths to make pregnancy safer. Br J Anaesth 2008; 100(1): 17-22.
        [http://dx.doi.org/10.1093/bja/aem344] [PMID: 18070784]

[6]   Williamson RM, Mallaiah S, Barclay P. Rocuronium and sugammadex for rapid sequence induction of obstetric general anaesthesia. Acta Anaesthesiol Scand 2011; 55(6): 694-9.
        [http://dx.doi.org/10.1111/j.1399-6576.2011.02431.x] [PMID: 21480829]

[7]   Kessell G, Trapp JN. Rocuronium and sugammadex for rapid sequence induction of obstetric general anaesthesia. Acta Anaesthesiol Scand 2012; 56(3): 394.
        [http://dx.doi.org/10.1111/j.1399-6576.2011.02530.x] [PMID: 22221068]

[8]   Devroe S, Van de Velde M, Rex S. General anesthesia for caesarean section. Curr Opin Anaesthesiol 2015; 28(3): 240-6.
        [http://dx.doi.org/10.1097/ACO.0000000000000185] [PMID: 25827280]

[9]   Mushambi MC, Kinsella SM, Popat M, *et al.* Obstetric Anaesthetists' Association and Difficult Airway Society guidelines for the management of difficult and failed tracheal intubation in obstetrics. Anaesthesia 2015; 70(11): 1286-306.
        [http://dx.doi.org/10.1111/anae.13260] [PMID: 26449292]

[10]   Onwochei DN, Halpern S, Balki M. Teamwork assessment tools in obstetric emergencies. Simul Healthc 2017; 12(3): 165-76.
        [http://dx.doi.org/10.1097/SIH.0000000000000210] [PMID: 28009653]

[11]   Dillon SJ, Kleinmann W, Seasely A, *et al.* How personality affects teamwork: a study in multidisciplinary obstetrical simulation. Am J Obstet Gynecol MFM 2021; 3(2): 100303.
        [http://dx.doi.org/10.1016/j.ajogmf.2020.100303] [PMID: 33383231]

[12]   Shroff R, Thompson ACD, McCrum A, Rees SGO. Prospective multidisciplinary audit of obstetric general anaesthesia in a District General Hospital. J Obstet Gynaecol 2004; 24(6): 641-6.
        [http://dx.doi.org/10.1080/01443610400007877] [PMID: 16147603]

[13]   Kodali BS, Chandrasekhar S, Bulich LN, Topulos GP, Datta S. Airway changes during labor and delivery. Anesthesiology 2008; 108(3): 357-62.

[http://dx.doi.org/10.1097/ALN.0b013e31816452d3] [PMID: 18292672]

[14]   Plaat F, Wray S. Role of the anaesthetist in obstetric critical care. Best Pract Res Clin Obstet Gynaecol 2008; 22(5): 917-35.
[http://dx.doi.org/10.1016/j.bpobgyn.2008.06.006] [PMID: 18723402]

[15]   Hess PE. What's New in Obstetric Anesthesia. Anesth Analg 2017; 124(3): 863-71.
[http://dx.doi.org/10.1213/ANE.0000000000001681] [PMID: 28212182]

[16]   Boutonnet M, Faitot V, Katz A, Salomon L, Keita H. Mallampati class changes during pregnancy, labour, and after delivery: can these be predicted? Br J Anaesth 2010; 104(1): 67-70.
[http://dx.doi.org/10.1093/bja/aep356] [PMID: 20007793]

[17]   Cheung KL, Lafayette RA. Renal physiology of pregnancy. Adv Chronic Kidney Dis 2013; 20(3): 209-14.
[http://dx.doi.org/10.1053/j.ackd.2013.01.012] [PMID: 23928384]

[18]   Kepley JM, Bates K, Mohiuddin SS. Physiology, Maternal Changes. En: StatPearls [Internet]. Treasure Island (FL): StatPearls Publishing; 2021.

[19]   Tan EK, Tan EL. Alterations in physiology and anatomy during pregnancy. Best Pract Res Clin Obstet Gynaecol 2013; 27(6): 791-802.
[http://dx.doi.org/10.1016/j.bpobgyn.2013.08.001] [PMID: 24012425]

[20]   Hill CC, Pickinpaugh J. Physiologic changes in pregnancy. Surg Clin North Am 2008; 88(2): 391-401, vii.
[http://dx.doi.org/10.1016/j.suc.2007.12.005] [PMID: 18381119]

[21]   Costantine MM. Physiologic and pharmacokinetic changes in pregnancy. Front Pharmacol 2014; 5: 65.
[http://dx.doi.org/10.3389/fphar.2014.00065] [PMID: 24772083]

[22]   Frederiksen MC. Physiologic changes in pregnancy and their effect on drug disposition. Semin Perinatol 2001; 25(3): 120-3.
[http://dx.doi.org/10.1053/sper.2001.24565] [PMID: 11453606]

[23]   Quinn AC, Milne D, Columb M, Gorton H, Knight M. Failed tracheal intubation in obstetric anaesthesia: 2 yr national case–control study in the UK. Br J Anaesth 2013; 110(1): 74-80.
[http://dx.doi.org/10.1093/bja/aes320] [PMID: 22986421]

[24]   Wang T, Sun S, Huang S. The association of body mass index with difficult tracheal intubation management by direct laryngoscopy: a meta-analysis. BMC Anesthesiol 2018; 18(1): 79.
[http://dx.doi.org/10.1186/s12871-018-0534-4] [PMID: 29960594]

[25]   Uribe AA, Zvara DA, Puente EG, Otey AJ, Zhang J, Bergese SD. BMI as a Predictor for Potential Difficult Tracheal Intubation in Males. Front Med (Lausanne) 2015; 2: 38.
[http://dx.doi.org/10.3389/fmed.2015.00038] [PMID: 26137460]

[26]   Sinha A, Jayaraman L, Punhani D. Predictors of difficult airway in the obese are closely related to safe apnea time! J Anaesthesiol Clin Pharmacol 2020; 36(1): 25-30.
[http://dx.doi.org/10.4103/joacp.JOACP_164_19] [PMID: 32174653]

[27]   Izci B, Riha RL, Martin SE, *et al.* The upper airway in pregnancy and pre-eclampsia. Am J Respir Crit Care Med 2003; 167(2): 137-40.
[http://dx.doi.org/10.1164/rccm.200206-590OC] [PMID: 12411285]

[28]   Preston R, Jee R. Obstetric airway management. Int Anesthesiol Clin 2014; 52(2): 1-28.
[http://dx.doi.org/10.1097/AIA.0000000000000014] [PMID: 24667446]

[29]   Rucklidge MWM, Yentis SM. Obstetric difficult airway guidelines - decision-making in critical situations. Anaesthesia 2015; 70(11): 1221-5.
[http://dx.doi.org/10.1111/anae.13259] [PMID: 26449291]

[30]   Mushambi MC, Jaladi S. Airway management and training in obstetric anaesthesia. Curr Opin

Anaesthesiol 2016; 29(3): 261-7.
[http://dx.doi.org/10.1097/ACO.0000000000000309] [PMID: 26844863]

[31] Orphan Anaesthesia. Orphan Anaesthesia. A project of the German Society of Anesthesiology and Intensive Care Medicine. 2019.

[32] Mushambi MC, Athanassoglou V, Kinsella SM. Anticipated difficult airway during obstetric general anaesthesia: narrative literature review and management recommendations. Anaesthesia 2020; 75(7): 945-61.
[http://dx.doi.org/10.1111/anae.15007] [PMID: 32144770]

[33] Odor PM, Bampoe S, Moonesinghe SR, *et al.* General anaesthetic and airway management practice for obstetric surgery in England: a prospective, multicentre observational study. Anaesthesia 2021; 76(4): 460-71.
[http://dx.doi.org/10.1111/anae.15250] [PMID: 32959372]

[34] Hood DD, Dewan DM. Anesthetic and obstetric outcome in morbidly obese parturients. Anesthesiology 1993; 79(6): 1210-8.
[http://dx.doi.org/10.1097/00000542-199312000-00011] [PMID: 8267196]

[35] Nørskov AK, Rosenstock CV, Wetterslev J, Astrup G, Afshari A, Lundstrøm LH. Diagnostic accuracy of anaesthesiologists' prediction of difficult airway management in daily clinical practice: a cohort study of 188 064 patients registered in the Danish Anaesthesia Database. Anaesthesia 2015; 70(3): 272-81.
[http://dx.doi.org/10.1111/anae.12955] [PMID: 25511370]

[36] Riad W, Ansari T, Shetty N. Does neck circumference help to predict difficult intubation in obstetric patients? A prospective observational study. Saudi J Anaesth 2018; 12(1): 77-81.
[http://dx.doi.org/10.4103/sja.SJA_385_17] [PMID: 29416461]

[37] Rocke DA, Murray WB, Rout CC, Gouws E. Relative risk analysis of factors associated with difficult intubation in obstetric anesthesia. Anesthesiology 1992; 77(1): 67-73.
[http://dx.doi.org/10.1097/00000542-199207000-00010] [PMID: 1610011]

[38] Khan ZH, Kashfi A, Ebrahimkhani E. A comparison of the upper lip bite test (a simple new technique) with modified Mallampati classification in predicting difficulty in endotracheal intubation: a prospective blinded study. Anesth Analg 2003; 96(2): 595-9.
[http://dx.doi.org/10.1213/00000539-200302000-00053] [PMID: 12538218]

[39] Zieleskiewicz L, Pierrou C, Ragonnet B, *et al.* Pré-éclampsie sévère et hémorragie post-partum: apport de l'échographie « corps entier ». Can J Anaesth 2013; 60(8): 796-802.
[http://dx.doi.org/10.1007/s12630-013-9967-x]

[40] de Souza DG, Doar LH, Mehta SH, Tiouririne M. Aspiration prophylaxis and rapid sequence induction for elective cesarean delivery: time to reassess old dogma? Anesth Analg 2010; 110(5): 1503-5.
[http://dx.doi.org/10.1213/ANE.0b013e3181d7e33c] [PMID: 20418311]

[41] Van de Putte P, Perlas A. The link between gastric volume and aspiration risk. In search of the Holy Grail? Anaesthesia 2018; 73(3): 274-9.
[http://dx.doi.org/10.1111/anae.14164] [PMID: 29265172]

[42] Perlas A, Mitsakakis N, Liu L, *et al.* Validation of a mathematical model for ultrasound assessment of gastric volume by gastroscopic examination. Anesth Analg 2013; 116(2): 357-63.
[http://dx.doi.org/10.1213/ANE.0b013e318274fc19] [PMID: 23302981]

[43] Fulkerson JS, Moore HM, Anderson TS, Lowe RF Jr. Ultrasonography in the preoperative difficult airway assessment. J Clin Monit Comput 2017; 31(3): 513-30.
[http://dx.doi.org/10.1007/s10877-016-9888-7] [PMID: 27156094]

[44] Zheng BX, Zheng H, Lin XM. Ultrasound for predicting difficult airway in obstetric anesthesia. Medicine (Baltimore) 2019; 98(46): e17846.

[http://dx.doi.org/10.1097/MD.0000000000017846] [PMID: 31725624]

[45] You-Ten KE, Desai D, Postonogova T, Siddiqui N. Accuracy of conventional digital palpation and ultrasound of the cricothyroid membrane in obese women in labour. Anaesthesia 2015; 70: 11.
[http://dx.doi.org/10.1111/anae.13167] [PMID: 26186092]

[46] Kristensen MS, Teoh WH, Rudolph SS. Ultrasonographic identification of the cricothyroid membrane: best evidence, techniques, and clinical impact. Br J Anaesth 2016; 117 (Suppl. 1): i39-48.
[http://dx.doi.org/10.1093/bja/aew176] [PMID: 27432055]

[47] Chou HC, Tseng WP, Wang CH, *et al.* Tracheal rapid ultrasound exam (T.R.U.E.) for confirming endotracheal tube placement during emergency intubation. Resuscitation 2011; 82(10): 1279-84.
[http://dx.doi.org/10.1016/j.resuscitation.2011.05.016] [PMID: 21684668]

[48] Weaver B, Lyon M, Blaivas M. Confirmation of endotracheal tube placement after intubation using the ultrasound sliding lung sign. Acad Emerg Med 2006; 13(3): 239-44.
[http://dx.doi.org/10.1197/j.aem.2005.08.014] [PMID: 16495415]

[49] Warner MA, Warner ME, Weber JG. Clinical significance of pulmonary aspiration during the perioperative period. Anesthesiology 1993; 78(1): 56-62.
[http://dx.doi.org/10.1097/00000542-199301000-00010] [PMID: 8424572]

[50] McDonnell NJ, Paech MJ, Clavisi OM, Scott KL. Difficult and failed intubation in obstetric anaesthesia: an observational study of airway management and complications associated with general anaesthesia for caesarean section. Int J Obstet Anesth 2008; 17(4): 292-7.
[http://dx.doi.org/10.1016/j.ijoa.2008.01.017] [PMID: 18617389]

[51] Haynes AB, Weiser TG, Berry WR, *et al.* A surgical safety checklist to reduce morbidity and mortality in a global population. N Engl J Med 2009; 360(5): 491-9.
[http://dx.doi.org/10.1056/NEJMsa0810119] [PMID: 19144931]

[52] Russell EC, Wrench I, Feast M, Mohammed F. Pre-oxygenation in pregnancy: the effect of fresh gas flow rates within a circle breathing system. Anaesthesia 2008; 63(8): 833-6.
[http://dx.doi.org/10.1111/j.1365-2044.2008.05502.x] [PMID: 18518865]

[53] Sellick BA. Cricoid pressure to control regurgitation of stomach contents during induction of anaesthesia. Lancet 1961; 278(7199): 404-6.
[http://dx.doi.org/10.1016/S0140-6736(61)92485-0] [PMID: 13749923]

[54] Ovassapian A, Salem MR. Sellick's maneuver: to do or not do. Anesth Analg 2009; 109(5): 1360-2.
[http://dx.doi.org/10.1213/ANE.0b013e3181b763c0] [PMID: 19843769]

[55] Birenbaum A, Hajage D, Roche S, *et al.* Effect of cricoid pressure compared with a sham procedure in the rapid sequence induction of anesthesia. jama surg 2019; 154(1): 9-17.
[http://dx.doi.org/10.1001/jamasurg.2018.3577] [PMID: 30347104]

[56] Connor CW, Saffary R, Feliz E. Performance of the Sellick maneuver significantly improves when residents and trained nurses use a visually interactive guidance device in simulation. Physiol Meas 2013; 34(12): 1645-56.
[http://dx.doi.org/10.1088/0967-3334/34/12/1645] [PMID: 24201217]

[57] Baker RD, Taylor RJ, Smurthwaite G, Kitchen GB, Mehmood I. Analysing deviation-from-target data: applying the correct force in sellick's maneuver. J biopharm stat 2015; 25(4): 619-34.
[http://dx.doi.org/10.1080/10543406.2014.920872] [PMID: 24906015]

[58] Hee HI, Wong CL, Wijeweera O, Sultana R, Sng BL. Sellick maneuver assisted real-time to achieve target force range in simulated environment—A prospective observational cross-sectional study on manikin. PLoS One 2020; 15(2): e0227805.
[http://dx.doi.org/10.1371/journal.pone.0227805] [PMID: 32045936]

[59] Stopar Pintaric T, Blajic I, Hodzovic I. Comparing videolaryngoscopes with direct laryngoscopy in obstetric patients. Int J Obstet Anesth 2020; 41: 119-20.
[http://dx.doi.org/10.1016/j.ijoa.2019.07.007] [PMID: 31445792]

[60]   Liu S-H, Shao L-J-Z, Xue F-S. Comparing videolaryngoscopes with direct laryngoscopy in obstetric patients. Int J Obstet Anesth 2020; 41: 118-9.
[http://dx.doi.org/10.1016/j.ijoa.2019.07.008] [PMID: 31445789]

[61]   Cook TM, Kelly FE. A national survey of videolaryngoscopy in the United Kingdom. Br J Anaesth 2017; 118(4): 593-600.
[http://dx.doi.org/10.1093/bja/aex052] [PMID: 28403414]

[62]   Howle R, Onwochei D, Harrison SL, Desai N. Comparison of videolaryngoscopy and direct laryngoscopy for tracheal intubation in obstetrics: a mixed-methods systematic review and meta-analysis. Can J Anaesth 2021; 68(4): 546-65.
[http://dx.doi.org/10.1007/s12630-020-01908-w] [PMID: 33438172]

[63]   Cook TM, Kelly FE. Time to abandon the 'vintage' laryngeal mask airway and adopt second-generation supraglottic airway devices as first choice. Br J Anaesth 2015; 115(4): 497-9.
[http://dx.doi.org/10.1093/bja/aev156] [PMID: 25995266]

[64]   Bick E, Bailes I, Patel A, Brain AIJ. Fewer sore throats and a better seal: why routine manometry for laryngeal mask airways must become the standard of care. Anaesthesia 2014; 69(12): 1304-8.
[http://dx.doi.org/10.1111/anae.12902] [PMID: 25303083]

[65]   Kristensen MS, Teoh WHL, Baker PA. Percutaneous emergency airway access; prevention, preparation, technique and training. Br J Anaesth 2015; 114(3): 357-61.
[http://dx.doi.org/10.1093/bja/aev029] [PMID: 25694555]

[66]   Douglas MJ, Preston RL. The obstetric airway: things are seldom as they seem. Can J Anaesth 2011; 58(6): 494-8.
[http://dx.doi.org/10.1007/s12630-011-9492-8] [PMID: 21455646]

[67]   Cook TM, Woodall N, Frerk C. Major complications of airway management in the UK: results of the Fourth National Audit Project of the Royal College of Anaesthetists and the Difficult Airway Society. Part 1: Anaesthesia. Br J Anaesth 2011; 106(5): 617-31.
[http://dx.doi.org/10.1093/bja/aer058] [PMID: 21447488]

[68]   Cook TM, Woodall N, Harper J, Benger J. Major complications of airway management in the UK: results of the Fourth National Audit Project of the Royal College of Anaesthetists and the Difficult Airway Society. Part 2: intensive care and emergency departments. Br J Anaesth 2011; 106(5): 632-42.
[http://dx.doi.org/10.1093/bja/aer059] [PMID: 21447489]

[69]   Mitchell V, Dravid R, Patel A, Swampillai C, Higgs A, Higgs A. Difficult Airway Society Guidelines for the management of tracheal extubation. Anaesthesia 2012; 67(3): 318-40.
[http://dx.doi.org/10.1111/j.1365-2044.2012.07075.x] [PMID: 22321104]

[70]   Odor PM, Bampoe S, Lucas DN, Moonesinghe SR, Andrade J, Pandit JJ. Protocol for direct reporting of awareness in maternity patients (DREAMY): a prospective, multicentre cohort study of accidental awareness during general anaesthesia. Int J Obstet Anesth 2020; 42: 47-56.
[http://dx.doi.org/10.1016/j.ijoa.2020.02.004] [PMID: 32139144]

[71]   Odor PM, Bampoe S, Lucas DN, *et al.* Incidence of accidental awareness during general anaesthesia in obstetrics: a multicentre, prospective cohort study. Anaesthesia 2021; 76(6): 759-76.
[http://dx.doi.org/10.1111/anae.15385] [PMID: 33434945]

[72]   Ma Y, Cao X, Zhang H, Ge S. Awake fiberoptic orotracheal intubation: a protocol feasibility study. J Int Med Res 2021; 49: (1).
[http://dx.doi.org/10.1177/0300060520987395] [PMID: 33472482]

[73]   Hezelgrave NL, Srinivas K, Ahmad I, Mascarenhas L. Use of awake oral fibreoptic intubation (AFOI) for caesarian section in a woman with Goldenhar Syndrome: a case report. Eur J Obstet Gynecol Reprod Biol 2011; 159(2): 479-80.
[http://dx.doi.org/10.1016/j.ejogrb.2011.08.004] [PMID: 21962463]

[74]   Chrimes NC. The Vortex: striving for simplicity, context independence and teamwork in an airway cognitive tool. Br J Anaesth 2015; 115(1): 148-9.
[http://dx.doi.org/10.1093/bja/aev047] [PMID: 26089469]

[75]   Chrimes N. The Vortex: a universal 'high-acuity implementation tool' for emergency airway management. Br J Anaesth 2016; 117 (Suppl. 1): i20-7.
[http://dx.doi.org/10.1093/bja/aew175] [PMID: 27440673]

[76]   Chrimes N, Higgs A, Rehak A. Lost in transition: the challenges of getting airway clinicians to move from the upper airway to the neck during an airway crisis. Br J Anaesth 2020; 125(1): e38-46.
[http://dx.doi.org/10.1016/j.bja.2020.04.052] [PMID: 32475685]

[77]   Bamber JH, Evans SA. The value of decision tree analysis in planning anaesthetic care in obstetrics. Int J Obstet Anesth 2016; 27: 55-61.
[http://dx.doi.org/10.1016/j.ijoa.2016.02.007] [PMID: 27026589]

[78]   Daga V, Mendonca C, Choksey F, Elton J, Radhakrishna S. Anaesthetic management of a patient with multiple pterygium syndrome for elective caesarean section. Int J Obstet Anesth 2017; 31: 96-100.
[http://dx.doi.org/10.1016/j.ijoa.2017.04.005] [PMID: 28684141]

[79]   Krom AJ, Cohen Y, Miller JP, Ezri T, Halpern SH, Ginosar Y. Choice of anaesthesia for category-1 caesarean section in women with anticipated difficult tracheal intubation: the use of decision analysis. Anaesthesia 2017; 72(2): 156-71.
[http://dx.doi.org/10.1111/anae.13729] [PMID: 27900760]

[80]   Ahmad I, El-Boghdadly K, Bhagrath R, Hodzovic I, McNarry AF, Mir F, *et al.* Difficult Airway Society guidelines for awake tracheal intubation (ATI) in adults. Anaesthesia 2019.
[PMID: 31729018]

[81]   Zaouter C, Calderon J, Hemmerling TM. Videolaryngoscopy as a new standard of care. Br J Anaesth 2015; 114(2): 181-3.
[http://dx.doi.org/10.1093/bja/aeu266] [PMID: 25150988]

[82]   Alhomary M, Ramadan E, Curran E, Walsh SR. Videolaryngoscopy vs. fibreoptic bronchoscopy for awake tracheal intubation: a systematic review and meta-analysis. Anaesthesia 2018; 73(9): 1151-61.
[http://dx.doi.org/10.1111/anae.14299] [PMID: 29687891]

[83]   Chiang JCS, Irwin MG, Hussain A, Tang YK, Hiong YT. Anaesthesia for emergency caesarean section in a patient with large anterior mediastinal tumour presenting as intrathoracic airway compression and superior vena cava obstruction. Case Rep Med 2010; 2010: 1-5.
[http://dx.doi.org/10.1155/2010/708481] [PMID: 20981348]

[84]   Roze des Ordons AL, Lee J, Bader E, *et al.* Cesarean delivery in a parturient with an anterior mediastinal mass. Can J Anaesth 2013; 60(1): 89-90.
[http://dx.doi.org/10.1007/s12630-012-9815-4] [PMID: 23132046]

[85]   Kusajima K, Ishihara S, Yokoyama T, Katayama K. Anesthetic management of cesarean section in a patient with a large anterior mediastinal mass: a case report. JA Clin Rep 2017; 3(1): 28.
[http://dx.doi.org/10.1186/s40981-017-0098-1] [PMID: 29457072]

[86]   Mahmood A, Mushambi M, Porter R, Khare M. Regional anaesthesia with extracorporeal membrane oxygenation backup for caesarean section in a parturient with neck and mediastinal masses. Int J Obstet Anesth 2018; 35: 99-103.
[http://dx.doi.org/10.1016/j.ijoa.2018.02.009] [PMID: 29631812]

[87]   Hendrie MA, Kumar MM. Airway obstruction, caesarean section and thyroidectomy. Int J Obstet Anesth 2013; 22(4): 340-3.
[http://dx.doi.org/10.1016/j.ijoa.2013.06.002] [PMID: 23993801]

CHAPTER 4

Anesthesia for Fetal Surgery

Marta Chacón Castillo[1,*], **Natalia Martos Gisbert**[1] and **Adriana Orozco Vinasco**[1]

[1] *Department of Anaesthesiology and Intensive Care. University Hospital Severo Ochoa, Leganes, Madrid, Spain*

Abstract: Fetal surgery has evolved in the last decades, mostly because of the technical advances in therapeutic and monitoring devices. The timing and mode of surgery depend on the disease to be treated. Local, neuraxial or general anesthesia can be used on the mother. In some cases, fetal analgesia and paralysis are needed.

The idea of treating the fetus as a patient has evolved in recent years, as a consequence of improvements in diagnostic imaging and surgical devices. In fetuses with congenital airway obstruction, intrapartum surgical correction or airway management can be performed while maintaining perfusion via the umbilical cord.

In 1980, maternal laparotomy and hysterotomy were proposed to treat fetuses with congenital and developmental abnormalities, and the prerequisites for maternal-fetal surgery were first formulated in 1982. They are still in use with some minor modifications. A multidisciplinary approach to fetal intervention is essential. Both obstetric and pediatric anesthesia is involved and it a close collaboration with surgical teams is necessary.

Keywords: Exit Procedure, Fetal Anesthesia, Fetal Surgery, Fetal Surgery Anesthesia, Maternal Anesthesia, Presto Procedure.

INTRODUCTION

The idea of treating the fetus as a patient has evolved in recent years, as a consequence of improvements in diagnostic imaging and surgical devices. The first fetal intervention was in 1963, when Liley performed an intraperitoneal blood transfusion for the treatment of erythroblastosis fetalis. In the 1980s, maternal laparotomy and hysterotomy were proposed to treat fetuses with congenital and developmental abnormalities.

* **Corresponding author Marta Chacón Castillo:** Department of Anaesthesiology and Intensive Care. University Hospital Severo Ochoa, Leganes, Madrid, Spain; E-mail: marta.chacon@gmail.com

Eugenio Daniel Martinez-Hurtado, Monica Sanjuan-Alvarez & Marta Chacon-Castillo (Eds.)
All rights reserved-© 2022 Bentham Science Publishers

Most fetal anomalies are not amenable to prenatal correction. However, some entities are better managed before they can cause irreversible organ damage [1]. In fetuses with congenital airway obstruction, intrapartum surgical correction or airway management can be performed while maintaining perfusion via the umbilical cord. The prerequisites for maternal-fetal surgery were first formulated in 1982, and are still in use with some minor modifications. They require the following [2]:

1. The ability to establish an accurate prenatal diagnosis.
2. A well-defined natural history of the disorder.
3. The presence of a correctable lesion which, if untreated, will lead to fetal demise, irreversible organ dysfunction before birth, or severe postnatal morbidity.
4. The absence of severe associated anomalies.
5. An acceptable risk-to-benefit ratio for both the mother and the fetus. Fetal anesthesia is the anesthetic provided to pregnant women, or the anesthesia administered directly to the fetus, or both.

A multidisciplinary approach to fetal intervention is essential. Both obstetric and pediatric anesthesia are involved and it is necessary to have a close collaboration with surgical teams. This chapter focuses on the different procedures that are currently performed and their anesthetic management.

PHYSIOLOGY

Fetomaternal physiology is explained in detail in chapter 1. The most important aspects with regard to the anesthetic procedure will be summarized here.

-*Maternal Physiology*:

- Higher sensitivity to anesthetic agents, including inhalational anesthetics, non-depolarizing muscle relaxants, and epidural anesthetics.
- Hemodynamic changes: decreased systemic vascular resistance with high cardiac output. Risk of supine hypotension with aortocaval compression. The increased sympathetic tone is important for maintenance of blood pressure: marked hypotension can ensue after the use of drugs with vasodilating properties, or neuraxial blocks (sympathectomy). Placental blood flow depends on maternal blood pressure, so mantaining the maternal hemodinamics is essential for the fetus' well-being.
- Higher O_2 consumption and reduction in functional residual capacity lead to rapid oxygen desaturation and hypoxia during apnea. Edema of the upper airway

and mucosal fragility can lead to upper airway bleeding and difficult airway management.

-*Fetal Physiology*:

- Fetal cardiac output is highly dependent on the heart rate. The exposure of the fetus to high doses of volatile anesthetics can cause myocardial depression and bradycardia. Fetal bradycardia can lead rapidly to hypoperfusion, hypoxia, and acidosis.
- The fetus' capacity for thermoregulation is minimal, and depends on maternal temperature. Active warming of the mother and fetus is very important, especially in open fetal surgery.
- The question of pain perception in the fetus remains controversial. However, fetuses exhibit hormonal and circulatory stress changes in response to noxious stimuli. The long-term effects of fetal pain are currently unknown. Besides pain control, fetal analgesia helps to inhibit fetal movement, prevent hormonal stress responses associated with poor fetal outcomes, and possibly prevent adverse effects on long-term neurodevelopment [1, 3, 4].

GENERAL MANAGEMENT IN ALL INSTANCES OF FETAL SURGERY

Regardless of the type and timing of the intervention, there are some common measures that must be taken in almost all women subjected to fetal surgery [3]:

- Aspiration prophylaxis with multiple agents.
- Left lateral tilt to avoid aortocaval compression.
- Restriction of maternal iv fluids to avoid pulmonary edema.
- Aggressive blood pressure management to maintain uteroplacental perfusion: start therapy as soon as blood pressure decrease is detected. Both ephedrine and phenylephrine can be used safely in pregnant patients.
- Postoperative pain control.
- Prevention of preterm labor.
- Available personnel and equipment in case of delivery.

TYPES OF FETAL INTERVENTIONS

Fetal interventions can be divided into minimally invasive, open mid-gestation, EXIT and PRESTO procedures.

Minimally Invasive Interventions

Minimally invasive interventions are the most frequently performed fetal surgical procedures. There is usually no need for hysterotomy: the uterine cavity is accessed with needles that are inserted percutaneously under ultrasound guidance (fetal image-guided surgery) or with small trocar sheaths (fetoscopy) (Fig. 1) [1, 5]. After minimally invasive interventions, vaginal delivery is feasible in the current and future pregnancies. In some instances, a laparotomy is necessary if an anterior placenta prevents a percutaneous approach. The timing of minimally invasive procedures is early gestation or mid-gestation.

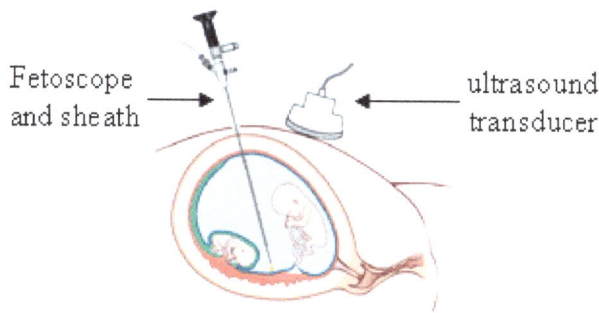

Fig. (1). Fetoscopy. US Government website, public domain.

The most frequent fetal procedures performed by minimally invasive approach are:

- *Lower Urinary Tract Obstruction* (*LUTO*): It is caused by posterior urethral valves or urethral obstruction, resulting in renal damage secondary to hydronephrosis, oligohydramnios and pulmonary hypoplasia. Perinatal mortality is as high as 90%, in these cases, and half of the survivors have severe renal dysfunction. The intervention is a vesicoamniotic shunt in order to open the urinary tract. When the cause is posterior urethral valves, fetal cystoscopy has shown promising results, with a higher survival rate and normal renal function in 75% of survivors [2].
- *Fetal Transfusion for Anemia*: Most common causes of fetal anemia are sensitization to Rh or other red blood cell antigens, hemorrhage, placental chorioangiomas and parvovirus infection. This condition is currently assessed by Doppler studies of the middle cerebral artery [4]. The transfusion is usually given into the umbilical vein near the placental end. In some cases, the intrahepatic portion of the umbilical vein must be used. The umbilical vein has no pain receptors, but in case of transfusion to the intrahepatic portion of the

vein, an intramuscular dose of fentanyl must be given to the fetus. The needle is inserted into the vein using ultrasound guidance. A blood sample is taken from the vein before the transfusion, to assess the degree of fetal anemia, and the amount of type O, Rh negative, irradiated, leukodepleted and CMV-negative, and packed RBCs are determined. Typically, fetal Hb levels decline slowly after the procedure, and multiple repeat procedures are needed until delivery.

- ***Twin-twin Transfusion Syndrome***: It is a complication of monochorionic twin pregnancy in which twins share unequal amounts of the placenta's blood supply resulting in the two fetuses growing at different rates. The recipient twin becomes hypervolemic with polyhydramnios and ventricular hypertrophy. The donor twin becomes hypovolemic with oligohydramnios. Both twins are at risk of death. The first therapeutic approach to this disorder was amnioreduction. By decreasing polyhydramnios, the risk for premature labor and maternal respiratory distress is reduced, and the lower hydrostatic pressure of the amniotic fluid improves placental perfusion. Fetoscopic laser coagulation is the best current prenatal intervention, which tries to balance blood perfusion between the two twins by ablating vascular anastomoses. It is performed under US guidance, and the most usual anesthetic technique is local infiltration of the abdominal wall, although neuraxial anesthesia can also be used.

- ***Congenital Diaphragmatic Hernia***: It is a condition characterized by a defect in the diaphragm leading to protrusion of abdominal contents into the thoracic cavity interfering with the normal development of the lungs. The fetal lung secretes a fluid into the amniotic cavity via the trachea. The procedure consists of placing a balloon in the fetal trachea between 27 weeks and 31 weeks gestation. The buildup of fluid promotes expansion and development of the lung and pushes the viscera into the abdomen. The balloon is removed before delivery, in the second fetoscopic procedure [1, 4].

- ***Heart Defects***: The most common congenital heart defect that can be treated prenatally is aortic valve stenosis. In this defect, blood flow is diverted through the low-resistance foramen ovale, which results in the underdevelopment of the left ventricle. The procedure is performed with real-time US guidance, and a cannula is inserted through the maternal abdominal wall, uterus and fetal chest into the left ventricle outlet. A coronary balloon catheter is positioned in the aortic annulus and inflated and deflated multiple times. The fetus should be positioned with the chest anterior, so in some cases, an external fetal version is needed. In this case, maternal general anesthesia may be preferred to obtain uterine relaxation. In the majority of cases, however, the procedure is performed under neuraxial or local anesthesia. Other cardiac defects that can be addressed in a similar fashion are pulmonary valve stenosis and intact or restrictive atrial septum.

- Other indications have been described, such as congenital cystic adenomatoid malformations, amniotic band syndrome or twin reversed arterial perfusion. All of them are performed by a minimally invasive, ultrasound-guided procedure.

Anesthetic Management

It depends on the duration of the procedure, surgical approach, position and maternal comorbidities, but most interventions are performed under neuraxial anesthesia, with or without intravenous sedation. A T4 level block is needed for most instances of uterine surgical manipulation [6]. Some procedures may be managed with local anesthetic infiltrations [5]. Certain cases may require fetal immobilization, which can be achieved by a remifentanil infusion (0,1 mcg/kg/min), improving operating conditions and maternal comfort. For more invasive fetal procedures, such as valvuloplasty or endoluminal tracheal occlusion, fetal immobilization may be ensured by an intramuscular fetal injection of rocuronium, fentanyl, and atropine [7].

Before the procedure, aspiration prophylaxis should be administered, although standard fasting is applied. Initially, tocolysis is not necessary [7].

Postoperative complications include hemorrhage, chorioamnionitis, sepsis, oligohydramnios and preterm labor. Maternal pulmonary edema can result from the irrigation of the uterine cavity with large volumes of fluid during fetoscopic surgery [8].

Open Midgestation Fetal Surgery

After induction of general anesthesia, a maternal laparotomy is performed followed by hysterotomy. Implantation of the placenta dictates the surgical approach. Profound uterus relaxation is required to perform the hysterotomy and expose the necessary anatomy of the fetus.

Most current open fetal indications are summarized next:

- *Myelomeningocele (MMC)* (Fig. **2**): Repairing a fetal MMC has shown better neurologic and functional scores and also a decrease in the need for ventriculoperitoneal shunt compared to postnatal repair [1, 9]. After laparotomy, the uterus is positioned so the hysterotomy will not injury the placental insertion. The myelomeningocele is exposed and repaired. Most surgical teams prefer an open technique. However, in order to decrease maternal morbidity, some groups advocate a fetoscopic approach to fetal MMC repair [7]. In these cases, premature delivery is almost universal.

• *Sacrococcygeal Teratoma (SCT):* Is the most common tumor presenting in newborns. They may grow rapidly and create a low resistance state [1], with high-output heart failure. In these cases, the tumor must be removed given that a mortality rate of almost 50% has been described.

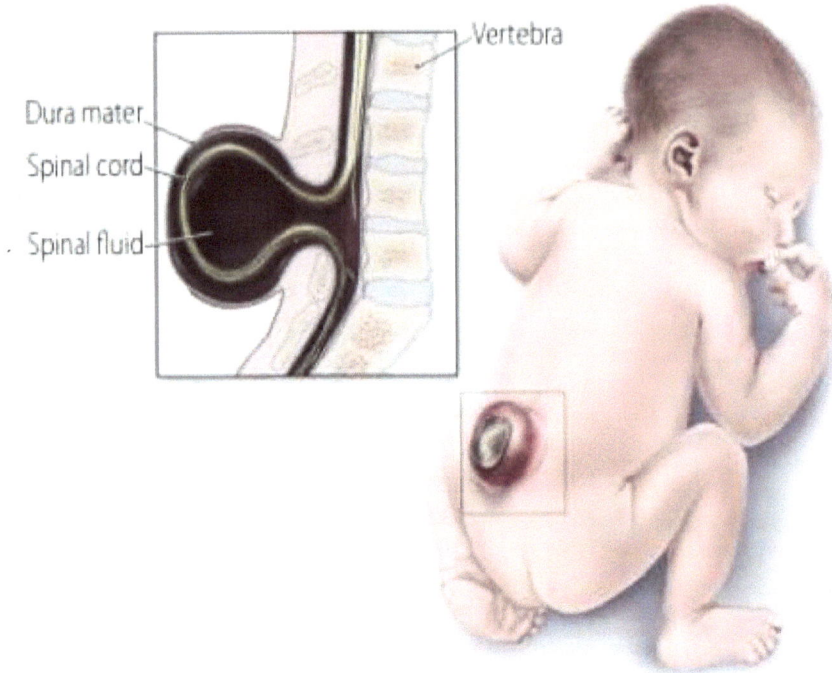

Spina Bifida (Open Defect)

Fig. (2). Content source: Division of Birth Defects and Developmental Disabilities, NCBDDD, Centers for Disease Control and Prevention.

Anesthetic Management

Open fetal surgeries are usually performed under maternal general anesthesia. Pure neuraxial techniques neither provide fetal anesthesia-analgesia nor uterine relaxation [6]. The placement of a lumbar epidural catheter is recommended for later use in the postoperative period. Epidural analgesia (with a combination of an opioid and a local anesthetic) is superior to parenteral analgesics. The epidural catheter should not be used until the end of the surgery, to avoid hemodynamic instability.

With a peripheral IV, rapid sequence induction and intubation take place. Placement of an arterial catheter for blood pressure monitoring and a second IV catheter is recommended. The use of fluids should be restricted to avoid maternal pulmonary edema and hemodynamic stability is achieved with vasopressors if necessary [8].

Open fetal surgery requires profound uterine relaxation. Originally, high doses of volatile agents (2 MAC) were used to achieve such relaxation [7]. However, fetal left ventricular dysfunction was frequent with this approach. Later, a new protocol was described which includes maintenance with intravenous anesthesia (propofol and remifentanil) and a lower desflurane concentration (1-1,5 MAC). In addition, a magnesium sulfate bolus after induction allows to reduce the dose of volatile agents. An infusion of magnesium sulfate is recommended to maintain postoperative tocolysis and oral nifedipine is continued till the end of the pregnancy [8]. Placental transfer of volatile anesthetics provides significant fetal anesthesia [1]. After exposure of the fetus, an intramuscular injection of fentanyl, rocuronium and atropine is given in order to avoid fetal movements.

Fetal echocardiography is performed to monitor heart rate and contractility. Umbilical artery doppler can also be measured. A pulse oximeter is placed in the fetus' hand under sterile conditions. A continuous infusion of warm saline into the uterus helps to keep the fetus warm and buoyant.

A high rate of maternal complications has been described: pulmonary edema, placental abruption, chorioamnionitis, preterm labor. After an open fetal surgery, cesarean delivery must be perfomed, and it is also recommended in future pregnancies.

Ex Utero Intrapartum Therapy (*EXIT*) and Procedure Requiring Second Team in the Operating Room (*PRESTO*) Procedures

The EXIT procedure is performed while the fetus is in the process of being delivered. During the intervention, fetal circulation is maintained, so oxygenation comes from the umbilical cord and placenta [7]. It is important that no ventilation of the lungs occurs until the umbilical cord is clamped.

The EXIT approach is used, more frequently, in cases of airway obstruction. Once the hysterotomy is done and the fetus is partially exposed, a quick direct laryngoscopy and endotracheal intubation are performed. Additional airway interventions are occasionally required such as rigid bronchoscopy, fiberoptic intubation, and tracheostomy [8].

If there is a reasonable chance that the newborn airway can be secured after birth or the mother is not a candidate for an EXIT procedure, a second surgery and anesthesia team is prepared to operate if necessary (PRESTO procedure). Close communication with both teams is essential, because treatment decisions are taken quickly after a newborn is delivered.

Current indications of EXIT/PRESTO procedures are summarized next:

- *Airway Obstruction*: An extrinsic airway obstruction (mass, micrognathia) may not produce development problems so it is not necessary to treat in the middle of gestation. The problems begin at birth, because airway obstruction impairs the newborn first breath. It can be treated with an EXIT procedure if the obstruction completely blocks the newborn´s airway or with a PRESTO procedure if a reasonable chance of breathing exists.
- *Lung Masses*: These include bronchopulmonary sequestration or congenital airway malformations. If the lung lesion is large, it is not possible to wait for a scheduled elective lobectomy. In these cases, an EXIT or a PRESTO thoracotomy is needed.

Anesthetic Management

Initial anesthesia management for the EXIT and PRESTO procedures is similar to open fetal surgeries. The mother receives general anesthesia (previous epidural catheter emplacement) and an arterial line and a central venous line must be considered [8]. Uterine and fetal relaxant protocol is the same as explained in the open surgery section. Fluid restriction is not necessary.

Fetal monitoring is essential before airway intubation and it may include echocardiography and pulse oximeter [7]. Depending on the magnitude of the procedure, a fetal PIV must be inserted for the administration of fluids and packed red blood cells. In the EXIT procedure, rapid reversal of uterine relaxation after clamping the umbilical cord is critical, so, at that moment, an oxytocin infusion must be started. Maternal complications are similar to cesarean delivery. Nevertheless, the neonatal complication rate is high and a mortality rate of 15% is described.

CONCLUSION

Fetal surgery anesthesia is a complex discipline, and it is rapidly evolving. The combination of maternal and fetal physiology and the surgical team's needs is a delicate balance that challenges the expertise of the anesthesiologist.

CONSENT FOR PUBLICATION

Not applicable.

CONFLICT OF INTEREST

The authors declare no conflict of interest, financial or otherwise.

ACKNOWLEDGEMENT

Declared none.

REFERENCES

[1]   Ferschl M, Rollins M. Anesthesia for fetal surgery and other fetal therapies. In: Gropper M, Ed. Miller's Anesthesia 9th ed. 2019; 2042-67.

[2]   Partridge EA, Flake AW. Maternal–fetal surgery for structural malformations. Best Pract Res Clin Obstet Gynaecol 2012; 26(5): 669-82.
[http://dx.doi.org/10.1016/j.bpobgyn.2012.03.003] [PMID: 22542765]

[3]   Sviggum HP, Kodali BS. Maternal anesthesia for fetal surgery. Clin Perinatol 2013; 40(3): 413-27.
[http://dx.doi.org/10.1016/j.clp.2013.05.012] [PMID: 23972748]

[4]   Rollins M. Anesthesia for Fetal Surgery and Other Intrauterine Procedures. In: Chestnut D, Ed. by Chestnut's Obstetric Anesthesia 6th ed. 2020; 132-50.

[5]   Lin EE, Tran KM. Anesthesia for fetal surgery. Semin Pediatr Surg 2013; 22(1): 50-5.
[http://dx.doi.org/10.1053/j.sempedsurg.2012.10.009] [PMID: 23395146]

[6]   Brusseau R, Mizrahi-Arnaud A. Fetal anesthesia and pain management for intrauterine therapy. Clin Perinatol 2013; 40(3): 429-42.
[http://dx.doi.org/10.1016/j.clp.2013.05.006] [PMID: 23972749]

[7]   Tran KM, Chatterjee D. New Trends in Fetal Anesthesia. Anesthesiol Clin 2020; 38(3): 605-19.
[http://dx.doi.org/10.1016/j.anclin.2020.05.006] [PMID: 32792187]

[8]   Ring LE, Ginosar Y. Anesthesia for fetal surgery and fetal procedures. clin perinatol 2019; 46(4): 801-16.
[http://dx.doi.org/10.1016/j.clp.2019.08.011] [PMID: 31653309]

[9]   Adzick NS, Thom EA, Spong CY, *et al.* A randomized trial of prenatal versus postnatal repair of myelomeningocele. N Engl J Med 2011; 364(11): 993-1004.
[http://dx.doi.org/10.1056/NEJMoa1014379] [PMID: 21306277]

CHAPTER 5

Regional and Parenteral Analgesia in Labour

Monir Kabiri Sacramento[1,*], Javier Alcázar Esteras[2], Patricia Alfaro de la Torre[3], Sergi Boada Pie[3] and **Miriam Sánchez Merchante[4]**

[1] *Department of Anesthesiology and Intensive Care, HM Hospital Universitario Madrid, Madrid, Spain*

[2] *Hospital Universitario de Torrejón de Ardoz, Madrid, Spain*

[3] *Hospital Joan XXIII, Tarragona, Spain*

[4] *Hospital Universitario Fundación Alcorcón, Madrid, Spain*

Abstract: Labour pain is a complex phenomenon involving subjective psychological factors and physiological neurohormonal factors. Many different factors contribute to the perception of pain: cultural factors, bond, and trust in the delivery team, being able to take their own decisions, relaxation ability, previous labour, anatomical and fetal-related factors. Pain relief is one of the elements involved in overall satisfaction but it is not the only one and is important to remember that pharmacological intervention is only a part of it.

Keywords: Combined Spinal-Epidural, Dural Puncture Epidural, Epidural Analgesia, Fentanyl, Labour, Neuraxial Analgesia, Opioids, Paracervical Block, Patient-Controlled Analgesia, Pethidine, Pudendal Nerve Block, Remifentanil, Spinal Analgesia, and Newborn Outcome.

INTRODUCTION

The experience and individual response to labour pain are different in every woman, influenced by her own circumstances, cultural background, support, environment, as well as many labour-related issues (onset of labour, position, instrumental delivery, episiotomy, *etc.*) [1, 2].

Pain relief can be achieved by numerous techniques, some of which require medical intervention (intravenous drugs, regional analgesia, nitrous oxide), while others do not (relaxation, hypnosis, acupuncture, reflexology, *etc*). Whatever method is chosen, it must be safe for both mother and baby and it should make the

---

[*] **Corresponding author Monir Kabiri Sacramento:** Department of Anesthesiology and Intensive Care. HM Hospital Universitario Madrid, Madrid, Spain.; Email: monirkabiri@gmail.com

Eugenio Daniel Martinez-Hurtado, Monica Sanjuan-Alvarez & Marta Chacon-Castillo (Eds.)
All rights reserved-© 2022 Bentham Science Publishers

birth experience as positive as possible. Pain is one of the factors with the most influence on labour and birth satisfaction [2].

Labour pain is a combination of visceral and somatic pain from uterine contractions and cervical dilatation, as well as from fetal descent through the pelvis, vagina and perineum. It is initially transmitted through T10-L1 roots, and as labour progresses it involves sacral roots S2-S4 (pudendal nerves) [3].

REGIONAL ANALGESIA

Regional analgesia for labour pain can include two groups of techniques. First, neuraxial techniques [4, 5], which are widely used, effective and safe, but are surrounded by many controversies yet to be clarified. Secondly, there are pelvic regional blocks that can be used to ease the pain, mainly during the second stage of labour [6, 7] (Table **1**).

Table 1. Techniques for regional analgesia for labour pain.

Technique	Advantages	Disadvantages
Continuous epidural analge sia (*CEA*)	- Continuous analgesia - No dural puncture - Adjustable dose	- Slow onset - Larger LA doses → higher risk of LAST, higher fetal exposition
Combined spinal-epidural analgesia (*CSE*)	- Rapid onset of analgesia - Wider sacral spread - Lower rate of epidural catheter misplacement	- Delayed verification of epidural catheter placement - Higher risk of postdural puncture headache (*PDPH*)
Dural Puncture Epidural (*DPE*)	- Faster onset - Better sacral spread - Lower incidence of asymmetrical block	- Increased risk for PDPH
Continuous spinal analgesia (*CSA*)	- Low dose of LA and opioid - Less hemodynamic impact - Rapid onset of analgesia	- Increased risk for PDPH - Risk of total spinal anaesthesia if spinal catheter mistaken for epidural catheter
Single shot spinal analgesia (*SSS*)	- Rapid onset of analgesia - Immediate sacral analgesia - Low LA dose	- Limited duration of action - Greater risk of maternal hypotension
Pudendal nerve block	- Less invasive technique - Low dose of LA	- Requires bilateral puncture - Limited duration of action
Paracervical block		- High risk of uterine artery puncture: fetal death, LA absorption

Pain and stress responses induce the release of corticotropin, cortisol, norepinephrine, beta-endorphins and epinephrine, all of which decrease uterine blood flow.

Pain reduction and sympathectomy caused by neural blockade result in lower levels of catecholamines and improvement in uteroplacental perfusion, especially in states of low uterine blood flow.

The ideal local anesthetic (*LA*) for labour should produce a reliable sensory block with no motor block, cause no tachyphylaxis and have a good safety profile so that inadvertent intravascular administration or overdose are harmless.

Neuraxial Analgesia

There are significant differences in the use of neuraxial analgesia for labour between different countries worldwide, and even between different hospitals in the same country.

Neuraxial analgesia in obstetrics includes spinal puncture, epidural catheter or a combination of both by a combined spinal epidural (*CSE*) technique [3 - 5].

Low dose LA, usually in combination with low dose opioid (fentanyl, sufentanil or morphine) is given by an initial bolus and different continued regimens to maintain analgesia through labour.

Neuraxial Techniques

-***Spinal Puncture***: The effect of a dural puncture and LA with or without adjuvant opioids (usually fentanyl, morphine or sufentanil) has a rapid onset but is limited by the duration of the LA/mixture administered. Hence, its use is limited to situations where a fast relief is required and a limited duration of the pain is expected, such as delivery. The low concentration of LA (bupivacaine 0,25%) is generally used in order to minimize hemodynamic effects and motor block.

- ***Standard Epidural Technique***: where a loss of resistance technique is used to identify the epidural space and a catheter is placed.

- The combined spinal-epidural (*CSE*) technique has shown several advantages over the epidural technique alone. It has a shorter onset of analgesia, as the initial dose is given in the subarachnoid space [4, 5, 8]. Even in the early stages, pain can be controlled by spinal opioids alone, with no sympathetic or motor block. It also allows better and faster sacral analgesia. It is associated with a lower rate of misplaced epidural catheters, but the verification of its proper placement and function is delayed by the initial spinal dose. It is also associated with a higher incidence of pruritus and possible higher risk of fetal bradycardia [5] (due to the rapid decrease in circulating catecholamines, which have a tocolytic effect, causing uterine tachysystole).

- The dural puncture epidural technique (*DPE*) is a modification of the CSE where there is a spinal puncture performed through the epidural needle but no intrathecal medication is injected. It appears to associate improved sacral analgesia with less hypotension, pruritus and uterine tachysystole [4, 5].

About the timing of analgesia over the course of labour, according to the American College of Obstetricians and Gynecologists, and the American Society of Anaesthesia, "*in the absence of medical contraindication, maternal request is sufficient medical indication for pain relief during labour*" [8]. Early or late initiation of epidural analgesia makes no significant difference in the duration of the second stage of labour or in the risk of instrumental delivery or C-section [4, 5].

Maintenance and Dosing of Epidural Analgesia

Low dose LA and opioid (fentanyl,sufentanil, morphine) mixture is the most common pharmacological strategy used for labour epidural analgesia. An initial bolus is given followed by a maintenance dose of a low concentration LA (bupivacaine 0.1%, ropivacaine 0.08-0.2%, levobupivacaine 0.05-0.125%). The addition of opioids to the LA allows for decreasing the concentration of the LA, resulting in a lower total dose of LA and sparing of the motor block (walking epidural or mobile epidural).

Spinal or epidural opioids alone can be a useful approach for high-risk patients who cannot tolerate the hemodynamic consequences of epidural or spinal sympathectomy. However, analgesia is incomplete, opioids can cause nausea and vomiting, sedation and respiratory depression, and they do not provide perineal relaxation.

Several maintenance regimes can be used: intermittent manual bolus, continuous epidural infusion, patient-controlled epidural analgesia, and programmed intermittent epidural bolus. They all require an infusion pump (except in the intermittent manual bolus technique) and the patient must be monitored and followed up regularly in order to identify and treat any possible complications [4, 5, 8].

-Intermittent manual bolus technique: Not routinely used nowadays as infusion pumps are widely available. An initial bolus is given and followed by manual boluses (8-12 ml) on recurrence of pain. Pain relief is intermittent, it requires frequent provider intervention and motor blockade is likely after several injections.

-Continuous epidural infusion: After the initial bolus, a continuous infusion of LA is delivered *via.* infusion pump. It provides more stable analgesia and hemodynamic stability with less breakthrough pain than the intermittent manual bolus technique. It still requires provider intervention in case an additional dose is needed. Total doses of LA are larger, which may condition a higher rate of instrumental deliveries [1, 4, 5].

-Patient-controlled epidural analgesia (PCEA): It allows the patient to partially control the dose of analgesia improving maternal satisfaction. It can be adjusted according to the pain and needs of the patient. It requires proper education of the parturient, leading to less clinician intervention, with a reduced total amount of LA and opioids and less motor blocks [1, 4, 5].

-Programmed intermittent epidural bolus (PIEB): A bolus of a pre-set volume of LA is administered at a pre-set time interval by a pump, with or without the possibility of extra boluses in case of uncontrolled pain [4, 5]. Compared to PCEA, it has shown to be a more stable analgesia, with better pain control and higher patient satisfaction, along with a reduction in supplemental boluses. The total consumption of LA is lower, with less motor blockade [1, 9, 10]. The mechanism of this improved analgesia is believed to be a greater medication spread in the epidural space. A potential disadvantage is the unintentional high blockade due to catheter migration into intrathecal space. Continuous automated administration or manual boluses are inherently safer than programmed intermittent boluses, as signs of catheter malposition can be suspected [9, 10].

Effects of Neuraxial Analgesia on Labour and Newborn

-Duration of labour: Many different factors are involved in the duration of labour which makes it difficult to establish the real influence of neuraxial analgesia alone [4, 5, 8]. However, some conclusions can be drawn from recent publications [11 - 14]:

- The second stage of labour is 15-30 minutes longer in patients with effective epidural analgesia, but can be prolonged up to two hours. The clinical significance and the risk of neonatal complications associated to this are yet to be established.
- Labour is faster when early neuraxial analgesia is administered compared to early systemic opioids and late neuraxial analgesia.
- Maintenance of epidural analgesia by intermittent bolus (*IEB*) is associated with shorter second-stage labour compared to continuous infusion or patient-controlled analgesia.

- *Instrumental delivery and C-section*: Again, many factors influence the outcome of labour, such as neuraxial technique, spontaneous or induced labour, LA concentration, fetal position, motor block, *etc* [3, 4]. Evidence does not seem to support that neuraxial analgesia increases the risk of caesarean section itself [4, 5, 8], but high concentration epidural analgesia is associated with lower rates of vaginal birth [9, 11]. When comparing neuraxial techniques, CSE shows a less instrumental delivery rate than epidural analgesia [4, 5]. No difference in caesarean delivery between patients receiving early or late neuraxial analgesia has been reported. On the other hand, the length of exposure to epidural analgesia is associated with non-spontaneous births in primiparous and multiparous women [12, 13, 15].

- *Maternal fever*: Patients receiving EA are more likely to present intrapartum fever (>38°C), but it has not been established whether this increased maternal temperature is caused by EA or obstetric management [9]. Epidural-related maternal fever occurs within 6 hours after initiating EA. The mechanism by which EA is associated with pyrexia is yet to be defined, being more likely a combination of several effects [9, 16, 17]:

- Altered thermoregulation secondary to autonomous response to EA: vasodilation in lower limbs and vasoconstriction in the upper part of the body leads to an unbalanced perception of warm and cold sensations. This causes a false response of the temperature centre, activating heat production [2, 12].
- Release of inflammatory non-infectious molecules through immunomodulation and cell injury that occurs during labour, involving IL-6 and TNF-α. The concentration of these molecules increases as analgesia time increases [17].
- Contribution of local anesthetics, with a higher incidence of intra and postpartum fever in higher concentration regimes, as the concentration of IL-6 and TNF-α increases with the concentration of LA and the duration of EA (from the fourth hour of exposition) [17].
- LA contributes to setting off a sterile inflammation mechanism driven by endogenous alarmins following tissue damage.

- *Newborn outcome*: Different factors may impact newborn outcomes during labour under EA, although it is difficult to establish if they are directly related to EA and its clinical significance.

- Placental perfusion may be compromised after the initiation of epidural analgesia. Fetal bradycardia after the initiation of EA can occur as a consequence of the hemodynamic effects of the EA (hypotension), which usually responds to intravenous fluids, Trendelenburg position and α-agonists [4, 5, 11, 18].

- Analgesia-mediated fetal bradycardia can ensue, due to a rapid decrease in circulating epinephrine concentration, as it has a tocolytic effect and its rapid withdrawal may contribute to uterine tachysystole, reducing placental perfusion time.

- LA and epidural opiates can be detected in umbilical venous plasma at the time of delivery and 24 hours after delivery in urine [11, 18]. Some studies reflect lower Apgar scores at 1 and 5 minutes after birth, with a higher proportion requiring resuscitation and neonatal intensive care unit admission, compared to absent or light analgesia [11, 14]. These effects are associated mainly with opioids.

- Maternal fever (secondary to EA, chorioamnionitis or placental inflammation) is associated with worse neonatal outcomes: low Apgar score, neonatal morbidity, encephalopathy, and thus requires more resuscitation and neonatal intensive care unit admission [4, 5, 17, 18].

- The prolongation of the second stage of labour and longer pushing periods are associated with an increased relative risk of neonatal complications and adverse maternal outcomes.

- *Maternal depression*: The severity and intensity of pain during labour and after childbirth is an important factor contributing to the development of maternal postpartum depression, which can affect the cognitive and emotional development of the child. Pain relief and EA reduce the risk of early maternal depression and even up to two years after childbirth. Even though there is still evidence needed to fully support this affirmation, EA can improve the child's neurocognitive development by decreasing postpartum depression [2, 11, 18, 19].

In conclusion, it is difficult to establish the direct cause-effect relationship between EA and different items on labour, childbirth and newborn outcomes. As many different variables are involved and different options for pain relief are available, it is difficult to compare them all [2, 19].

Regional Blocks for Labour Analgesia

When other analgesia strategies are not available (whatever the reason), we still can provide certain degree of analgesia by regional blocks in the late second stage of labour during vaginal birth.

Two main blocks can be performed: paracervical block (*PCB*) and pudendal nerve block (*PNB*). They can be used simultaneously as they target different structures.

Performing these blocks during the late second stage of labour, with or without a previous epidural technique for the first stage of labour analgesia, has several advantages: it shortens the duration of the second stage of labour, less additional boluses are required which reduce motor block, leading to a higher satisfaction [6].

Pudendal Nerve Block

This block is especially useful in the second stage of labour where the pain is due to the strain of the perineum and also for episiotomy or delivery lacerations. It can be useful for an urgent delivery with forceps, although it is a complex technique and it can be dangerous since it involves needle placement very close to the fetal head.

The pudendal nerve originates from sacral roots S2, S3, and S4 and it is composed of somatic, vegetative, motor, and sensory fibres. 30% of the fibres are autonomic and 70% somatic (50% sensitive and 20% motor). Three segments are distinguished: presacral region, infra-piriform canal and Alcock canal. Once the nerve passes under the ischial spine, it divides into its branches: lower rectal nerve, perineal nerve and dorsal nerve of the clitoris or penis. This block can be performed transvaginally by anatomical landmarks or under ultrasound guidance.

- *Ultrasound-guided block*: With the patient in lateral decubitus and legs slightly flexed, the probe must be placed in the imaginary line between the greater trochanter and the posterior ischiatic spine. Then it is displaced caudally parallel to this line, until the nerve is located next to the pudendal artery (Doppler mode), medial to the internal obturator muscle, and below the gluteus maximus [6, 20].

- *Transvaginal approach* [20, 21]: Traditionally, this block has been performed blindly by anatomical landmarks, with the patient in the lithotomy position. After palpating the ischial spine, the needle is introduced through the vaginal wall, directing it towards the spine until bone contact is made, followed by aspiration and injection. To block the lower rectal branch, the nerve can be localized by nerve stimulation, 1 cm laterally and 1 cm deep on both sides of the anal sphincter (at 3 and 6 o'clock), easy to do with the patient in leg loops. However, this block does not reach the perineal branch, which is responsible for the pain in this phase of labour.

This nerve is small and is invariably accompanied by its artery, so a small amount of 5-10 ml of LA is sufficient, always without a vasoconstrictor. The block must be performed bilaterally.

Paracervical Block

It is an old technique, described in 1926, which has not been shown to be useful for uterine interventionism such as hysteroscopies, endometrial biopsies, fractionated curettage, and aspiration-induced abortions, but it has been used in the first phase of labour, during cervical dilation [7, 21].

With the patient in the gynecological position, 10-15 ml of LA is injected at the base of the broad ligament, through both vaginal fornices (at 3 and 6 o'clock), extending through the uterus-vaginal plexus, blocking sympathetic and parasympathetic fibres [21, 22].

This blockage is of high risk due to the proximity of the uterine artery, and fetal deaths have been reported due to bradycardia secondary to LA absorption. Other reported complications are fetal head puncture, vaginal and urethral trauma and uterine hematoma. Its use is not recommended [21, 22].

PARENTERAL ANALGESIA

Labour pain relief when epidural analgesia is not possible (contraindication, maternal rejection, unavailability, comorbidities, *etc.*) can be managed by other methods, among which there are pharmacological and non-pharmacological methods. Different drugs (opioids, NSAIDs, nitrous oxide, *etc*) can be administered through different routes (intravenous, intramuscular, inhalation, subcutaneous, *etc*). It is important to know them all, as well as their safety and effectiveness profiles.

Opioids

The use of opioids for labour pain relief is widely extended, either alone or combined with other drugs. In middle and high-income countries, parenteral opioids are offered to almost half of the women in labour and around 25% of women in labour receive them [23]. In some hospitals, it can still be the standard procedure for labour pain relief [24]. Its use is controversial as it can have secondary effects both on the mother and the fetus: nausea and vomiting, drowsiness, respiratory depression, variations in the fetal heart rate and neonatal respiratory depression.

Different opioids are used depending on availability. Pethidine is the most widely used opioid, followed by fentanyl, morphine or remifentanil. Other opioids include meptazinol, diamorphine, nalbuphine, butorphanol, buprenorphine, pentazocine, tramadol, alfentanil and sufentanil. Some of them can be used on a single shot or scheduled basis; others can be used in patient-controlled regimens.

Even though neuraxial techniques provide a greater reduction in pain scores than intravenous opioids [7, 25], satisfaction rates are similar in both approaches. Obviously, risks associated with each technique and secondary effects are very different, making it essential that the patient makes an informed choice.

Effects on the baby [26, 27]: Opioids cross the placenta by passive diffusion, compromising fetal well-being during labour. General effects include the central nervous system depression, which causes respiratory depression, respiratory acidosis, and abnormal neurological behaviour. Opioids also affect the fetal heart rate and fetal variability, decrease fetal movements and inhibit suction, which combined with the decreased alertness can delay effective breastfeeding during the initial skin-to-skin moments.

These effects vary between the different agents, time of exposure, and fetal maturity, with premature neonates being highly sensitive.

Opioids Used in Labour Analgesia

- **Pethidine**: It is the most widely used opioid in the world as it is inexpensive and, in many countries [28], midwives are allowed to prescribe it without medical supervision [6]. It is given by intravenous or intramuscular injection in doses of 25-50 mg that can be repeated every 6 hours up to 100 mg. 50 mg or less of intravenous or intramuscular pethidine does not appear to affect the newborn APGAR scale [29]. Its administration is associated with maternal nausea and vomiting and maternal sedation. It can take up to 3 days for a newborn to eliminate pethidine and up to 6 days to eliminate its metabolite norpethidine from its system [29].

- **Fentanyl**: A common approach is patient-controlled intravenous analgesia, although its use is being reduced in favour of remifentanil PCA. It can also be used in single or repeated intravenous or subcutaneous shots. Intravenous repeated doses of fentanyl are associated with low APGAR scores in up to 44% of neonates [30]. Typical settings for a fentanyl PCA are 25 mcg every 10-15 minutes with an hourly lockout of 100 mcg [31].

- **Remifentanil**: Its rapid onset of action, short duration, and elimination mechanism with no accumulation have made it more popular in the last years. It has been proven less effective than epidural analgesia in pain relief [7, 32, 33] but it is a useful and reliable alternative when not contraindicated [34]. There is no significant economic difference between the two [32], but the side effects, and the need to monitor and pay close attention to the patient are limiting factors for its implementation [35].

Side effects include nausea and vomiting, respiratory depression, maternal sedation, respiratory arrest, and effects on the newborn [36]. Special attention should be paid to the patient, with continuous measurement of the heart rate, peripheral oxygen saturation, arterial pressure and exhaled CO_2. It is usually recommended to add supplemental oxygen [36, 37], but this is being questioned as hyperoxia can increase respiratory depression [38]. To reduce maternal risks and newborn repercussions, it has been proposed that the administration of remifentanil is based on programs that take into consideration the mother's respiratory parameters and heart rate [39, 40].

Remifentanil-PCA has been associated with lower maternal fever than epidural-PCA [41]. Also, remifentanil has been used for the external cephalic version, providing pain control with no difference on the outcome [42, 43]. Different PCA regimes can be programmed with two main strategies [44 - 47]:

- Continuous infusion (0,025-0,1 µg/kg/min).
- Continuous infusion (0,025-0,05 µg/kg/min) with additional boluses (0,025 µg/kg, lockout time 2 minutes and maximum dose of 3 mg of remifentanil every 4 hours).
- Some authors (RemiPCA SAFE Network) defend the use of no continuous infusion with 10-30 mcg bolus on a 2-minute lockout time.

-Morphine: Its use has been replaced by regional techniques or short-acting opioids [7].

-Tramadol: It is less frequently used during labour, and if so, it is usually given intramuscularly. Higher incidence of nausea, vomiting and maternal sedation, though no effects on the newborn have been observed. No major benefits over paracetamol or other opioids have been observed [48].

-Butorphanol: This is uncommonly used, it can provide a light analgesic effect, more significant during the first hours of the first phase of labour [49].

-Meptazinol: It is not very commonly used nowadays [50].

Ketamine

Ketamine can be helpful in certain patients [51] but should not be the first option of treatment.

In 2020, the French health authorities (Haute Autorité de Santé - HAS), in collaboration with the National Board of Gynecology and Obstetricians (Collège National des Gynécologues et Obstetriciens Français - CNGOF) and the French

Midwife Board (Collège National des Sages-femmes de France - CNSF) have excluded the use of ketamine from the recommended drugs as an alternative to neuraxial analgesia for labour [52].

It can be useful in very specific scenarios, usually prior to delivery or as adjuvant to regional anesthesia [51]. Low doses of ketamine (10-15 mg) have analgesic properties without sedation. Higher doses (1 mg/kg) can be associated with hypertonic uterine contractions as well as neurologic side effects [53].

Non-Steroidal Anti-Inflammatory Drugs (*NSAIDs*)

Only acetaminophen is safe to use during labour (and pregnancy) as any other type of non-steroid anti-inflammatory agent can promote closure of the fetal ductus arteriosus and can suppress uterine contractions.

Dipyrone (metamizole) is not teratogenic but there is certain evidence of fetal toxicity in the form of fetal renal insufficiency and narrowing of the ductus arteriosus. This is why its use is contraindicated in the third trimester [25]. In addition, its metabolites are excreted through breast milk. Therefore, if used during lactation, it is suggested to discard breast milk for 48 hours after a single dose of dipyrone [51, 54].

Comparison Between Different Parenteral Medications

There are many options for opioid administration, but it is difficult to establish if one is better than the rest of them, as each hospital uses different strategies and each patient experiences pain differently. However, some comparisons have been published [25, 30, 31, 36, 37, 47, 51, 53 - 63].

- There is no difference between intravenous or intramuscular pethidine concerning pain management but there is difference in patient satisfaction and feeling of freedom [56].
- Pethidine has a superior analgesic effect than tramadol and placebo [29].
- Pethidine is not superior to acetaminophen (paracetamol) [29] or dipyrone (metamizole) [53].
- Pethidine is less effective than epidural analgesia [62] and other opioids as fentanyl or diamorphine [29].
- Pethidine has shown a higher efficacy than tramadol for labour pain management with lower rates of nausea and fatigue [58, 59].
- No major benefits of tramadol over paracetamol or other opioids have been observed [29].
- Nitrous oxide has a higher initial pain relief (30 minutes) than pethidine, but this

advantage disappears at 60 minutes after administration [55].

- The use of nitrous oxide combined with meperidine can significantly reduce pain and meperidine doses without increasing maternal or neonatal complications [64].
- Pethidine has a higher conversion rate to regional analgesia than remifentanil PCA (41% *vs* 16%) [37].
- Fentanyl PCA is associated with higher maternal satisfaction, less sedation and lower interference with breastfeeding than pethidine [30].
- Intravenous fentanyl and intramuscular pethidine have a similar pain relief profile, though fentanyl may have higher fetal side effects (lower APGAR score and higher needs of neonatal resuscitation and naloxone) [31].
- Intrapartum fentanyl seems to have less interference on breastfeeding initiation than intramuscular meperidine [26].
- Low dose morphine and paracetamol have a similar effect in visual analogic scale (*VAS*) measurement initially, but higher requirements of rescue analgesia are needed with paracetamol [60, 65].
- Ketamine can provide better pain control than meperidine, with less nausea and vomiting and higher APGAR score in the newborn, but also higher hallucination rates [53].
- The use of paracetamol with epidural analgesia does not modify the VAS scores but reduces the epidural needs during the first hour and there are lower requirements of additional boluses [54].
- Remifentanil-PCA is significantly superior to intramuscular pethidine for labour pain control with a higher maternal satisfaction [37].
- Remifentanil-PCA is associated to a higher maternal satisfaction than any other intramuscular or intravenous opioids [57].

CONCLUSION

There are so many factors involved in labour pain that comparing different analgesia techniques and pharmacological regimens is difficult. Epidural analgesia is still the technique with the higher satisfaction rates. Programmed intermittent epidural bolus is the most advantageous maintenance regimen: higher satisfaction, lower doses of LA, less motor block. Patients receiving EA are more likely to present intrapartum fever. Epidural analgesia is associated to less maternal depression.

Remifentanil can be a safe alternative to epidural analgesia as long as safety recommendations are followed. The use of ketamine during labour is not recommended as an alternative to epidural analgesia.

CONSENT FOR PUBLICATION

Not applicable.

CONFLICT OF INTEREST

The authors declare no conflict of interest, financial or otherwise.

ACKNOWLEDGEMENT

Declared none.

REFERENCES

[1]   Xu J, Zhou J, Xiao H, *et al.* A Systematic Review and Meta-Analysis Comparing Programmed Intermittent Bolus and Continuous Infusion as the Background Infusion for Parturient-Controlled Epidural Analgesia. Sci Rep 2019; 9(1): 2583.
[http://dx.doi.org/10.1038/s41598-019-39248-5] [PMID: 30796286]

[2]   Lim G. A review of the impact of obstetric anesthesia on maternal and neonatal out- comes:24.

[3]   Kelly A, Tran Q. The optimal pain management approach for a laboring patient: a review of current literature. Cureus 2017; 9(5): e1240.
[http://dx.doi.org/10.7759/cureus.1240] [PMID: 28620569]

[4]   Meng ML, Smiley R. Modern Neuraxial Anesthesia for Labor and Delivery. F1000 Res 2017; 6: 1211.
[http://dx.doi.org/10.12688/f1000research.11130.1] [PMID: 28781763]

[5]   Gupta S, Partani S. Neuraxial techniques of labour analgesia. Indian J Anaesth 2018; 62(9): 658-66.
[http://dx.doi.org/10.4103/ija.IJA_445_18] [PMID: 30237590]

[6]   Xu J, Zhou R, Su W, *et al.* Ultrasound-guided bilateral pudendal nerve blocks of nulliparous women with epidural labour analgesia in the second stage of labour: a randomised, double-blind, controlled trial. BMJ Open 2020; 10(8): e035887.
[http://dx.doi.org/10.1136/bmjopen-2019-035887] [PMID: 32843515]

[7]   Mody SK, Farala JP, Jimenez B, Nishikawa M, Ngo LL. Paracervical Block for Intrauterine Device Placement Among Nulliparous Women. Obstet Gynecol 2018; 132(3): 575-82.
[http://dx.doi.org/10.1097/AOG.0000000000002790] [PMID: 30095776]

[8]   Miles ETC, Stone JP. Pain relief during labour. Lancet 2019; 394(10198): e14.
[http://dx.doi.org/10.1016/S0140-6736(19)30709-3] [PMID: 31262492]

[9]   Tzeng IS, Kao MC, Pan PT, *et al.* A Meta-Analysis of Comparing Intermittent Epidural Boluses and Continuous Epidural Infusion for Labor Analgesia. Int J Environ Res Public Health 2020; 17(19): 7082.
[http://dx.doi.org/10.3390/ijerph17197082] [PMID: 32992642]

[10]   Munro A, George RB. Programmed Intermittent Epidural Boluses (PIEB): A Superior Technique for Maitenance of Labor Analgesia. Turk J Anaesthesiol Reanim 2017; 45(2): 67-9.
[http://dx.doi.org/10.5152/TJAR.2017.09032] [PMID: 28439434]

[11]   Anim-Somuah M, Smyth RM, Cyna AM, Cuthbert A. Epidural versus non-epidural or no analgesia for pain management in labour 2018.

[12]   Li CJ, Xia F, Xu SQ, Shen XF. Concerned topics of epidural labor analgesia: labor elongation and maternal pyrexia: a systematic review. Chin Med J (Engl) 2020; 133(5): 597-605.
[http://dx.doi.org/10.1097/CM9.0000000000000646] [PMID: 32032081]

[13]   Garcia-Lausin L, Perez-Botella M, Duran X, *et al.* Relation between Length of Exposure to Epidural Analgesia during Labour and Birth Mode. Int J Environ Res Public Health 2019; 16(16): 2928. [http://dx.doi.org/10.3390/ijerph16162928] [PMID: 31443209]

[14]   Biel FM, Marshall NE, Snowden JM. Maternal Body Mass Index and Regional Anaesthesia Use at Term: Prevalence and Complications. Paediatr Perinat Epidemiol 2017; 31(6): 495-505. [http://dx.doi.org/10.1111/ppe.12387] [PMID: 28833337]

[15]   Zheng H, Zheng BX, Lin XM. The Trend of Labor Analgesia in the World and China: A Bibliometric Analysis of Publications in Recent 30 Years. J Pain Res 2020; 13: 517-26. [http://dx.doi.org/10.2147/JPR.S232132] [PMID: 32214842]

[16]   Ando H, Makino S, Takeda J, *et al.* Comparison of the labor curves with and without combined spinal-epidural analgesia in nulliparous women- a retrospective study. BMC Pregnancy Childbirth 2020; 20(1): 467. [http://dx.doi.org/10.1186/s12884-020-03161-x] [PMID: 32799848]

[17]   Zhou X, Li J, Deng S, Xu Z, Liu Z. Ropivacaine at different concentrations on intrapartum fever, IL-6 and TNF-α in parturient with epidural labor analgesia. Exp Ther Med. 019 Mar 17(3): 1631-6.

[18]   Liu ZH, Wang DX. Potential impact of epidural labor analgesia on the outcomes of neonates and children. Chin Med J (Engl) 2020; 133(19): 2353-8. [http://dx.doi.org/10.1097/CM9.0000000000000900] [PMID: 32541360]

[19]   Lim G, Farrell LM, Facco FL, Gold MS, Wasan AD. Labor Analgesia as a Predictor for Reduced Postpartum Depression Scores. Anesth Analg 2018; 126(5): 1598-605. [http://dx.doi.org/10.1213/ANE.0000000000002720] [PMID: 29239949]

[20]   Kale A, Usta T, Basol G, Cam I, Yavuz M, Aytuluk HG. Comparison of Ultrasound-Guided Transglu-teal and Finger-Guided Transvaginal Pudendal Nerve Block Techniques: Which One is More E☐ective? Int Neurourol J. 31 de diciembre de ;2019 :(4)23 310-20.

[21]   Kongwattanakul K, Rojanapithayakorn N, *et al.* Anaesthesia/analgesia for manual removal of retained placenta. Cochrane Pregnancy and Childbirth Group, editor. Cochrane Database of Systematic Reviews. June 2020.https://doi.wiley.com/ 10.1002/14651858.CD013013.pub2

[22]   Chin J, Kaneshiro B, Elia J, Raidoo S, Savala M, Soon R. Buffered lidocaine for paracervical blocks in first-trimester abortions: a randomized controlled trial 2020. [http://dx.doi.org/10.1016/j.conx.2020.100044]

[23]   Smith LA, Burns E, Cuthbert A. Parenteral opioids for maternal pain management in labour. Cochrane Libr 2018; 2018(6): CD007396. [http://dx.doi.org/10.1002/14651858.CD007396.pub3] [PMID: 29870574]

[24]   Staikou C, Makris A, Theodoraki K, *et al.* Current Practice in Obstetric Anesthesia and Analgesia in Public Hospitals of Greece: A 2016 National Survey. Balkan Med J 2018; 35(5): 394-7. [http://dx.doi.org/10.4274/balkanmedj.2018.0083] [PMID: 29914232]

[25]   Babaoğlu G, Kiliçaslan B, Ankay Yilbaş A, Çelebĭoğlu B. Effects of different analgesic methods used for vaginal delivery on mothers and fetuses. Turk J Med Sci 2020; 50(4): 930-6. [http://dx.doi.org/10.3906/sag-1911-61] [PMID: 32394678]

[26]   Fleet JA, Jones M, Belan I. The influence of intrapartum opioid use on breastfeeding experience at 6 weeks post partum: A secondary analysis. Midwifery 2017; 50: 106-9. [http://dx.doi.org/10.1016/j.midw.2017.03.024] [PMID: 28411530]

[27]   Hemati Z, Abdollahi M, Broumand S, Delaram M, Namnabati M, Kiani D. Association between newborns' breastfeeding behaviors in the first two hours after birth and drugs used for their mothers in labor. iran J child neurol 2018; 12(2): 33-40. [PMID: 29696044]

[28]   Nunes R, Colares P, Montenegro J. Is Pethidine Safe during Labor? Systematic Review. Rev Bras

Ginecol Obstet 2017; 39(12): 686-91.
[http://dx.doi.org/10.1055/s-0037-1604065] [PMID: 28666300]

[29]   Wong SSC, Cheung CW. Analgesic Efficacy and Adverse Effects of Meperidine in Managing Post-operative or Labor Pain: A Narrative Review. Pain Physician 2020; 28.

[30]   Rezk M, El-Shamy ES, Massod A, Dawood R, Habeeb R. The safety and acceptability of intravenous fentanyl versus intramuscular pethidine for pain relief during labour. Clin Exp Obstet Gynecol 2015; 42(6): 781-4.
[http://dx.doi.org/10.12891/ceog1991.2015] [PMID: 26753485]

[31]   Fleet J, Belan I, Jones MJ, Ullah S, Cyna AM. A comparison of fentanyl with pethidine for pain relief during childbirth: a randomised controlled trial. BJOG 2015; 122(7): 983-92.
[http://dx.doi.org/10.1111/1471-0528.13249] [PMID: 25558983]

[32]   Freeman L, Middeldorp J, van den Akker E, *et al.* An economic analysis of patient controlled remifentanil and epidural analgesia as pain relief in labour (RAVEL trial); a randomised controlled trial. PLoS One 2018; 13(10): e0205220.
[http://dx.doi.org/10.1371/journal.pone.0205220] [PMID: 30307986]

[33]   Lee M, Zhu F, Moodie J, Zhang Z, Cheng D, Martin J. Remifentanil as an alternative to epidural analgesia for vaginal delivery: A meta-analysis of randomized trials. J Clin Anesth 2017; 39: 57-63.
[http://dx.doi.org/10.1016/j.jclinane.2017.03.026] [PMID: 28494909]

[34]   Van de Velde M. Remifentanil Patient-Controlled Intravenous Analgesia for Labor Pain Relief. Anesth Analg 2017; 124(4): 1029-31.
[http://dx.doi.org/10.1213/ANE.0000000000001693] [PMID: 28319538]

[35]   Messmer AA, Potts JM, Orlikowski CE. A prospective observational study of maternal oxygenation during remifentanil patient-controlled analgesia use in labour. Anaesthesia 2016; 71(2): 171-6.
[http://dx.doi.org/10.1111/anae.13329] [PMID: 26617275]

[36]   Stourac P, Kosinova M, Harazim H, *et al.* The analgesic efficacy of remifentanil for labour. Systematic review of the recent literature. Biomed Pap Med Fac Univ Palacky Olomouc Czech Repub 2016; 160(1): 30-8.
[http://dx.doi.org/10.5507/bp.2015.043] [PMID: 26460593]

[37]   Wilson MJA, MacArthur C, Hewitt CA, *et al.* Intravenous remifentanil patient-controlled analgesia versus intramuscular pethidine for pain relief in labour (RESPITE): an open-label, multicentre, randomised controlled trial. Lancet 2018; 392(10148): 662-72.
[http://dx.doi.org/10.1016/S0140-6736(18)31613-1] [PMID: 30115484]

[38]   Dahan A, Douma M, Olofsen E, Niesters M. High inspired oxygen concentration increases the speed of onset of remifentanil-induced respiratory depression. Br J Anaesth 2016; 116(6): 878-9.
[http://dx.doi.org/10.1093/bja/aew130] [PMID: 27199320]

[39]   Leong WL, Sng BL, Zhang Q, Han NLR, Sultana R, Sia ATH. A case series of vital signs-controlled, patient-assisted intravenous analgesia (VPIA) using remifentanil for labour and delivery. Anaesthesia 2017; 72(7): 845-52.
[http://dx.doi.org/10.1111/anae.13878] [PMID: 28418067]

[40]   Weiniger CF, Carvalho B, Stocki D, Einav S. Analysis of Physiological Respiratory Variable Alarm Alerts Among Laboring Women Receiving Remifentanil. Anesth Analg 2017; 124(4): 1211-8.
[http://dx.doi.org/10.1213/ANE.0000000000001644] [PMID: 27870644]

[41]   Lu G, Yao W, Chen X, Zhang S, Zhou M. Remifentanil patient-controlled versus epidural analgesia on intrapartum maternal fever: a systematic review and meta-analysis. BMC Pregnancy Childbirth 2020; 20(1): 151.
[http://dx.doi.org/10.1186/s12884-020-2800-y] [PMID: 32164593]

[42]   Burgos J, Pijoan JI, Osuna C, *et al.* Increased pain relief with remifentanil does not improve the success rate of external cephalic version: a randomized controlled trial. Acta Obstet Gynecol Scand

2016; 95(5): 547-54.
[http://dx.doi.org/10.1111/aogs.12859] [PMID: 26830687]

[43]   Khaw KS, Lee SWY, Ngan Kee WD, *et al.* Randomized trial of anaesthetic interventions in external cephalic version for breech presentation. Br J Anaesth 2015; 114(6): 944-50.
[http://dx.doi.org/10.1093/bja/aev107] [PMID: 25962611]

[44]   Ohashi Y, Baghirzada L, Sumikura H, Balki M. Remifentanil for labor analgesia: a comprehensive review. J Anesth 2016; 30(6): 1020-30.
[http://dx.doi.org/10.1007/s00540-016-2233-y] [PMID: 27619509]

[45]   Melber AA, Jelting Y, Huber M, *et al.* Remifentanil patient-controlled analgesia in labour: six-year audit of outcome data of the RemiPCA SAFE Network (2010–2015). Int J Obstet Anesth 2019; 39: 12-21.
[http://dx.doi.org/10.1016/j.ijoa.2018.12.004] [PMID: 30685299]

[46]   Van de Velde M, Carvalho B. Remifentanil for labor analgesia: an evidence-based narrative review. Int J Obstet Anesth 2016; 25: 66-74.
[http://dx.doi.org/10.1016/j.ijoa.2015.12.004] [PMID: 26777438]

[47]   Murray H, Hodgkinson P, Hughes D. Remifentanil patient-controlled intravenous analgesia during labour: a retrospective observational study of 10 years' experience. Int J Obstet Anesth 2019; 39: 29-34.
[http://dx.doi.org/10.1016/j.ijoa.2019.05.012] [PMID: 31230993]

[48]   Kaur Makkar J, Jain K, Bhatia N, Jain V, Mal Mithrawal S. Comparison of analgesic efficacy of paracetamol and tramadol for pain relief in active labor. J Clin Anesth 2015; 27(2): 159-63.
[http://dx.doi.org/10.1016/j.jclinane.2014.08.008] [PMID: 25434500]

[49]   Yadav J, Regmi MC, Basnet P, Guddy KM, Bhattarai B, Poudel P. Butorphanol in Labour Analgesia. JNMA J Nepal Med Assoc 2018; 56(214): 940-4.
[http://dx.doi.org/10.31729/jnma.3905] [PMID: 31065139]

[50]   Singer J, Jank A, Amara S, Stepan P, Kaisers U, Hoehne C. Efficacy and Effects of Parenteral Pethidine or Meptazinol and Regional Analgesia for Pain Relief during Delivery. A Comparative Observational Study. Geburtshilfe Frauenheilkd 2016; 76(9): 964-71.
[http://dx.doi.org/10.1055/s-0042-111009] [PMID: 27681521]

[51]   Potter J, Perez-Velasco D, Maxymiv NG, Graham J, Faircloth A, Thakrar S. A combination of inhaled nitrous oxide and low-dose ketamine infusion for labor analgesia. J Clin Anesth 2019; 57: 64-5.
[http://dx.doi.org/10.1016/j.jclinane.2019.02.019] [PMID: 30875519]

[52]   Ducloy-Bouthors A-S, *et al.* Normal childbirth: physiolo- gic labor support and medical procedures. Guidelines of the French National Authority for Health [HAS] - Mother's wellbeing and regional or systemic analgesia for labor. Gynécol Obstét Fertil Sénol 2020; 48(12): 891-906.33011380.

[53]   El-Halwagy A, Fathy S, Dawood A. Intranasal Ketamine vs. Intramuscular Pethidine in Labor Pain Analgesia. J Anesth Clin Res 2017; 8.

[54]   Nunes R, Primo A. Pethidine in Low Doses versus Dipyrone for Pain Relief in Labor: A Randomized Controlled Trial. Rev Bras Ginecol Obstet 2019; 41(2): 084-9.
[http://dx.doi.org/10.1055/s-0038-1676509] [PMID: 30786304]

[55]   Mobaraki N, Yousefian M, Seifi S, Sakaki M. A Randomized Controlled Trial Comparing Use of Enthonox With Pethidine for Pain Relief in Primigravid Women During the Active Phase of Labor. Anesth Pain Med 2016; 6(4): e37420.
[http://dx.doi.org/10.5812/aapm.37420] [PMID: 27843776]

[56]   Fleet JA, Jones M, Belan I. Taking the alternative route: Women's experience of intranasal fentanyl, subcutaneous fentanyl or intramuscular pethidine for labour analgesia. Midwifery 2017; 53: 15-9.
[http://dx.doi.org/10.1016/j.midw.2017.07.006] [PMID: 28735031]

[57]   Weibel S, Jelting Y, Afshari A, *et al.* Patient-controlled analgesia with remifentanil versus alternative

parenteral methods for pain management in labour. Cochrane Libr 2017; 2017(4): CD011989.
[http://dx.doi.org/10.1002/14651858.CD011989.pub2] [PMID: 28407220]

[58]   Keskin HL, Aktepe Keskin E, Avsar AF, Tabuk M, Caglar GS. Pethidine versus tramadol for pain
       relief during labor. Int J Gynaecol Obstet 2003; 82(1): 11-6.
       [http://dx.doi.org/10.1016/S0020-7292(03)00047-X] [PMID: 12834936]

[59]   Jain S, Arya VK, Gopalan S, Jain V. Analgesic efficacy of intramuscular opioids versus epidural
       analgesia in labor. Int J Gynaecol Obstet 2003; 83(1): 19-27.
       [http://dx.doi.org/10.1016/S0020-7292(03)00201-7] [PMID: 14511868]

[60]   Ankumah NE, Tsao M, Hutchinson M, *et al.* Intravenous Acetaminophen versus Morphine for
       Analgesia in Labor: A Randomized Trial. Am J Perinatol 2017; 34(1): 38-43.
       [PMID: 27182992]

[61]   Süğür T, Kızılateş E, Kızılateş A, İnanoğlu K, Karslı B. Labor analgesia: Comparison of epidural pa-
       tient-controlled analgesia and intravenous patient-controlled analgesia. Agri Agri Algoloji Derneginin
       Yayin Organidir J Turk Soc Algol. 2020; 32(1): 8-18.

[62]   Freeman LM, Bloemenkamp KW, Franssen MT, *et al.* Patient controlled analgesia with remifentanil
       versus epidural analgesia in labour: randomised multicentre equivalence trial. BMJ 2015; h846.
       [http://dx.doi.org/10.1136/bmj.h846] [PMID: 25713015]

[63]   Moran VH, Thomson G, Cook J, *et al.* Qualitative exploration of women's experiences of
       intramuscular pethidine or remifentanil patient-controlled analgesia for labour pain. BMJ Open 2019;
       9(12): e032203.
       [http://dx.doi.org/10.1136/bmjopen-2019-032203] [PMID: 31874879]

[64]   Sharifian Attar A, Shirinzadeh Feizabadi A, Jarahi L, Shirinzadeh Feizabadi L, Sheybani S. Effect of
       Entonox on reducing the need for Pethidine and the Relevant Fetal and Maternal Complications for
       Painless Labor. Electron Physician 2016; 8(12): 3325-32.
       [http://dx.doi.org/10.19082/3325] [PMID: 28163844]

[65]   Gupta K, Mitra S, Kazal S, Saroa R, Ahuja V, Goel P. I.V. paracetamol as an adjunct to patient-
       controlled epidural analgesia with levobupivacaine and fentanyl in labour: a randomized controlled
       study. Br J Anaesth 2016; 117(5): 617-22.
       [http://dx.doi.org/10.1093/bja/aew311] [PMID: 27799176]

CHAPTER 6

Local Anesthetics and Adjuvants for Labor: Local Anesthetic Systemic Toxicity

Patricia Alfaro de la Torre[1,*], **Monir Kabiri Sacramento**[2], **Irene Riquelme Osado**[3] and **Rosa Fernández García**[4]

[1] *Hospital Joan XXIII, Tarragona, Spain*

[2] *Department of Anesthesiology and Intensive Care, HM Hospital Universitario Madrid, Madrid, Spain*

[3] *Hospital Sanitas La Moraleja, Madrid, Spain*

[4] *Hospital Universitario Príncipe de Asturias, Madrid, Spain*

Abstract: The choice of drugs used during labor is almost as important as the analgesic technique selected since effective pain relief contributes directly to satisfaction: the better the pain relief, the higher the satisfaction. Although bupivacaine has traditionally been the most widely used local anesthetic, L-bupivacaine and ropivacaine have similar action profiles with a lower risk of cardiovascular and neurologic toxicity and especially less motor blockade, when used under low-concentration strategies. The use of adjuvants, especially opioids, allows us to improve the analgesic quality while reducing the total dose of local anesthetics, although their use should be individualized, and patients should be monitored and treated for side effects if they appear.

Keywords: Anesthetic Complications, Body Distribution, Bupivacaine, Dosage, Drugs, Fat Emulsions, Intralipid, Levobupivacaine, Lidocaine, Liposomal Bupivacaine, Lipid Emulsion, Lipid Shuttle, Lipid Sink, Local Anesthetic, Local Anesthetic Systemic Toxicity, Metabolism, Pharmacokinetics, Procaine, Regional Anesthesia, Ropivacaine, Tetracaine, Toxicity.

INTRODUCTION

Local anesthetics (*LA*) are a group of pharmacological agents that block the conduction of electrical nerve impulses, temporarily and predictably, causing a loss of sensitivity, that can affect any nervous structure, including the CNS.

The ideal LA for obstetric analgesia should have a good safety profile when acci-

---

* **Corresponding author Patricia Alfaro de la Torre:** Department of Anesthesiology and Intensive Care, HM Hospital Universitario Madrid, Spain; Email: doloralfaro@gmail.com

Eugenio Daniel Martinez-Hurtado, Monica Sanjuan-Alvarez & Marta Chacon-Castillo (Eds.)
All rights reserved-© 2022 Bentham Science Publishers

dentally overdosed or administered intravenously, produce a reliable sensory block, have no motor block, and no tachyphylaxis.

MECHANISM OF ACTION OF LOCAL ANESTHETICS

Local anesthetics inhibit the propagation of the nerve impulse by reducing the permeability of the voltage-dependent sodium channel, blocking the initial phase of the action potential. The lower sodium influx depresses excitability, the rate of depolarization, and therefore the amplitude of the action potential. To do this, local anesthetics must cross the nerve membrane, since their fundamental pharmacological action is carried out on the cytoplasmic side of the sodium channel [1].

The interruption of the afferent transmission of the painful stimuli that is achieved with neuraxial sensory block allows to achieve adequate anesthesia or analgesia, depending on the local anesthetic used and its dose. Since the effect of LAs varies depending on the size of the nerve and the amount of myelin around it, a differential block of fibers occurs following this chronology:

1. Increased skin temperature, and vasodilation (blocking of autonomous B and SC fibers).
2. Loss of thermal sensation, and pain relief (Aδ and C fiber block).
3. Loss of proprioception (AΥ fibers).
4. Loss of touch and pressure sensation (Aβ fibers).
5. Loss of motor skills (Aα fibers).

The recovery from these neurological effects follows the reverse order of its onset. The differential blocking of the different types of fibers according to their thickness and amount of myelin can not only be explained by the differences between the layers of myelin, but also by the electrophysiological properties of the ion channel.

Properties and Implications of Local Anesthetics

Physiochemical properties of local anesthetics vary between them, defining their differences. These properties include potency, latency and duration of action.

Potency is determined by the liposolubility of the molecule. To exert their pharmacological action, local anesthetics must permeate the nerve membrane, which is 90% lipidic. There is a positive correlation between the liposolubility coefficient of the local anesthetics and their potency. Another factor that affects both the anesthetic potency and the duration of action is the vasodilator and redistribution power to the tissues, an intrinsic property of each local anesthetic

(Lidocaine is more vasodilator than mepivacaine and ropivacaine is more vasoconstrictor than bupivacaine) [1].

The onset of action or latency is highly conditioned by the pKa of each drug. The percentage of the non-ionized portion is inversely proportional to the pKa of the anesthetic (Table **1**). It is the main indicator that sets the beginning of action for the local anesthetic.

Table 1. Local Anesthetics doses of administration.

DRUG	BUPIVACAINE	L-BUPIVACAINE	ROPIVACAINE	LIDOCAINE	MEPIVACAINE
ANALGESIC	0.0625-0.2%	0.0625-0.25%	0.1-0.2%	0.75%	0.75%
ANESTHETIC	0.5%	0.5%	0.5-0.75%	2-5%	2%
MAX. DOSE (mg/kg)	2'5	2	2	4'5	5
ONSET (min)	10-30	10-12	6-7	5-10	10-15
DURATION (min)	280-480	240-360	180-480	120-240	180-360
pKa	8.1	8.1	8	7.9	7.6

Local anesthetics are highly protein-bound molecules, which correlate with their duration of action, where highly lipid-soluble local anesthetics have a longer duration of action. This is partly explained by the fact that said binding capacity determines the percentage of free ionized and non-ionized form and, therefore, its effect, as the non-bound fraction of the molecules are the ones responsible for the action of the local anesthetic [2].

In low plasmatic protein states, such as pregnancy, neonates or hypoproteinemia, local anesthetic systemic toxicity events can be seen, as the free active fraction is increased. We must have these hypoproteinemia states in mind as we estimate both the administered dose and the administration time.

The pH of the organism also determines the percentage of the anesthetics protein binding. Acidosis situations generate a marked decrease in the said fixation of the local anesthetic to plasma proteins, causing an increase in the drug free fraction, which can also lead to systemic toxicity. This is especially relevant with bupivacaine, whose free drug concentration can increase from 5% to 30% just because of the presence of acidosis [3].

Placental transfer of bupivacaine seems to occur by a passive diffusion mechanism, rather than active transport, and appears to be influenced by maternal and fetal plasma protein binding capacity, fetal pH, and placental performance.

Anyhow, lidocaine and bupivacaine, in clinical doses through the epidural or subarachnoid route, rarely affect the APGAR and Newborn Adaptive Capacity tests, except when they are administered under adverse pathophysiological situations (acidosis) or paracervically [4].

Animal studies on uteroplacental hemodynamics have shown that both ropivacaine and bupivacaine, which present a similar placental diffusion rate, have minimal effects when administered in usual epidural doses, and are not harmful to either mother or fetus.

DIFFERENCES BETWEEN LOCAL ANESTHETICS AND THEIR EFFECTS

Lidocaine

Compared to the others, it has a very fast onset of action and a short duration but produces greater motor blockage. Its placental diffusion is large and in the presence of acidosis, greater accumulation may occur in the fetus, especially in premature babies (caused by the decrease in plasma proteins). Lidocaine causes tachyphylaxis from the 4th or 5th dose administered. It is very useful in short deliveries, urgent cesarean sections or to check the effectiveness of an epidural catheter.

Mepivacaine

Its dosage should be adjusted according to age, weight and the physical condition of each patient. Children and the elderly require a lower dose than adults and in obstetrics, it should be reduced by 30% taking into account the altered anatomical characteristics of the epidural space and the greater sensitivity to local anesthetics during pregnancy. It is an intermediate-acting anesthetic, with a rapid onset.

In addition, it has a certain degree of vasoconstrictor activity, which allows to reduce the total dose and generally dispenses with the use of additional vasoconstrictors in its administration. It is very useful in short deliveries and emergency cesarean sections.

Bupivacaine

Derived from mepivacaine, it is four times more powerful than lidocaine. It is the most toxic of the amides. Long-term local anesthetic is indicated in subarachnoid anesthesia to perform interventions on the lower extremities, perineum, lower abdomen and obstetrics [5].

For years, it has been the most widely employed LA in labor and delivery. It has a long duration (due to its high pKa), with high protein binding capacity, low rate of placental diffusion, and a high capacity for sensory blockade with little motor blockade when administered at lower concentrations (0.125-0.2%). Its greatest disadvantage is its potential cardiotoxic effect, to which pregnant patients are more susceptible.

Levobupivacaine

It is the levorotatory enantiomer of bupivacaine, equipotent with it but with less cardiovascular and neurotoxicity as well as less motor blocking capacity. It is 19% more powerful than ropivacaine and is currently the most widely used drug for continuous infusions in labor analgesia [5, 6]. When used at concentrations of 0.0625%, it even allows the ambulation of the woman during labor (walking epidural).

Ropivacaine

The latest generation LA is marketed in its pure enantiomeric form (S) in order to improve the safety profile of this type of drug (lower cardiotoxicity and adverse effects at the central nervous system level). It has intrinsic vasoconstrictor action. The duration of the motor block is slightly shorter than bupivacaine's [6]. Ropivacaine and bupivacaine are not equipotent (0.15% ropivacaine is equivalent to 0,1% bupivacaine), and do not have a superior sensory-motor differential block. As being more lipophilic, they have a selective action on sensory fibers (A-delta and C), making it more difficult for them to penetrate large myelinated fibers (A-alfa).

LOCAL ANESTHETICS ADJUVANTS

Opioids

The analgesic effect of an opioid is due to its plasma absorption and redistribution, regardless of the place of administration, hence its use must be individualized since its systemic side effects can counteract its analgesic benefits.

The intrathecal behavior of opioids does not obey the relative potency of their intravenous administration: sufentanil is thousand times more potent than morphine when administered intravenously, but intrathecally it is only 10 times more potent; the potency of fentanyl would be 2-4 times more than morphine at the intrathecal level while at the intravenous level, it would be 100 times higher.

Therefore, the selectivity of opioids at the spinal level and the duration of their postoperative analgesic effects together with a minimum effective dose that reduces the rate of side effects should be our goal.

Administered epidurally (alone, with no LA), they provide pain relief in the first phase of labor but not in the second (which is why they should not always be used by the protocol, but rather adapt their use to the patient's situation). The most common side effects include pruritus and nausea/vomiting, and very exceptionally, respiratory depression.

Combined with LA, their synergic effect allows to reduce the dose of LA, with less motor block, the shorter onset of action and a longer effect [7]. Adding a lipid-soluble opioid (*e.g.*, fentanyl, sufentanil) to the LA enhances intraoperative anesthesia by reducing the total dose of LA, reducing hypotension, nausea, and vomiting [7].

Fentanyl

Fentanyl is by far the most widely used, in an initial epidural bolus dose of 50 µg together with LA and in perfusion of LA at a concentration of 1-2 µg /ml. The addition of fentanyl to the spinal LA in a caesarean section increases the duration and improves the analgesic effects without increasing the motor block for up to 6 hours with no fetal repercussion. The optimal dose of 15 µg is also not exempted from the pruritus that many patients develop.

Morphine

Morphine is a water-soluble opioid that confers postoperative analgesia with or without fentanil in the spinal single-shot mix or for epidural analgesia before catheter removal after delivery [8]. It is considered the gold standard for epidural opioids with a longer half-life up to 24-36 h. The intrathecal dose is 1/10 of the calculated epidural route and it is recommended not to exceed 10 mg. per day. Patients should be monitored for respiratory depression as morphine has a double phasic absorption, with a late peak at 12 hours after administration.

Meperidine (Pethidine)

Meperidine and its derivatives possess pharmacological properties similar to those of LAs (including hyperbaricity when used intrathecally) and a liposolubility similar to morphine (cephalic diffusion). Although one of its advantages is reducing the tremors associated with neuraxial techniques, it requires high effective doses that produce a higher incidence of side effects compared to other opioids.

Pure spinal opioid's administration alone could be very useful in high risk patients (hypovolemia, aortic stenosis, Fallot tetralogy, pulmonary hypertension) since, with the exception of meperidine, they do not cause motor or sympathetic block.

Adrenaline

Due to the increased sensitivity of the pregnant patient and the consequent increased risks, the administration of epinephrine in the epidural test dose is not clear. The administration of epinephrine 1: 200000 in combination with LA should not be used routinely as recent studies have not demonstrated its efficacy. If used, it should not exceed a dose of 2-4 ml and should not be used but during epidural catheter placement [9].

Bicarbonate

Sodium bicarbonate has traditionally been added to LAs in order to alkalize the mixture and thus accelerate the onset of action of the drug. But nevertheless, the effects of alkalization of LAs are not entirely clear. According to bibliographic reviews, the addition of bicarbonate provides few benefits, and the main drawback is the precipitation of the mixture. Its use is not recommended.

Other Local Anesthetics Additives

There are many additives under study that we did not include because their use in this setting is off-label (dexamethasone, dexmedetomidine, buprenorphine) [10 - 12]. Despite this and the absence of FDA approval, the use of clonidine is quite widespread since, when added to LA, it seems to extend almost a hundred minutes the long-lasting pain-relieving effect of the LA. The estimated effective and safe dose is 100-150 µg, higher doses are associated with a higher incidence of side effects such as dizziness, hypotension and bradycardia [10]. These cardiovascular effects must be especially taken into consideration as they can have an important repercussion on the fetus.

POSSIBLE DOSES OF ADMINISTRATION

Depending on the phase of delivery that we are assisting, the requirements will be different. The situation must always be individualized and assessed, based on the analgesic or anesthetic requirements, the patient's comorbidities and the need for an emergency action (labor/cesarean section/emergency) (Tables **1** and **2**). Low dose strategies minimize hemodynamic effects, motor block, placental drug transfer, LA toxicity and opioids' side-effects [13].

Table 2. Opioids doses of administration.

DRUG	MORFINE	MEPERIDINE	FENTANIL	SUFENTANIL
INTRATECAL	0.1-0.3 mg	10-15 mg	10-25 µg	3-10 µg
EPIDURAL	2-5 mg	50-100 mg	50-150 µg	10-20 µg
RELATIVE LIPO-SOLUBILITY	1	30	600	1200
ONSET (min)	15-30	5-10	5-10	5-15
DURATION (h)	4-24	4-6	1-3	2-6
MEDULAR SELECTIVITY Epidural/ Intratecal	++++ / ++++	? / ?	-- / ++	- / ++

Low dose strategies of epidural LA are not associated with a prolonged duration of the second stage of labor or an increased instrumental birth rate.

General recommendations for the use of LA in labor:

Epidural Catheter for Labor

Test Dose: The traditional concept of a test dose appears inappropriate in obstetric population as it is more likely to cause complications than to avoid them. In view of the contemporary practice of low-dose–low-concentration epidural, the analgesic dose itself or a fraction of it may be considered as an appropriate test dose [9]. The most commonly used drugs are 2-3 ml. of bupivacaine 0.25% or lidocaine 1-2% with adrenaline 1: 200.000 through the catheter.

Initial Bolus: Given that, a T10-L1 level must be reached to be effective, it is usually necessary to administer an initial bolus of 6-10 ml. of LA and 5 ml. increments spaced 2-5 minutes apart until the desired sensory level is achieved.

Combined Epidural-Spinal Technique

Analgesia onset is faster and with lower maternal hypotension and opioid side effects. A dose of opioid, alone or with a small dose of LA, usually less than 5 mg (bupivacaine, l-bupivacaine, ropivacaine), is administered into the spinal space and the epidural catheter is then placed, so that analgesia over the sacral roots is established almost immediately, providing better analgesia in the first 30 minutes compared to epidural alone [14].

The benefits of sacral analgesia improvement compared to epidural analgesia alone, result in less pruritus, hypotension, supplemental epidural doses, and uterine tachysystole than combined spinal-epidural analgesia [15].

Patient-Controlled/Continuous/Intermittent Perfusion

Basically, for low dose LA perfusions (preparations of L-bupivacaine 0.125-0.0625% or ropivacaine 0.2-0.1%) to which low dose opioids are added if considered necessary, such as 2 µg/ml fentanyl, the infusion rate is usually 5 to 15 ml/h [16]. Additional boluses can be programmed and administered on demand if needed.

Caesarean Section

There is great variability worldwide in the procedure, and many facts need to be taken into consideration (level of emergency, prior epidural, hemodynamic situation, *etc.*) when evaluating the need for general anesthesia versus reconversion of an epidural technique.

In case we consider reconversion of epidural analgesia to anesthesia, we will need to administer a potent LA with a fast onset at an anesthetic dose. These may be some possibilities/examples of conversion doses from epidural analgesia to anesthesia for intrapartum cesarean delivery:

- Lidocaine 2-5%: - 7-10 ml
- Mepivacaine 2%: 8-10 ml
- Ropivacaine / L-bupivacaine 0.75%: 7-10 ml

If there is no epidural catheter or we are facing a programmed c-section, single-shot spinal anesthesia may be possible for cesarean delivery. In contrast to epidural anesthesia, as the total local anesthetic dose required is lower; there is virtually no risk for local anesthetic systemic toxicity and fetal drug transfer is minimal.

The effective dose for hyperbaric bupivacaine in 95% of patients (ED95) is 13 mg when administered with intrathecal fentanyl (10-25 µg) and morphine (50-200 µg). Higher doses (*e.g.*, 15 mg) are associated with a longer duration, but also with higher sensory blockade and a higher incidence and degree of hypotension [17].

Every dose must be individualized in each patient according to their height and weight, comorbidities and considering the physiological changes that take place in the epidural and subarachnoid spaces in the pregnant patient (higher pressure, dilated veins, higher intake), which will generally lead us to a lower dose than the ED95.

LOCAL ANESTHETIC SYSTEMIC TOXICITY (*LAST*)

Manifestations of LA toxicity can appear/manifest between 30 seconds and 60 minutes after injection, usually within the first 5 minutes. They include subjective symptoms of CNS excitement such as auditory changes, numbness, metallic taste, and agitation that can then progress/evolve to seizures and/or CNS depression (coma, respiratory arrest).

In classic descriptions of LAST (Fig. **1**), cardiac toxicity does not occur without preceding CNS toxicity [18].

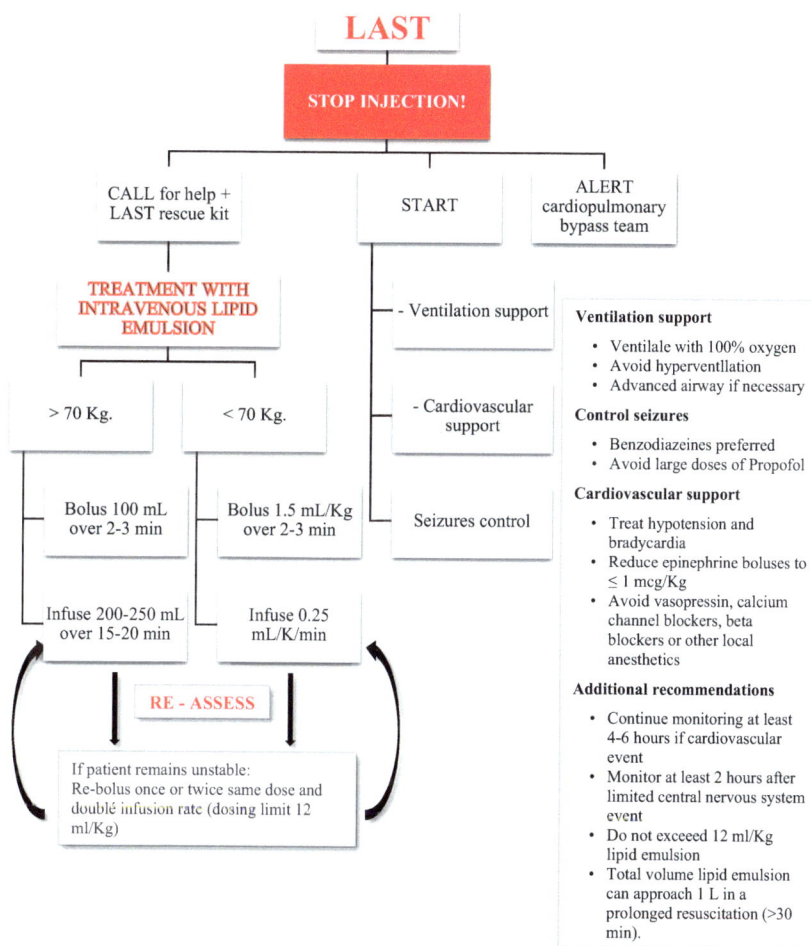

Fig. (1). Local Anesthetic Systemic Toxicity (LAST) protocol treatment. Based in NYSORA (New York School of Regional Anesthesia) proposed protocol.

The prevention of this complication is essential, with all the measures that we have at our disposal, as well as always using the minimum concentration of LA and all possible caution in its administration [19]. In order to prevent and recognize early signs and symptoms of last, the patient should be always monitored while performing techniques using LA. Also, aspiration prior to injection allows to minimize the risk of intravascular administration of LA. The total dose should be given slowly and fractioned if larger volumes are to be given.

One of the peculiarities of this syndrome is its immense variability in the clinical forms in which it can appear, hence its early recognition is extremely important, as treatment consists of supportive measures, controlling seizures and maintaining cardiovascular stability/function.

Treatment with intravenous lipid emulsion (*ILE*) has been accepted in the most recent guidelines despite presenting many unanswered responses [20] (Fig. **2**). Its main indication is cardiac arrest or shock refractory to conventional measures that are a direct consequence of the toxic effect of local anesthetics, calcium antagonists, beta-blockers, cyclic antidepressants, antipsychotics and other highly lipid-soluble toxins [21].

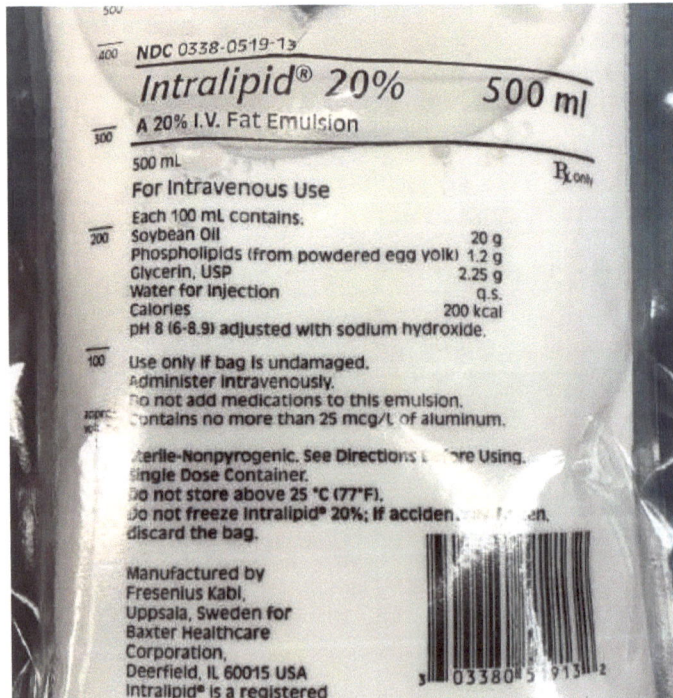

Fig. (2). Intralipid 20% (intravenous lipid emulsion) composition.

The mechanism of action of ILE consists of:

1. Binding the free plasma fraction of LA (high affinity for bupivacaine due to its lipophilic nature). It is a *"sponge"* effect, where the high liposolubility of the plasmatic ILE would cause an immediate mobilization of the toxin from the tissue deposit, in this case, the cardiovascular system, towards the extracellular space, would reduce the concentration of the toxin in the target organ by increasing the plasmatic concentration. Ultimately, what the ILE does is modify the volume of distribution of the toxin.

2. Interaction with the sodium channel. It seems that fatty acids could activate some ion channels and / or unblock some adrenergic receptors, which would explain the therapeutic effect observed in toxicity caused by by some calcium antagonists such as (verapamil) sodium pump blocking antidepressants (clomipramine) and beta-blockers (propranolol).

3. It collaborates with the metabolism of the mitochondria, in particular of the cardiomyocytes, and specifically on the ATPases, which are the subset of enzymes capable of producing dephosphorylation, that is, the hydrolysis of adenosine triphosphate (*ATP*) into adenosine diphosphate (*ADP*) and a free phosphorus ion (phosphate ion).

The updated AORN Clinical Guide for the Care of the Patient Receiving Local Anesthesia provides guidance on perioperative care evaluations and interventions for patients receiving local anesthesia [21].

This guide addresses patient evaluation, the importance of having a general understanding of the local agent being used, recommended monitoring requirements, and possible adverse events, including those that are life-threatening. An American Society of Regional Anesthesia (*ASRA*) LAST checklist was studied based on studies and experience updated in 2020 with simple recommendations for prevention and treatment of LAST [22] (Fig. **3**).

CONCLUSION

There is a greater likelihood of systemic toxicity from local anesthetics in those patients who are short in stature, have less muscle mass, in those who are extremely old, and in those with pre-existing cardiac disease or carnitine deficiency.

Approximately half of the cases present without seizures, and only present with cardiovascular involvement with cardiovascular toxicity, or present clinically late.

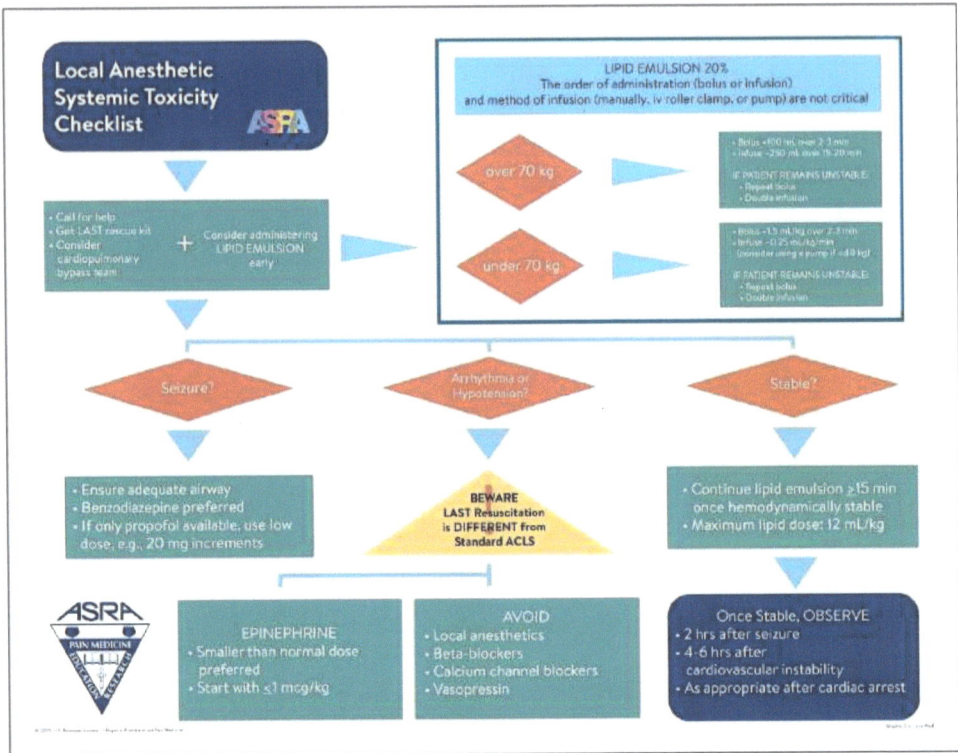

Fig. (3). Checklist for Treatment of Local Anesthetic Systemic Toxicity [22].

- The incidence of toxicity increases when the anesthetic is injected near vascularized areas. It is highest with paravertebral injections, followed by upper and lower extremity injections.
- Prevention of LAST-related morbidity requires optimization of the entire regional anesthesia care process, including proper patient selection, choice of nerve block, drug and dose to be used, and adequate monitoring, which must be complete. This preparation should include the preparation of a kit for the treatment of LAST, as well as the periodic practice of simulation.
- Prevention also includes awareness and education of non-anesthesiologists on the appropriate use of LAs and the risks that their use may entail, including the management of LAST.

CONSENT FOR PUBLICATION

Not applicable.

CONFLICT OF INTEREST

The authors declare no conflict of interest, financial or otherwise.

ACKNOWLEDGEMENT

Declared none.

REFERENCES

[1]   Lirk Philipp, Picardi Susanne, Hollmann Markus W. Local anaesthetics: 10 essentials, European Journal of Anaesthesiology: November 2014; 31(11): 575-85.

[2]   Zink Wolfgang, Graf Bernhard M. 2. Zink, Wolfgang; Graf, Bernhard M The toxicity of local anesthetics: the place of ropivacaine and levobupivacaine, Current Opinion in Anaesthesiology: October 2008; 21(5): 645-50.

[3]   Lim G, Facco FL, Nathan N, Waters JH, Wong CA, Eltzschig HK. A review of the impact of obstetric anesthesia on maternal and neonatal outcomes. anesthesiology 2018; 129(1): 192-215.
       [http://dx.doi.org/10.1097/ALN.0000000000002182] [PMID: 29561267]

[4]   Eduardo Adolfo Casini Pasaje transplacentario de drogas. Simposio sobre Obstetricia y Anestesia. Rev Arg Anest 2000; 58(6): 345-57.

[5]   Veering BT, Burm AG, Feyen HM, Olieman W, M Souverijn JH, Van Kleef JW. Pharmacokinetics of bupivacaine during postoperative epidural infusion: enantioselectivity and role of protein binding. Anesthesiology 2002; 96(5): 1062-9.
       [http://dx.doi.org/10.1097/00000542-200205000-00006] [PMID: 11981143]

[6]   Casati A, Putzu M. Bupivacaine, levobupivacaine and ropivacaine: are they clinically different? Baillieres Best Pract Res Clin Anaesthesiol 2005; 19(2): 247-68.
       [http://dx.doi.org/10.1016/j.bpa.2004.12.003] [PMID: 15966496]

[7]   Dahlgren G, Hultstrand C, Jakobsson J, Norman M, Eriksson EW, Martin H. Intrathecal sufentanil, fentanyl, or placebo added to bupivacaine for cesarean section. Anesth Analg 1997; 85(6): 1288-93.
       [http://dx.doi.org/10.1213/00000539-199712000-00020] [PMID: 9390596]

[8]   Palmer CM, Emerson S, Volgoropolous D, Alves D. Dose-response relationship of intrathecal morphine for postcesarean analgesia. Anesthesiology 1999; 90(2): 437-44.
       [http://dx.doi.org/10.1097/00000542-199902000-00018] [PMID: 9952150]

[9]   Massoth C, Wenk M. Epidural test dose in obstetric patients. Curr Opin Anaesthesiol 2019; 32(3): 263-7.
       [http://dx.doi.org/10.1097/ACO.0000000000000721] [PMID: 30985339]

[10]   Lavand'homme PM, Roelants F, Waterloos H, Collet V, De Kock MF. An evaluation of the postoperative antihyperalgesic and analgesic effects of intrathecal clonidine administered during elective cesarean delivery. Anesth Analg 2008; 107(3): 948-55.
       [http://dx.doi.org/10.1213/ane.0b013e31817f1595] [PMID: 18713912]

[11]   Brummett CM, Williams BA. Additives to local anesthetics for peripheral nerve blockade. Int Anesthesiol Clin 2011; 49(4): 104-16.
       [http://dx.doi.org/10.1097/AIA.0b013e31820e4a49] [PMID: 21956081]

[12]   Brummett CM, Amodeo FS, Janda AM, Padda AK, Lydic R. Perineural dexmedetomidine provides an increased duration of analgesia to a thermal stimulus when compared with a systemic control in a rat sciatic nerve block. Reg Anesth Pain Med 2010; 35(5): 427-31.
       [http://dx.doi.org/10.1097/AAP.0b013e3181ef4cf0] [PMID: 20814283]

[13]   Wang TT, Sun S, Huang SQ. effects of epidural labor analgesia with low concentrations of local

anesthetics on obstetric outcomes. anesth analg 2017; 124(5): 1571-80.
[http://dx.doi.org/10.1213/ANE.0000000000001709] [PMID: 27828798]

[14] Goodman SR, Smiley RM, Negron MA, Freedman PA, Landau R. A randomized trial of breakthrough pain during combined spinal-epidural versus epidural labor analgesia in parous women. Anesth Analg 2009; 108(1): 246-51.
[http://dx.doi.org/10.1213/ane.0b013e31818f896f] [PMID: 19095858]

[15] Chau A, Bibbo C, Huang CC, *et al.* Dural Puncture Epidural Technique Improves Labor Analgesia Quality With Fewer Side Effects Compared With Epidural and Combined Spinal Epidural Techniques. Anesth Analg 2017; 124(2): 560-9.
[http://dx.doi.org/10.1213/ANE.0000000000001798] [PMID: 28067707]

[16] Meng ML, Smiley R. Modern Neuraxial Anesthesia for Labor and Delivery. F1000 Res 2017; 6: 1211.
[http://dx.doi.org/10.12688/f1000research.11130.1] [PMID: 28781763]

[17] Garry M, Davies S. Failure of regional blockade for caesarean section. Int J Obstet Anesth 2002; 11(1): 9-12.
[http://dx.doi.org/10.1054/ijoa.2001.0903] [PMID: 15321571]

[18] Neal JM, Bernards CM, Butterworth JF IV, *et al.* ASRA practice advisory on local anesthetic systemic toxicity. Reg Anesth Pain Med 2010; 35(2): 152-61.
[http://dx.doi.org/10.1097/AAP.0b013e3181d22fcd] [PMID: 20216033]

[19] Neal JM, Woodward CM, Harrison TK. The american society of regional anesthesia and pain medicine checklist for managing local anesthetic systemic toxicity. reg anesth pain med 2018; 43(2): 150-3.
[http://dx.doi.org/10.1097/AAP.0000000000000726] [PMID: 29356775]

[20] Fencl JL. Guideline implementation: local anesthesia. AORN J 2015; 101(6): 682-92.
[http://dx.doi.org/10.1016/j.aorn.2015.04.014] [PMID: 26025744]

[21] Paneta M, Waring WS. Literature review of the evidence regarding intravenous lipid administration in drug-induced cardiotoxicity. Expert Rev Clin Pharmacol 2019; 12(7): 591-602.
[http://dx.doi.org/10.1080/17512433.2019.1621163] [PMID: 31106655]

[22] Neal JM, Neal EJ, Weinberg GL. American Society of Regional Anesthesia and Pain Medicine Local Anesthetic Systemic Toxicity checklist: 2020 version. Reg Anesth Pain Med 2021; 46(1): 81-2.
[http://dx.doi.org/10.1136/rapm-2020-101986] [PMID: 33148630]

CHAPTER 7

Anesthesia for Cesarean Section

Mónica San Juan Álvarez[1,*], **Adriana Orozco Vinasco**[1], **Marta Chacón Castillo**[1] and **Juan José Correa Barrera**[1]

[1] Department of Anesthesiology and Critical Care, Hospital Universitario Severo Ochoa, Madrid, Spain

Abstract: Caesarean section is the most frequently performed surgery in adults, with a total of 20 million procedures per year. More than 70% of cases are due to lack of labor progression, fetal distress, breech presentation or previous cesarean section.

Obstetric anesthesia practice has substantially changed over the last 20 years. The main cause of this is the introduction of regional techniques to the detriment of general anesthesia, which has reduced maternal mortality due to complications such as gastric aspiration or difficulty in orotracheal intubation. In general, we can affirm that regional anesthesia is the most frequently used anesthetic technique for cesarean section, reserving general anesthesia for urgent or life-threatening situations.

Keywords: Cesarean Section, COVID-19, General Anesthesia, Hypotension, Spinal Anesthesia.

INTRODUCTION

An estimated of 20 million cesarean sections are performed worldwide every year, being the most frequent abdominal surgery carried out in adults [1].

In the USA, cesarean section is the most common surgical procedure, being performed approximately one million times per year [2]. More than 70% of cesarean sections are due to lack of labor progression, fetal distress, breech presentation or previous cesarean section.

Obstetric mortality related to anesthesia has dropped to the seventh leading cause of maternal mortality in the USA, and it accounts for 1-3 maternal deaths/million births in both the USA and the UK [3, 4].

The reduction in mortality has been associated with an increase in the use of

---
[*] **Corresponding author Mónica San Juan Álvarez:** Department of Anesthesiology and Critical Care, Hospital Universitario Severo Ochoa, Madrid, Spain; Email: sanjuanmo@gmail.com

Eugenio Daniel Martinez-Hurtado, Monica Sanjuan-Alvarez & Marta Chacon-Castillo (Eds.)
All rights reserved-© 2022 Bentham Science Publishers

regional techniques as opposed to general anesthesia. The use of the latter for cesarean section has decreased notably, being reserved for situations in which, either because of the urgency of the surgery, the woman's personal history, or failure of a regional technique, general anesthesia is the last alternative.

REGIONAL ANESTHESIA FOR CESAREAN SECTION

Complications of Regional Anesthesia

It is the most commonly used technique for cesarean section. Regarding neuraxial anesthesia, epidural anesthesia requires a longer time from its administration until the skin incision can be made (Table **1**), and it provides poorer intraoperative analgesia than the spinal technique (Table **2**). The latter, due to its rapidity of action, allows an earlier start of surgery and is the most frequently used anesthesia technique for cesarean section.

Table 1. Features of epidural anesthesia.

INDICATIONS	CONTRAINDICATIONS
- Elective or urgent cesarean section with previously established epidural block.	- Those inherent to epidural anesthesia. - Maternal refusal. - Emergent cesarean section (life-threatening situations).
ADVANTAGES	**DISADVANTAGES**
- Reduces the risk of bronchoaspiration and complications derived from orotracheal intubation difficulty. - Less administration of drugs with depressant effect on the fetus compared to general anesthesia. - Less arterial hypotension compared to intradural anesthesia. - Possibility of postoperative analgesia. - Allows the mother to enjoy childbirth.	- Long latency time. - Risk of arterial hypotension. - Risk of technique failure.

A sensory blockade level above T10 impedes cesarean-dependent somatic sensations. Elimination of visceral pain by peritoneal stimulation and uterus manipulation requires more extensive anesthesia. Only when an anesthesia level above T5 is achieved, women will be reliably pain-free during cesarean section.

The most frequently used local anesthetics are bupivacaine, levobupivacaine, and lidocaine. Opioids such as fentanyl or sufentanil can be added to enhance intraoperative analgesia. In the case of epidural anesthesia, 3-4 mg of morphine chloride can be administered through the catheter to ensure adequate postoperative analgesia.

Cardiovascular Effects

Maternal arterial hypotension is defined as a systolic blood pressure < 100 mmHg or a decrease in systolic blood pressure greater than 20% from its baseline level [5]. The importance of arterial hypotension after regional anesthesia is that it can cause adverse events in both mother and fetus. Maternal symptoms such as nausea, vomiting or dyspnea frequently accompany severe arterial hypotension. Adverse effects on the fetus, such as a low Apgar test score or umbilical acidosis, are related to the severity and duration of arterial hypotension.

Table 2. Features of spinal anesthesia.

INDICATIONS	CONTRAINDICATIONS
- Urgent cesarean section without previous epidural block. - Scheduled cesarean section.	- Those inherent to spinal anesthesia. - Maternal refusal.
ADVANTAGES	**DISADVANTAGES**
- Short latency. - Reduces the risk of bronchoaspiration and orotracheal intubation difficulty. - Simple technique with a low failure rate. - Allows the mother to enjoy childbirth.	- Increased risk of arterial hypotension when compared to epidural anesthesia. - Risk of postdural puncture headache.

The duration of the hemodynamic event is more important than its severity. A drop in maternal blood pressure of ≥ 30% does not affect the newborn need for oxygen [6], but arterial hypotension longer than 4 minutes is associated with neurological changes at 4-7 days of life [7].

Hemodynamic changes following neuraxial anesthesia result from the sympathetic nervous system block added to inferior vena cava compression by the gravid uterus, especially if the patient is in the supine position. The speed and extent of the sympathetic blockade, and thus the severity of hypotension, are direct consequences of the onset and spread of the local anesthetic in the neuraxial space. This explains the lower incidence of arterial hypotension in the epidural technique when compared to the spinal technique; in the former, the onset of the block is slower, allowing compensatory mechanisms to be activated.

Once spinal anesthesia has been performed, all efforts must be directed to prevent maternal arterial hypotension. A 15° left tilt of the patient is used to lessen the hemodynamic effect of aortocaval compression by the pregnant uterus. Leg compression has been shown to be more effective than its absence, but its benefit depends on the degree of compression employed.

Maternal crystalloid preloading is considered minimally effective in preventing arterial hypotension during neuraxial anesthesia. Colloid preloading is more effective in preventing hemodynamic changes. It also reduces the severity of these changes and the need for vasopressor agents. Crystalloid co-loading is more effective in reducing arterial hypotension and vasopressor requirements than preloading [8, 9]. Colloid co-loading is as effective as preloading, so surgery should not be delayed because of colloid administration [10].

Once arterial hypotension is established, a vigorous treatment should be performed combining fluids, uterus lateral displacement and vasopressor agents [11]. Vasopressors with an α-agonist effect are the best choice to reverse the hemodynamic effects of spinal anesthesia. Phenylephrine is the drug with the best evidence for this use [12]. Ephedrine is an indirectly acting agonist agent, which shows α- and β-agonist effects. Although its administration is associated with lower neonatal pH values, no differences have been found in Apgar test scores compared to phenylephrine [13]. Phenylephrine prophylactic administration has shown benefit by reducing both arterial hypotension and nausea and vomiting. Kuhn et al. demonstrated that an initial 0.25 mcg/kg phenylephrine bolus followed by an 0.25 mcg/kg/min infusion maintains adequate blood pressure during cesarean section without adverse events [14].

Nausea and Vomiting

Intraoperative nausea and vomiting incidence can reach 80%. The main anesthetic cause is arterial hypotension. Activation of the vomiting center in the brain occurs due to reduction in cerebral perfusion following arterial hypotension. Studies show that arterial hypotension is accompanied by a decrease in cerebral blood flow and cerebral oxygenation [15]. As a matter of fact, oxygen administration reduces nausea occurrence.

Post-Dural Puncture Headache

Accidental post-dural puncture headache is an adverse effect of epidural anesthesia occurring in 1.5% of all cases, and it is the main cause of prolonged hospital stay. Post-dural puncture headache may also complicate a spinal technique with an incidence of 0.4-4.6%. The epidural hematic patch is the gold standard treatment for severe headaches.

Central Nervous System Infections

In regular anesthetic practice, the infection incidence after regional anesthesia is very low (1/10.000 anesthetics) and is limited, in most cases, to catheter colonization or skin superficial inflammation without major clinical consequences. Serious infectious complications after neuraxial anesthesia are rare as long as the technique indications and contraindications, as well as strict aseptic measures, are respected.

Accidental Puncture of a Blood Vessel

In pregnant women at term, its incidence is 10-12%. It can lead to systemic toxicity, incomplete analgesia or epidural hematoma.

GENERAL ANESTHESIA FOR CESAREAN SECTION

Advantages of general anesthesia include rapid induction, airway control and hemodynamic stability. Disadvantages encompass maternal bronchoaspiration hazard, problems related to airway management and risk of intraoperative maternal awakening. General anesthesia is associated with an increased need for newborn resuscitation and a lower Apgar test score at five minutes, compared to newborns after regional block.

The patient should be placed in the supine position on the operating table and the uterus displaced to the left. The head, neck, and shoulders should remain in the "*sniffing position*" for proper airway management and the obstetrics airway algorithms must be followed. These algorithms and guidelines will be discussed in another chapter.

Induction of General Anesthesia

After routine patient monitoring, she should be preoxygenated with 100% oxygen through a perfectly sealed facemask. The preferred way to perform preoxygenation is with 3 minutes tidal volume technique. If, due to the emergency, this time is unavailable, the woman will be asked to perform 4-8 forced vital capacity breaths.

Rapid sequence induction is the gold standard for induction of anesthesia. Only skilled personnel should perform the Sellick maneuver, as it may hinder laryngoscopy and compromise intubation [16].

Classically thiopental (4-5 mg/kg) has been the induction agent of choice for cesarean section. Nevertheless, the use of propofol (2-3 mg/kg) is becoming widespread as it reduces the cardiovascular response to laryngoscopy. Neuromuscular relaxants facilitate intubation and improve surgical conditions. Succinylcholine (1 mg/kg) is the most commonly used agent in the setting of rapid sequence induction. Similar intubation conditions can be achieved with high doses (1-1.2 mg/kg) of rocuronium. It should be highlighted that the use of magnesium sulfate in pregnant women enhances non-depolarizing neuromuscular relaxant activity. Opioids should be first given after umbilical cord clamping to avoid neonatal respiratory depression. Remifentanil (0.1-1.3 mcg/kg), a very short-acting opioid, remains an option in women with risk factors, as it may attenuate the hypertensive response to laryngoscopy.

Bronchoaspiration

Anatomical and metabolic changes, along with an increased incidence of gastroesophageal reflux and more aggressive airway manipulation because of difficult orotracheal intubation, result in a higher risk of pulmonary aspiration.

The following medication can be administered to prevent damage in case pulmonary aspiration of gastric content occurs:

- *Sodium citrate* (**30 mL**): given orally immediately before cesarean section neutralizes the acidity of the stomach contents.
- *Ranitidine*: is an H_2 blocker that reduces gastric acid secretion, increasing the stomach pH.
- *Metoclopramide*: increases the tone of the lower esophageal sphincter and thus reduces reflux and regurgitation.

Maintenance of Anesthesia

The objectives sought during the conduct of anesthesia in the pregnant patient are:

- Adequate maternal and fetal oxygenation, maintaining normocapnia.
- Proper anesthesia depth to avoid intraoperative awakening.
- Minimal effects on uterine contractility.
- Avoid adverse events in the newborn.

Maternal inspired oxygen concentration affects fetal oxygenation, so that the latter is maximal when the inspired oxygen fraction is 1. Mechanical ventilation should aim for maternal normocapnia. Hypocapnia can cause uterine artery vasoconstriction as well as a left shift of the hemoglobin dissociation curve, compromising fetal oxygenation. At the other extreme, hypercapnia can cause maternal tachycardia.

Inhalation agents are the most commonly used agents for the maintenance of general anesthesia during cesarean section. No halogenated agent has been shown to be superior to any other for maintenance during surgery. These agents' requirements are reduced by 25% to 40% in pregnant patients [17]. Anesthesiologists tend to reduce the halogenated volatile agent dose for fear of neonatal depression and uterine atony. These drugs cause uterine musculature relaxation in a dose-dependent manner. Therefore, higher doses are associated with a risk of uterine atony and obstetric hemorrhage. However, reducing their administration increases the risk of intraoperative awakening.

A strategy would be the administration of 50% nitrous oxide in combination with a volatile agent at doses of 0.5-0.7 MAC (avoiding concentrations higher than 1 MAC) until birth and then the concentration of the former increases while reducing the halogenated agent once opioids have been administered, in order to diminish uterine atony occurrence.

The use of bispectral index (*BIS*) monitoring is encouraged to avoid the occurrence of intraoperative awakening. Values between 40-60 are recommended. Midazolam can also be administered after umbilical cord clamping. Propofol crosses readily the placental barrier and produces dose-dependent neonatal depression, but it can be an alternative in those cases at risk of uterine atony.

The patient should be awakened slightly reclined on the operating table. We must ensure that the patient's response to verbal commands and airway protective reflexes maintenance are adequate.

Antibiotic Prophylaxis

Endometritis prevention is greater if the antibiotic is administered before the surgical incision is made rather than after umbilical cord clamping. The antibiotic of choice varies according to the center. For example, cefazolin can be the initial choice, and, in case of allergy, clindamycin and gentamicin can be prescribed.

Deep Vein Thrombosis

Women are at high risk of deep vein thrombosis in the puerperium, and this risk is even greater after cesarean section than after vaginal delivery. Regional anesthesia seems to provide some protection against this pathology [18].

After a cesarean section, postpartum thrombotic risk should be assessed individually and, if necessary, prophylaxis with low molecular weight heparin should be started 6-8 hours after delivery.

ACUTE POSTOPERATIVE PAIN

Obstetric patients differ from the rest of the surgical population because of concern about possible fetal exposure to drugs administered to the mother and specific postoperative needs, including breastfeeding and newborn care.

Adequate analgesia after cesarean section promotes maternal-filial bonding, patient satisfaction, and early ambulation. Pregnancy increases the risk of deep vein thrombosis 5-10 times compared to the non-obstetric population and this risk increases even more in the postnatal period. Deep vein thrombosis has a multifactorial etiology, but there is no doubt that patient immobilization is a very important component.

Maternal pain relief allows breastfeeding to be initiated more promptly. The first hours after birth are decisive for the beginning of breastfeeding and the time to the first intake is crucial. Failure to initiate breastfeeding is associated with postpartum depression occurrence. Postpartum pain is a limitation for early breastfeeding introduction, not only as a result of a woman's discomfort, but also because it can decrease serotonin levels, causing anxiety and low mood that interferes with the success of the technique [19].

ANESTHETIC MANAGEMENT FOR CESAREAN SECTION IN COVID-19 PATIENT

Obstetric management of the patient diagnosed with COVID-19 differs from the rest of the population because of the possibility of patient cardiopulmonary involvement and for protection of all the personnel implicated in the process. The approach to these patients should be multidisciplinary, ensuring proper protection and care of the patient and healthcare professionals, and avoiding nosocomial transmission of the coronavirus [20].

In this setting, general anesthesia is a high-risk procedure and, therefore it is not the first choice for these patients' anesthetic management. Hence, neuraxial anesthesia performed by an expert anesthesiologist is recommended [21]. If general anesthesia is necessary, the most experienced anesthesiologist should perform it. In case of difficult intubation, the use of video laryngoscopes and second-generation supraglottic devices is encouraged. Intubation should be confirmed by capnography. For extubation, it is advisable to prevent the woman from coughing and to establish a physical barrier by covering the patient with plastic to hinder aerosol transmission.

CONCLUSION

Cesarean section is the most frequent abdominal surgery carried out in adults. Regional anesthesia is the most commonly used technique for cesarean section. The use of general anesthesia has decreased because of the risk of maternal bronchoaspiration and the problems related to airway management.

Hemodynamic changes following neuraxial anesthesia result from the sympathetic nervous system block. Intraoperative nausea and vomiting incidence can reach 80% and the main cause is arterial hypotension.

The risk of bronchoaspitarion during the induction of general anesthesia is the result of the anatomical and metabolic changes during pregnancy, an increased incidence of gastroesophageal reflux and the manipulation of the airway because of the difficult intubation.

The neuroaxial anesthesia performed by an expert anesthesiologist is recommended for cesarean section in COVID-19 patient.

CONSENT FOR PUBLICATION

Not applicable.

CONFLICT OF INTEREST

The authors declare no conflict of interest, financial or otherwise.

ACKNOWLEDGEMENT

Declared none.

REFERENCES

[1]   Betrán AP, Merialdi M, Lauer JA, *et al.* Rates of caesarean section: analysis of global, regional and national estimates. Paediatr Perinat Epidemiol 2007; 21(2): 98-113.
[http://dx.doi.org/10.1111/j.1365-3016.2007.00786.x] [PMID: 17302638]

[2]   Berghella V, Baxter JK, Chauhan SP. Evidence-based surgery for cesarean delivery. Am J Obstet Gynecol 2005; 193(5): 1607-17.
[http://dx.doi.org/10.1016/j.ajog.2005.03.063] [PMID: 16260200]

[3]   Lyons G. Saving mothers' lives: confidential enquiry into maternal and child health 2003-5. Int J Obstet Anesth 2008; 17(2): 103-5.
[http://dx.doi.org/10.1016/j.ijoa.2008.01.006] [PMID: 18308550]

[4]   D'Angelo R. Anesthesia-related maternal mortality: a pat on the back or a call to arms? Anesthesiology 2007; 106(6): 1082-4.
[http://dx.doi.org/10.1097/01.anes.0000267587.42250.29] [PMID: 17525579]

[5]   Kinsella SM, Carvalho B, Dyer RA, *et al.* International consensus statement on the management of hypotension with vasopressors during caesarean section under spinal anaesthesia. Anaesthesia 2018; 73(1): 71-92.
[http://dx.doi.org/10.1111/anae.14080] [PMID: 29090733]

[6]   Maayan-Metzger A, Schushan-Eisen I, Todris L, Etchin A, Kuint J. Maternal hypotension during elective cesarean section and short-term neonatal outcome. Am J Obstet Gynecol 2010; 202(1): 56.e1-5.
[http://dx.doi.org/10.1016/j.ajog.2009.07.012] [PMID: 19716536]

[7]   Hollmen AI, Jouppila R, Koivisto M, *et al.* Neurologic activity of infants following anesthesia for

cesarean section. Anesthesiology 1978; 48(5): 350-6.
[http://dx.doi.org/10.1097/00000542-197805000-00009] [PMID: 646154]

[8] Dyer RA, Farina Z, Joubert IA, *et al.* Crystalloid preload versus rapid crystalloid administration after induction of spinal anaesthesia (coload) for elective caesarean section. Anaesth Intensive Care 2004; 32(3): 351-7.
[http://dx.doi.org/10.1177/0310057X0403200308] [PMID: 15264729]

[9] Kee WDN, Khaw KS, Ng FF. Prevention of hypotension during spinal anesthesia for cesarean delivery: an effective technique using combination phenylephrine infusion and crystalloid cohydration. Anesthesiology 2005; 103(4): 744-50.
[http://dx.doi.org/10.1097/00000542-200510000-00012] [PMID: 16192766]

[10] Mercier FJ. Cesarean delivery fluid management. Curr Opin Anaesthesiol 2012; 25(3): 286-91.
[http://dx.doi.org/10.1097/ACO.0b013e3283530dab] [PMID: 22459983]

[11] Dahlgren G, Granath F, Wessel H, Irestedt L. Prediction of hypotension during spinal anesthesia for cesarean section and its relation to the effect of crystalloid or colloid preload. Int J Obstet Anesth 2007; 16(2): 128-34.
[http://dx.doi.org/10.1016/j.ijoa.2006.10.006] [PMID: 17276668]

[12] Heesen M, Stewart A, Fernando R. Vasopressors for the treatment of maternal hypotension following spinal anaesthesia for elective caesarean section: past, present and future. Anaesthesia 2015; 70(3): 252-7.
[http://dx.doi.org/10.1111/anae.13007] [PMID: 25583307]

[13] Lee A, Ngan Kee WD, Gin T. A quantitative, systematic review of randomized controlled trials of ephedrine versus phenylephrine for the management of hypotension during spinal anesthesia for cesarean delivery. Anesth Analg 2002; 94(4): 920-6.
[http://dx.doi.org/10.1097/00000539-200204000-00028] [PMID: 11916798]

[14] Kuhn JC, Hauge TH, Rosseland LA, Dahl V, Langesæter E. Hemodynamics of phenylephrine infusion versus lower extremity compression during spinal anesthesia for cesarean delivery: a randomized, double-blind, placebo-controlled study. Anesth Analg 2016; 122(4): 1120-9.
[http://dx.doi.org/10.1213/ANE.0000000000001174] [PMID: 26991619]

[15] Hirose N, Kondo Y, Maeda T, Suzuki T, Yoshino A. Relationship between regional cerebral blood volume and oxygenation and blood pressure during spinal anesthesia in women undergoing cesarean section. J Anesth 2016; 30(4): 603-9.
[http://dx.doi.org/10.1007/s00540-016-2165-6] [PMID: 27011334]

[16] Lyons G, Akerman N. Problems with general anaesthesia for Caesarean section. Minerva Anestesiol 2005; 71(1-2): 27-38.
[PMID: 15711504]

[17] Gambling DR, Sharma SK, White PF, Van Beveren T, Bala AS, Gouldson R. Use of sevoflurane during elective cesarean birth: a comparison with isoflurane and spinal anesthesia. Anesth Analg 1995; 81(1): 90-5.
[PMID: 7598289]

[18] Lie B, Juul J. Effect of epidural vs. general anesthesia on breastfeeding. Acta Obstet Gynecol Scand 1988; 67(3): 207-9.
[http://dx.doi.org/10.3109/00016348809004203] [PMID: 3176938]

[19] Watkins S, Meltzer-Brody S, Zolnoun D, Stuebe A. Early breastfeeding experiences and postpartum depression. Obstet Gynecol 2011; 118(2): 214-21.
[http://dx.doi.org/10.1097/AOG.0b013e3182260a2d] [PMID: 21734617]

[20] Du Y, Wang L, Wu G, Lei X, Li W, Lv J. Anesthesia and protection in an emergency cesarean section for pregnant woman infected with a novel coronavirus: case report and literature review. J Anesth 2020; 34(4): 613-8.
[http://dx.doi.org/10.1007/s00540-020-02796-6] [PMID: 32430561]

[21]   Guasch E, Brogly N, Manrique S. Recomendaciones prácticas en la paciente obstétrica con infección por COVID-19. Rev Esp Anestesiol Reanim 2020; 67(8): 438-45.
[http://dx.doi.org/10.1016/j.redar.2020.06.009]

Recent Advances in Anesthesiology, 2022, *Vol. 4*, 111-131

Locoregional Anesthesia Comments in the Obstetric Patient and Eventual Complications

María Mercedes García Domínguez[1,*], **Carlos Hugo Salazar Zamorano**[2], **Eugenio Martínez Hurtado**[1] and **Miriam Sánchez Merchante**[3]

[1] *Hospital Universitario Infanta Leonor, Madrid, Spain*

[2] *Hospital Universitario 12 de Octubre, Madrid, Spain*

[3] *Hospital Universitario Fundación Alcorcón, Madrid, Spain*

Abstract: Labor pain is associated with increased stress response and when it is excessive, it may lead to hypoxemia and fetal acidosis. The most important factor in obstetric analgesia is the desire for pain relief by the patient and neuraxial analgesia is the mainstay procedure in labor and in anesthesia for cesarean delivery. Continuous lumbar epidural analgesia is the mainstay of neuraxial labor analgesia. There are other methods, such as intrathecal block or combined spinal-epidural, that can be useful in specific cases. Despite being the safest and most effective method, the epidural labor analgesia may have some complications. Other therapies include bilateral paracervical block and pudendal block, which provide rapid onset analgesia (2–5 min). Although useful, they require training and are risky in cases of placental insufficiency or prematurity.

Keywords: Adverse Reactions, Central and Peripheral Blocks, Labor Pain, Local Anesthetics, Neuroaxial Analgesia.

INTRODUCTION

In 2018 in Western Europe, there were 5 million living births (birth rate of 9.7/1000 inhabitants) and nearly 28% of these had cesarean delivery (*CD*); Northern Europe had lower figures (for instance less than 10% CD in Scandina*via*), Southern Europe with higher figures was close to 28% CD [1]. Meanwhile in the same year 2018, there were 372.777 births in Spain, 90.3% from mothers under 40 years of age and 9.7% from mothers aged 40 or over (birth rate of 7.9/1.000 inhabitants) [2].

---

* **Corresponding author María Mercedes García Domínguez:** Department of Anesthesiology and Intensive Care. Hospital Universitario Infanta Leonor, Madrid, Spain; Email: mercedes_4_91@hotmail.com

Eugenio Daniel Martinez-Hurtado, Monica Sanjuan-Alvarez & Marta Chacon-Castillo (Eds.)
All rights reserved-© 2022 Bentham Science Publishers

Nearly 15.1% of these had instrumental vaginal delivery (*ID*) and 26.23% had cesarean delivery (*CD*), although 70%-80% were low risk pregnancies at the start of labor [3].

This epidemiological context determines to a greater or lesser extent, the assistance of the anesthesiologists during parturition. The incidence of analgesic epidural in childbirth in Spain varies greatly from region to region and from one type of hospital to another; it ranges between 30%-75% [4, 5].

In North America (USA, Canada), births with epidural average to 60-70% [6] and in France, nearly 80% [7].

PAIN AND LABOR ANALGESIA

Pain during labor and delivery is common. Most women describe labor pain as severe or most severe [8] and only 15% refer it as light to moderate pain [9]. It is of utmost important to have in mind that labour pain is not associated with a pathological event but rather with a physiological process that has psychological and cultural aspects as well [10].

MECHANISM OF PAIN

Although a large description of the mechanisms involved in labour pain [10 - 12] is out of the scope of this article, so a short summary is presented. Uterine contractions (first stage of labour) produce pain from mechanical distention of the lower uterine segment and cervix. It is transmitted through the hypogastric plexuses and the dorsal nerve roots of T10-L1 nerves to the spinal cord. It is mainly the visceral pain type (slow conduction and poorly localized) that is referred to the abdomen, lower back and rectum and readily susceptible to central neural blockade.

During the second stage of labour, the stretching of the lower birth canal by the fetal head descent produces pain in the thighs, legs, vagina, perineum and rectum; it is mainly somatic pain type (S2-S4 nerve roots, predominantly pudendal nerve dependent) with sharp, intense and well localized features and a little less susceptible to neural blockade.

CONSEQUENCES OF PAIN

Severe labor pain is associated with increased stress response generally innocuous during the course of an uncomplicated labor, but when excessive (extreme pain), it may lead to hypoxemia and fetal acidosis from increased plasma catecholamines and decreased oxygen transfer from the mother to the fetus (decreased placental perfusion plus leftward shift of oxygen-hemoglobin dissociation curve from hyperventilation caused by pain), and even to incoordinate uterine activity and dysfunctional labor [11 - 16]. Besides it may also be related in some cases to postpartum depression events [17, 18].

LABOR ANALGESIA

The most important factor in obstetric analgesia is the desire for pain relief by the patient and neuraxial analgesia is the mainstay procedure in labor and in anesthesia for cesarean delivery [19]. The change from epidural analgesia to epidural anesthesia in the event of cesarean delivery allows to avoid general anesthesia and it is associated with a higher risk of difficult tracheal intubation [20 - 23]. In fact, neuraxial blockades in obstetrics are associated with lower morbidity and mortality compared to general anesthesia in CD [24 - 27].

Neuraxial Obstetric Analgesia

Neuraxial analgesia techniques are the most effective and safe means to relieve pain throughout parturition; they are the method of choice for the relief of labor pain and should be available to all women in labor (ACOG level of evidence I a, A grade recommendation) [19, 28 - 31]. Theses techniques lead to lower pain scores and patients are more satisfied with neuraxial analgesia than with any other labor analgesia schedule [12, 32].

Indications [11, 28, 29, 31, 33]

- *Patient Request*: Always with anamnesis and eventual physical and analytical examination. In women at high risk of developing anesthetic complications, antepartum anesthetic evaluation is recommended.
- *Obstetric Specific Clinical Situations*: Such as dynamic dystocia (increased catecholamines due to pain can interfere with uterine coordination); some cases of preterm parturition; difficult breech delivery; instrumental vaginal birth; some cases of twin and multiple pregnancy; some cases of previous uterine surgery.
- *Medical Indications*: Such as preeclampsia (spinal analgesia leads to 15%-25% mean reduction in high blood pressure values) (ACOG B grade of recommendation); many cases of severe heart and/or lung diseases; retinal detachment; some cases of cerebral vascular diseases; cases of contraindicated general anesthesia.

Contraindications [11, 28, 29, 31, 33]

- Refusal by the patient, misunderstanding or non-acceptance of the procedure.
- Local anesthetic and/or opioid alergy.
- Severe hypotension unresponsive to treatment including shock and severe hemorrhage.

- Heart disease with limited cardiac output such as severe aortic stenosis (partial contraindication, neuraxial analgesia according to risk/benefit ratio for each patient).
- Neurological diseases with increased intracranial pressure; seizures.
- The immunocompromised patient (partial contraindication, risk: benefit ratio for each particular patient; see bellow).
- *Infection*: local (site of puncture) infection is an absolute contraindication. Nevertheless in systemic infections and or immunosupressed patients, the risk of central nervous system infection after neuraxial puncture is low (0.007%-0.6%) so a strict contraindication regarding this procedure should be assessed in each particular case and the risk–benefit ratio should prevail especially if antibiotic treatment has been started; nonetheless disseminated intravascular coagulation disorder associated to sepsis is a contraindication to neuraxial procedures [34].
- *Platelets disorders*: pregnant women with platelets between 50.000 and 100.000/μl are potential candidates after individual evaluation (ACOG B Grade recommendation). Although a specific lower-limit platelet count for adequate clotting prior to placement of a neuraxial catheter or needle has not been established, in low platelet counts cases, the epidural benefits have to outweigh the risks. Likewise if Ticagrelor (5 days wait), clopidogrel (5-7 days wait), Prasugrel (7 days wait) or Ticlopidine (10 days wait) has been used the respective day, span wait is mandatory before epidural puncture [28, 35 - 38].
- *Anticoagulant treatment*: spinal analgesia may be accomplished in patients with standard heparin treatment if they have a normal activated partial thromboplastin time (*aPTT*).

Patients with prophylactic doses of standard heparin or under treatment with low-dose aspirin have no contraindication. Patients with low molecular weight heparins (*LMWH*) treatment may have anticoagulant activity that is not reflected in the aPTT test and may be at risk of spinal or epidural hematomas so these patients can only receive spinal analgesia 24 hours after the last dose of LMWH and it will not be resumed until 24 hours after removing the catheter.

Patients with prophylactic low molecular weight heparins (*LMWH*) will receive spinal analgesia 12 hours after the last dose of LMWH and it will not be resumed until 12 hours after removing the catheter.

Patients with warfarin/coumadin treatment need an INR Prothrombine Time lower than 1,5 for neuraxial technique (1,5 INR PT means 45% activity of factor VII, the minimum safety limit is 55% that is INR PT 1,4).

DOACs (the new direct oral anticoagulants) are not regularly used in pregnant patients but if used, there should be a 48h last dose timespan.

As a general rule, whenever a patient is under the effects of some anticoagulant treatment, it is advisable to favor the spinal technique over the epidural and perform the procedure with as limited manipulation as possible [39, 40].

- Inherited bleeding disorders: the most common is Von Willebrand Disease; though desmopressin and/or factor VIII and cryoprecipitate may be used as treatment, each case has to be assessed individually according to the severity of the bleeding disorder and the risk/benefit ratio [41].
- Tatoos in the site of puncture may be a relative contraindication (if regional anesthesia is recommended, it may be avoided either by a small scalpel incision or by puncturing in a non-tattooed area if possible) [42].
- Vertebral deformities and similar pathologies; dysraphism (neural tube defects) may be relative contraindication.
- Progressive neurological diseases may be relative contraindication.

According to the specific technique neuraxial obstetric analgesia may be epidural, spinal, combined spinal-epidural or dural puncture epidural.

Epidural

- Continuous lumbar epidural analgesia with diluted local anesthetics is the mainstay of neuraxial labor analgesia [28, 31]. It can be performed as intermittent boluses, as continuous infusion (ECI - Epidural Continuous Infusion), as patient self-controlled dosing (*PCEA* - Patient controlled epidural analgesia) or as automatic bolus dosing (*PIEB* - Programmed intermittent epidural boluses). The latter, PIEB, seems to lead to greater maternal satisfaction, lower local anesthetic (*LA*) doses, less breakthrough pain, and fewer rescue boluses [43, 44].
- In laboring patients, epidural puncture at the L3–L4 interspace is the most common [41]. The patient is placed either in lateral decubitus or sitting position (according to maternal comfort as well as anesthesiologist preference), the intervertebral space is palpated, the epidural space is identified and after negative aspiration (no blood, no cerebrospinal fluid [*CSF*]), an adequate test dose of LA is injected and an infusion catheter is placed; then an initial fractioned bolus of low dose LA is injected and a programed perfusion is started afterwards [43, 45].
- Ultrasound may help in case of difficult identification of anatomical structures [46 - 48]. Most often ultrasonography is a preprocedural tool used to aid the operator in the assessment of particular anatomy circumstances such as patients with morbid obesity, derangements of spinal anatomy (scoliosis, spinal stenosis, or history of spinal instrumentation), patients in whom identification of specific vertebral levels might be warranted (preexisting disc herniation or nerve root

compression at a specific interspace), epidural depth assessment among others [49, 50].

- The identification of epidural space may be accomplished either with air or saline solution and it seems that there is no significant difference among them when the anesthesiologist is trained in both techniques [51, 52]. Inspite some isolated cases of pneumoencephalum with air have been reported [53], it is recommend to use the technique which anesthesiologists are most comfortable with [54].

- The test dose in epidural analgesia for labor is controversial. The regular test dose should include a small dose of LA and epinephrine to rule out intrathecal and/or intravascular injection; although the latter has been claimed as an eventual risk in reduction in uteroplacental circulation [55] there has been no report of adverse neonatal outcomes after intravenous injection of an epinephrine-containing test dose [56]. Lidocaine 2% 2 ml (or 1,5% 3 ml) with epinephrine 5 mcg/ml is the most common mixture used (intrathecal lidocaine would produce fast and evident spinal block; intravenous epinephrine would produce transient tachycardia) [57 - 60].

Ropivacaine and bupivacaine have shown to be less effective as the test dose [61]. The addition of epinephrine to the test dose should be highlighted for it is sensitive but not specific and means that a certain percentage of positive responses do not represent a true intravascular placement of the epidural needle or catheter for uterine contractions may produce transient increase of heart frequency as well [62, 63]. Nevertheless in cesarean delivery, the epidural injection of critical amounts of local anesthetic may be life-threatening if the injection is misplaced [64] so the test dose is mandatory [57].

- *Previous and periodic aspiration of injectate*: the test dose must always be accompanied by previous and periodic gentle aspirations. Inadvertent intravascular injection in obstetric patients may reach up to 7%-8% of cases and intrathecal sitement occurs approximately in 0.6-2.7% of cases and is usually detected by the exit of cerebrospinal fluid through the needle or catheter (please see Comments on Epidural bellow). Gentle aspiration followed by an adequate test dose in epidural anesthesia for cesarean delivery and careful observation of the patient in epidural labor analgesia is of utmost importance for the identification of an incorrectly placed catheter and the avoidance of deleterious effects [57].

LOCAL ANESTHETICS AND ADJUVANTS

- Bupivacaine and ropivacaine are the most commonly local anesthetics (*LA*) used for labor analgesia [54, 65]. Levobupivacaine may also be used though there seems to be no additional benefit in this context [66, 67]. The LA are used in low concentrations (0.0625% - 0,125% bupivacaine or 0,2% Ropivacaine) mixed with opioids (mainly low dose fentanyl: 50-100 mcg in the initial bolus; 1-2 mcg/ml in the perfusion mixture - or sufentanyl 5-10 mg initial bolus; 0.1-0.4 mcg/ml in the perfusion mixture) providing adequate pain relief while preserving motor function, short latency, decreased adverse side effects, no significant effect on uterine activity and uteroplacental perfusion, minimal risk of toxicity for mother and fetus and high level of maternal satisfaction [68 - 70].

- Supplementing analgesia with larger volumes of the prepared mixture or more concentrated solutions of local anesthetic may be necessary for vaginal delivery [71, 72].

- Fentanyl (and sufentanyl) by acting on endogenous opioid spinal receptors contribute to the analgesic effect allowing a reduction in the dose of LA [73], however their moderate analgesic effects (more effective on visceral pain) are not enough for adequate labor analgesia when given alone except on early labor pain (initial first stage of labor) [74]. These opioids also help to reduce shivering from epidural LA [75, 76]. Their high lipophilic feature makes them the most suitable opioids in labor analgesia [77].

- Epinephrine in low doses (1.25 mcg-5 mcg/ml: 1: 80.000-1:200.000) is sometimes an adjunct to the mixture of local anesthetics. It shortens the latency time and prolongs the duration of epidural bupivacaine analgesia [71, 78] for it enhances its effect by nearly 30% probably by stimulation of alpha-adrenergic receptors in the spinal cord [79]; there seems to be a slight enhancement of epidural opioids effect as well [80]. But its drawback is that epinephrine also increases the intensity of motor blockade [81, 82]. Regardless of these effects, the administration of an epidural epinephrine- containing local anesthetic solution at the concentrations aforementioned does not adversely affect intervillous blood flow [83] or neonatal outcomes [78, 82].

- Clonidine, dexmetomidine, and neostigmine have been used in selected patients leading to increase LA analgesic effect but there are also secondary effects that have to be controlled (bradycardia, hypotension, maternal sedation, emesis, etc.); besides they have shown no advantage to the lipid soluble opioids.

MAINTENANCE OF ANALGESIA

The frequent maintenance of local anesthetic mixture includes the use of bupivacaine from 0.05% to 0.125% or ropivacaine 0,2% plus fentanyl 1-2 mcg/ml as mentioned above [84]. The maintenance has evolved from intermittent boluses by medical/midwife staff (5-12 ml low dose LA boluses periodically according to obtained analgesia) to continuous infusion that led to less variability in the quality of analgesia (for instance 7-12 ml/h of LA plus extra bolus for breakthrough pain) to patient-controlled epidural analgesia - PCEA (patient controlled epidural analgesia) with and without associated continuous infusion rate, for instance 4-7 ml/h local anesthetic plus patient controlled boluses of 5-8 ml with a set lockout interval - or as automatic intermittent epidural bolus dosing of local anesthetics - PIEB - (Programmed intermittent epidural boluses) [43, 44, 85 - 87].

It seems that PIEB leads to greater maternal satisfaction, lower LA dose, less breakthrough pain, and fewer rescue boluses [43, 44].

Spinal (Intrathecal)

Single-shot intrathecal block can provide analgesia for immediate delivery; the usual dose (2.5 mg bupivacaine plus 25 mcg fentanyl) lasts up to two hours in duration [88] and provides a rapid effect onset, minimal motor block, little/no risk of systemic LA toxicity and minimal/no drug transfer to the fetus. Larger doses (for instance 5-11 mg of bupivacaine) are suitable for cesarean delivery. Spinal analgesia/anesthesia may lead to transient hypotension that is more frequent and severe than with the epidural technique [89].

Combined Spinal-Epidural Technique

The combined spinal-epidural technique (*CSE*) [41, 90] introduced in obstetrics in 1984 [91] is another analgesic/anesthetic option. It consist of an initial intrathecal injection after the epidural space has been identified (for instance 1-2 mg bupivacaine plus 5-15 mgc fentanyl by means of a 25-27 gauge pencil point tip spinal needle) followed by the insertion of an epidural catheter to prolong the effect as needed.

The CSE can be either needle through needle technique (*NTN*) or separate needle technique (*SNT*). Analgesia is obtained faster while keeping the minimal motor block with no differences in obstetric outcomes as compared to the plain epidural technique [92, 93] but it may be more challenging when the epidural space has been correctly identified but the dural sac can not be adequately reached [94].

Although there have been no clear impact on obstetric or neonatal outcomes [72], some cases of fetal bradycardia [95] and increases in uterine hypertonus [96] have been associated with the CSE technique; the mechanism by which it occurs is unclear though a rapid decrease in plasma catecholamines from the fast analgesic effect has been claimed.

The main difference between labor CSE and labour epidural is this increased risk of transient hypotension and fetal bradycardia that requires intervention (5% in epidural analgesia, 31% in CSE analgesia), while there is no difference in the unintentional dural puncture, incidence of PDPH, rescue analgesia requirements, maternal satisfaction scores and mode of delivery [96 - 98]. There have been concerns of increased possibility of migration of the epidural catheter tip [99] but such an event would only happen after multiple dural punctures [100].

COMMETS ON EPIDURAL OBSTETRIC ANALGESIA

Epidural obstetric analgesia has no impact on the incidence of cesarean section or neonatal Apgar scores [84, 101 - 103]. It does not increase the length of the first stage of labor although it does prolong to some extent (mean of 15-20 minutes) the second stage [32, 104] and, an important issue, it is not associated with an increase in instrumented vaginal delivery when given during the expulsive phase [105] as was previously assumed [32].

Despite being the safest and most effective method, the epidural labor analgesia may have some complications:

- During the parturition period:
  - Paresthesias during the procedure (21%-50%): paresthesias during catheter treading in the epidural space is very common (21%-50%) but this very rarely leads to neural damage (see below) [106].
  - *Shivering* (18%): shivering associated to neuraxial anesthesia has not been clearly understood but it seems that there is a non-thermoregulatory shivering triggered by a reduction in sensed body temperature and hormonal factors may also play a role in it [102, 107]. Epidural administration of epinephrine seems to increase shivering and the etiology of this response is unknown.
  - Lateralized analgesia (16.4%) that may need a partial pull back of the catheter or even replacing it to accomplish adequate analgesia [108]. It occurs when the catheter moves laterally in the epidural space and the anesthetic effect is not uniform; this can be avoided by limiting the length of catheter within the epidural space to 3 cm. or so but this may increase the risk for outward migration of the catheter over time for laboring women change position frequently [102]. Rarely, it may also be caused by the presence of the Plica Mediana Dorsalis (a septum) within part of the epidural space.
  - *Arterial hypotension* (2.5%- 20%): neuraxial anesthesia sympathetic blockade produces peripheral vasodilation from decreased systemic vascular resistance that may lead to hypotension up to 10% in epidural analgesia and 10%-20% in intrathecal technique [89, 109, 110]. Intravenous administration of 0.5 to 1.5 L crystalloid solutions either prior ("*pre-load*") or concurrent

("*co-load*") with the epidural anesthesia/analgesia does not always prevent the presence and severity of this event [111 - 113].

When maternal blood pressure falls in excess of 20% of the preblock level and/or a new fetal heart rate abnormalities appears, a rapid correction with intravenous fluids and/or vasopressor should be applied (phenylephrine, ephedrine or similar drug) to avoid deleterious effects on the fetus as the placental perfusion depends on mean arterial blood pressure [31, 110, 114].

• *Vessel puncture* (5%-8%): vessel puncture and inadvertent intravascular injection in obstetric patients range from 4.9% to 8% (mainly with rigid nylon catheters), higher than 2.8% rate in non-pregnant patients [61, 62, 115], and it decreases to 0.6% - 2.3% with aspiration before the injection [57, 58].

Moreover, the aspiration of a multi-orifice epidural catheter for blood has 98% sensitivity for detection of an intravascular location [55]. Nevertheless inspite of an accidental intravascular injection, the low-dose/low-concentration solutions of local anesthetics used in labor analgesia do not cause systemic toxicity [55, 57, 116].

• *Ineffective analgesia* (1%-12%): ineffective analgesia is mostly associated with a failure of epidural catheter. The failure figures range between 6% in CSE epidural catheters to12% in plain epidural analgesia catheter disfunction [58, 117]. Nevertheless these figures are clearly reduced to 1,2% and 2% respectively when only expert staff preforms the epidural analgesia (no anesthesiology trainees participate in the procedure) [118]. A partial pull back of the catheter may be of help but many times it has to be replaced to obtain adequate analgesia [108].

Once the epidural catheter disfunction has been ruled out, supplemental local anesthetic bolus may be needed in case of breakthrough pain develops either with the same diluted concentration of local anesthetic (if inadequate block extension is detected, that is bupivacaine 0.0625%-0.125%) or with higher local anesthetic concentrations (if there is adequate block extension but more intense analgesia is required, that is bupivacaine 0.125%-0.25%) [71, 72].

• *Difficult technique* (5.2%): factors like obesity, spinal deformity and others.

• *Inadvertent intrathecal placement*: Inadvertent intrathecal placement occurs approximately in 0.6-2.7% of cases and is usually detected by the exit of cerebrospinal fluid through the needle or catheter [57, 97, 119]. Again, multiorifice epidural catheter has very high sensitivity for CSF aspiration when placed intrathecally [55].

• Gentle aspiration followed by an appropriate test dose, in epidural anesthesia for cesarean section, and careful observation of the patients in epidural labor analgesia increase the likelihood that an incorrectly placed catheter will be detected and that a harmful reaction to local anesthetics will be avoided [57].

• Re-siting the epidural catheter in a different interspace eliminates the problem of mistaking an intrathecal catheter for an epidural catheter. However, local anesthetics or opioids injected through the epidural catheter may pass through the dural puncture site and into the subarachnoid space, resulting in unexpectedly high neuroblockade [120, 121].

• During the postpartum period, there occur short term lumbar pain (18.5%), urinary retention (3.4%), post-dural puncture headache (1.4%) and peripheral neuropathy (0.9%) though permanent maternal injury is clearly low (1 in 80.000) [28, 122, 123].

Nevertheless it has to be kept in mind that combined spinal-epidural analgesia is associated with a higher rate of adverse reactions [95, 96, 124].

A total of 2.399 pregnant patients who had undergone neuraxial blockade were evaluated. Neurologic complications that occurred in these patients were divided into lower limb paresthesias (0.3%), transient radicular irritation (0.1%), and post-dural puncture headache (3%).

The patients who stayed more than 60 min in gynecological position showed an odds ratio of evolution with lower limb paresthesias of 1.75 and patients who stayed more than 120min showed an odds ratio of 2.1, but without statistical significance [23, 24, 125].

A total of 1.37 million women received an epidural for childbirth, reported in 27 articles. Most information (85% of women) was in larger (> 10.000 women) studies published after 1990, with risk estimates as follows: epidural hematoma, 1 in 168.000, deep epidural infection, 1 in 145.000; persistent neurologic injury, 1 in 240.000; and transient neurologic injury, 1 in 6.700. Earlier and smaller studies produced significantly higher risk estimates for transient neurologic injury plus injury of unknown duration [126].

Regardless of the technique used, the safe practice for the administration of epidural analgesia in labor requires initial catheter aspiration, gradual dose increases and continuous monitoring during and after catheter placement in order to detect any sign of anesthetic toxicity, bearing in mind that an epidural analgesia infusion that has been working well and stops having the desired effect may be an indication of catheter migration [116, 127].

If the epidural catheter should migrate into a vein during the continuous epidural infusion of a dilute solution of local anesthetic, it is unlikely that the patient will have symptoms of local anesthetic toxicity; rather, the level of anesthesia will regress [55, 128].

Aspiration of multi-orifice catheters is 98% sensitive in identifying their intravascular location, the sensitivity of aspiration is significantly lower for single-orifice catheters [55].

Other Therapies

Other therapies include bilateral paracervical block and pudendal block, which provide rapid onset analgesia (2–5 min); although useful, require training and are risky in cases of placental insufficiency or prematurity [129].

Paracervical Block

The puncture of local anesthetics in the uterovaginal cul-de-sac is useful in relieving pain produced in the period of dilation, although it is less effective during delivery [130].

Although its efficacy is endorsed by 4 randomized clinical trials (level of evidence Ia, grade of recommendation A) [131], it is not a highly recommended procedure because its use has been associated with the appearance of fetal bradycardia [131], in addition, its efficacy is short-lived and technique is ineffective in 10-30% of cases [132].

Pudendal Block

Blocking the internal pudendal nerves with its 3 perineal branches produces analgesia during labor delivery, a period in which pain is largely caused by pelvic distention [130].

These nerves can be accessed *via* the perineal or transvaginal route; the latter is one of the choices as it is easier, faster, passes through less tissue and uses less anesthesia. By placing the patient in the usual position of vaginal delivery, the needle directed by the middle and index fingers is inserted into the vagina, laterally and slightly medially and posteriorly to the ischial spine, resting on the supraspinatus ligament. Long (12-15 cm) and jacketed needles are usually used to avoid tissue damage during their introduction, from which the needle protrudes about 15mm. Before injecting the local anesthetic, it should be aspirated to rule out accidental puncture of the pudendal vessels [132].

This technique is highly effective in delivery, easy to administer, does not require subsequent monitoring, and reduces the tear frequency [132].

CONCLUSION

The incidence of analgesic epidural in childbirth in Spain ranges between 30%-75%. Severe labor pain is associated with increased stress response, and may lead to hypoxemia and fetal acidosis. Neuraxial analgesia techniques are the most effective and safe means to relieve pain throughout parturition. Continuous lumbar epidural analgesia is the mainstay of neuraxial labor analgesia. Epidural obstetric analgesia has no impact on the incidence of cesarean section nor does it increase the length of first stage of labor. The epidural labor analgesia may have some complications during the delivery or postpartum period. Bupivacaine and ropivacaine are the most commonly local anesthetics used for labor analgesia. Supplementing analgesia may be necessary for vaginal delivery. Single-shot intrathecal block can provide analgesia for immediate delivery. Combined spinal-epidural technique is another analgesic/anesthetic option but has no clear impact on hypotension and bradycardia fetal and increases in uterine hypertonus. Other therapies such as bilateral paracervical block and pudendal block provide rapid onset analgesia but require training and are risky in some cases.

CONSENT FOR PUBLICATION

Not applicable.

CONFLICT OF INTEREST

The authors declare no conflict of interest, financial or otherwise.

ACKNOWLEDGEMENT

Declared none.

REFERENCES

[1]   De Benito E. Desciende la tasa de natalidad en España en el 2018.

[2]   Desciende la tasa de natalidad en España en el 2020. Disponible en: https://datosmacro.expansion.com/demografia/natalidad/espana

[3]   Pais E. El 15% de los bebes en España se extraen usando instrumental externo en el parto. 26 de noviembre de 2018. Disponible en: https://elpais.com/sociedad/2018/11/26/actualidad/1543226984_467761.html

[4]   Instituto Nacional Estadistica. Nacimientos por tipo de parto, tiempo de gestación y grupo de edad de

la madre 2015.

[5]   Uso y procedimiento de la anestesia epidural durante el trabajo de parto. 30 de agosto de 2019.

[6]   Declercq ER, Sakala C, Corry MP, *et al.* Listening to Mothers III: Pregnancy and Childbirth. 2013.

[7]   Blondel B, Gonzalez L, Raynaud P, Golberg E. Institut national de la santé de la rechereche médicale 2017.

[8]   Costa-Martins JM, Pereira M, Martins H, Moura-Ramos M, Coelho R, Tavares J. Attachment styles, pain, and the consumption of analgesics during labor: a prospective observational study. J Pain 2014; 15(3): 304-11.
        [http://dx.doi.org/10.1016/j.jpain.2013.12.004] [PMID: 24393700]

[9]   Bonica JJ, McDonald JS. The pain and childbirth. The management of pain. 1990; 1313-43.

[10]   Lowe NK. The nature of labor pain. Am J Obstet Gynecol 2002; 186(5) (Suppl Nature): S16-24.
        [http://dx.doi.org/10.1016/S0002-9378(02)70179-8] [PMID: 12011870]

[11]   Brownridge P. The nature and consequences of childbirth pain. Eur J Obstet Gynecol Reprod Biol 1995; 59 (Suppl.): S9-S15.
        [http://dx.doi.org/10.1016/0028-2243(95)02058-Z] [PMID: 7556828]

[12]   Camann W. Pain, Pain Relief, Satisfaction and Excellence in Obstetric Anesthesia: A Surprisingly Complex Relationship. Anesth Analg. febrero de 2017; 124(2): 383-5.

[13]   Hawkins JL. Epidural analgesia for labor and delivery. N Engl J Med 2010; 362(16): 1503-10.
        [http://dx.doi.org/10.1056/NEJMct0909254] [PMID: 20410515]

[14]   Abboud TK, Sarkis F, Hung TT, *et al.* Effects of epidural anesthesia during labor on maternal plasma beta-endorphin levels. Anesthesiology 1983; 59(1): 1-5.
        [http://dx.doi.org/10.1097/00000542-198307000-00001] [PMID: 6305238]

[15]   Lederman RP, Lederman E, Bruce W Jr, McCann DS. Anxiety and epinephrine in multiparous women in labor: Relationship to duration of labor and fetal heart rate pattern. Am J Obstet Gynecol 1985; 153(8): 870-7.
        [http://dx.doi.org/10.1016/0002-9378(85)90692-1] [PMID: 4073158]

[16]   Levinson G, Shnider SM, deLorimier AA, Steffenson JL. Effects of maternal hyperventilation on uterine blood flow and fetal oxygenation and acid-base status. Anesthesiology 1974; 40(4): 340-7.
        [http://dx.doi.org/10.1097/00000542-197404000-00007] [PMID: 4594570]

[17]   Ding T, Wang DX, Qu Y, Chen Q, Zhu SN. Epidural labor analgesia is associated with a decreased risk of postpartum depression: a prospective cohort study. Anesth Analg 2014; 119(2): 383-92.
        [http://dx.doi.org/10.1213/ANE.0000000000000107] [PMID: 24797120]

[18]   Waldenström U, Bergman V, Vasell G. The complexity of labor pain: experiences of 278 women. J Psychosom Obstet Gynaecol 1996; 17(4): 215-28.
        [http://dx.doi.org/10.3109/01674829609025686] [PMID: 8997688]

[19]   Bucklin BA, Hawkins JL, Anderson JR, Ullrich FA. Obstetric anesthesia workforce survey: twenty-year update. Anesthesiology 2005; 103(3): 645-53.
        [http://dx.doi.org/10.1097/00000542-200509000-00030] [PMID: 16129992]

[20]   Quinn AC, Milne D, Columb M, Gorton H, Knight M. Failed tracheal intubation in obstetric anaesthesia: 2 yr national case–control study in the UK. Br J Anaesth 2013; 110(1): 74-80.
        [http://dx.doi.org/10.1093/bja/aes320] [PMID: 22986421]

[21]   Creanga AA, Syverson C, Seed K, Callaghan WM. Pregnancy-Related Mortality in the United States, 2011–2013. Obstet Gynecol 2017; 130(2): 366-73.
        [http://dx.doi.org/10.1097/AOG.0000000000002114] [PMID: 28697109]

[22]   Hawkins JL, Chang J, Palmer SK, Gibbs CP, Callaghan WM. Anesthesia-related maternal mortality in the United States: 1979-2002. Obstet Gynecol 2011; 117(1): 69-74.

[http://dx.doi.org/10.1097/AOG.0b013e31820093a9] [PMID: 21173646]

[23]   Preston R. The role of combined spinal epidural analgesia for labour: is there still a question? Can J Anaesth 2007; 54(1): 9-14.
[http://dx.doi.org/10.1007/BF03021893] [PMID: 17197462]

[24]   Loubert C, Hinova A, Fernando R. Update on modern neuraxial analgesia in labour: a review of the literature of the last 5 years. Anaesthesia 2011; 66(3): 191-212.
[http://dx.doi.org/10.1111/j.1365-2044.2010.06616.x] [PMID: 21320088]

[25]   Blanshard HJ, Cook TM. Use of combined spinal-epidural by obstetric anaesthetists. Anaesthesia 2004; 59(9): 922-3.
[http://dx.doi.org/10.1111/j.1365-2044.2004.03918.x] [PMID: 15310368]

[26]   Rawal N. Combined spinal-epidural anaesthesia. Curr Opin Anaesthesiol 2005; 18(5): 518-21.
[http://dx.doi.org/10.1097/01.aco.0000182565.25057.b3] [PMID: 16534286]

[27]   Côrtes CA, Sanchez CA, Oliveira AS, Sanchez FM. Labor analgesia: a comparative study between combined spinal-epidural anesthesia *versus* continuous epidural anesthesia. Rev Bras Anestesiol 2007; 57(1): 39-51.
[PMID: 19468617]

[28]   ACOG. Practice Bulletin. Obstetric analgesia and anesthesia. Int J Gynecol Obstet 2002; 78: 321-35.
[http://dx.doi.org/10.1016/S0020-7292(02)00268-0] [PMID: 12452132]

[29]   ACOG Committee Opinion #295: pain relief during labor. Obstet Gynecol. julio de 2004; 104(1): 213.

[30]   Jones L, Othman M, Dowswell T, *et al.* Pain management for women in labour: an overview of systematic reviews. Cochrane Database Syst Rev 2012; (3): CD009234.
[PMID: 22419342]

[31]   Practice Guidelines for Obstetric Anesthesia. Anesthesiology 2016; 124(2): 270-300.
[http://dx.doi.org/10.1097/ALN.0000000000000935] [PMID: 26580836]

[32]   Anim-Somuah M, Smyth RMD, Jones L. Epidural *versus* non-epidural or no analgesia in labour. Cochrane Libr 2011; 12(12): CD000331.
[http://dx.doi.org/10.1002/14651858.CD000331.pub3] [PMID: 22161362]

[33]   Progresos de obstetricia y ginecología 2009; 52(6): 374-83.

[34]   Gimeno AM, Errando CL. Neuraxial Regional Anaesthesia in Patients with Active Infection and Sepsis: A Clinical Narrative Review. Turk J Anaesthesiol Reanim. febrero de 2018; 46(1): 8-14.
[http://dx.doi.org/10.5152/TJAR.2018.12979]

[35]   Horlocker TT, Vandermeulen E, Kopp SI, *et al.* Regional Anesthesia in the Patient Receiving Antithrombotic or Thrombolytic Therapy: American Society of Regional Anesthesia and Pain Medicine Evidence-Based Guidelines (Fourth Edition). Reg Anesth Pain Med. 2018; 43: 263-309.

[36]   Collins J, Bowles L, MacCallum PK. Prevention and management of venous thromboembolism in pregnancy. Br J Hosp Med. diciembre de 2016; 77(12): C194-200.
[http://dx.doi.org/10.12968/hmed.2016.77.12.C194]

[37]   Collins P, Abdul-Kadir R, Thachil J. Subcommittees on Women' s Health Issues in T, Haemostasis, on Disseminated Intravascular C. Management of coagulopathy associated with postpartum hemorrhage: guidance from the SSC of the ISTH. J Thromb Haemost. enero de 2016; 14(1): 205-10.

[38]   Narouze S, Benzon HT, Provenzano D, *et al.* Interventional Spine and Pain Procedures in Patients on Antiplatelet and Anticoagulant Medications (Second Edition): Guidelines From the American Society of Regional Anesthesia and Pain Medicine, the European Society of Regional Anaesthesia and Pain Therapy, the American Academy of Pain Medicine, the International Neuromodulation Society, the North American Neuromodulation Society, and the World Institute of Pain. Reg. Anesth. Pain Med. abril de 2018; 43(3): 225-62.

[39]   Butwick AJ, Carvalho B. Anticoagulant and antithrombotic drugs in pregnancy: what are the

anesthetic implications for labor and cesarean delivery? J Perinatol 2011; 31(2): 73-84.
[http://dx.doi.org/10.1038/jp.2010.64] [PMID: 20559281]

[40]   Vandermeuelen E, Kopp SI, *et al.* Regional Anesthesia in the Patient Receiving Antithrombotic or Thrombolytic Therapy: American Society of Regional Anesthesia and Pain Medicine Evidence-Based Guidelines (Fourth Edition). Reg Anesth Pain Med. 2018; 43: 263-309.

[41]   https://www.nysora.com/regional-anesthesia-for-specific-surgical-procedures/abdomen/epi-ural-anesthesia-analgesia/

[42]   Raynaud L, Mercier FJ, Auroy Y, Benhamou D. Analgésie par voie péridurale et tatouage lombaire : que faire? Ann Fr Anesth Reanim 2006; 25(1): 71-3.
[http://dx.doi.org/10.1016/j.annfar.2005.07.081] [PMID: 16386402]

[43]   Actualización de los protocolos asistenciales de la sección de anestesia obstétrica de la SEDAR. 2o EDICIÓN. 2016; 16.

[44]   Onuoha OC. Epidural Analgesia for Labor: Continuous Infusion *versus* Programmed Intermittent Bolus. Anesthesiology clinics. marzo de 2017.

[45]   https://fpm.ac.uk/sites/fpm/files/documents/2020-09/Epidural-AUG-2020-FINAL.pdf

[46]   Perlas A, Chaparro LE, Chin KJ. Lumbar neuraxial ultrasound for spinal and epidural anesthesia: a systematic review and meta-analysis. Reg Anesth Pain Med 2016; 41(2): 251-60.
[http://dx.doi.org/10.1097/AAP.0000000000000184] [PMID: 25493689]

[47]   Arzola C, Mikhael R, Margarido C, Carvalho JCA. Spinal ultrasound *versus* palpation for epidural catheter insertion in labour. Eur J Anaesthesiol 2015; 32(7): 499-505.
[http://dx.doi.org/10.1097/EJA.0000000000000119] [PMID: 25036283]

[48]   Perna P, Gioia A, Ragazzi R, Volta CA, Innamorato M. Can pre-procedure neuroaxial ultrasound improve the identification of the potential epidural space when compared with anatomical landmarks? A prospective randomized study. Minerva Anestesiol 2017; 83(1): 41-9.
[http://dx.doi.org/10.23736/S0375-9393.16.11399-9] [PMID: 27701372]

[49]   Creaney M, Mullane D, Casby C, Tan T. Ultrasound to identify the lumbar space in women with impalpable bony landmarks presenting for elective caesarean delivery under spinal anaesthesia: a randomised trial. Int J Obstet Anesth 2016; 28: 12-6.
[http://dx.doi.org/10.1016/j.ijoa.2016.07.007] [PMID: 27641088]

[50]   Gupta D, Srirajakalidindi A, Soskin V. Dural puncture epidural analgesia is not superior to continuous labor epidural analgesia. Middle East J Anaesthesiol. octubre de 2013; 22(3): 309-16.

[51]   Segal S, Arendt KW. A retrospective effectiveness study of loss of resistance to air or saline for identification of the epidural space. Anesth Analg 2010; 110(2): 558-63.
[http://dx.doi.org/10.1213/ANE.0b013e3181c84e4e] [PMID: 19955501]

[52]   Brogly N, Guasch E, Alsina E, García C, Puertas L, *et al.* Epidural Space Identification With Loss of Resistance Technique for Epidural Analgesia During Labor: A Randomized Controlled Study Using Air or Saline-New Arguments for an Old Controversy 2018.
[http://dx.doi.org/10.1213/ANE.0000000000002593]

[53]   Nistal-Nuño B, Gómez-Ríos MÁ. Case Report: Pneumocephalus after labor epidural anesthesia. F1000 Res 2014; 3: 166.
[http://dx.doi.org/10.12688/f1000research.4693.1] [PMID: 25210618]

[54]   Nathan N, Wong CA. Spinal, Epidural, and Caudal Anesthesia: Anatomy, Physiology, and Technique 2009; 249.

[55]   Norris MC, Ferrenbach D, Dalman H, *et al.* Does epinephrine improve the diagnostic accuracy of aspiration during labor epidural analgesia? Anesth Analg 1999; 88(5): 1073-6.
[PMID: 10320171]

[56]   Mulroy M, Glosten B. The epinephrine test dose in obstetrics: note the limitations. Anesth Analg

1998; 86(5): 923-5.
[http://dx.doi.org/10.1213/00000539-199805000-00001] [PMID: 9585269]

[57]   Camorcia M. Testing the epidural catheter. Curr Opin Anaesthesiol 2009; 22(3): 336-40.
[http://dx.doi.org/10.1097/ACO.0b013e3283295281] [PMID: 19342949]

[58]   Pan PH, Bogard TD, Owen MD. Incidence and characteristics of failures in obstetric neuraxial analgesia and anesthesia: a retrospective analysis of 19,259 deliveries. Int J Obstet Anesth 2004; 13(4): 227-33.
[http://dx.doi.org/10.1016/j.ijoa.2004.04.008] [PMID: 15477051]

[59]   Abraham RA, Harris AP, Maxwell LG, Kaplow S. The efficacy of 1.5% lidocaine with 7.5% dextrose and epinephrine as an epidural test dose for obstetrics. Anesthesiology 1986; 64(1): 116-8.
[http://dx.doi.org/10.1097/00000542-198601000-00022] [PMID: 3942321]

[60]   Colonna-Romano P, Padolina R, Lingaraju N, Braitman LE. Diagnostic accuracy of an intrathecal test dose in epidural analgesia. Can J Anaesth 1994; 41(7): 572-4.
[http://dx.doi.org/10.1007/BF03009994] [PMID: 8087903]

[61]   Owen MD, Gautier P, Hood DD. Can ropivacaine and levobupivacaine be used as test doses during regional anesthesia? Anesthesiology 2004; 100(4): 922-5.
[http://dx.doi.org/10.1097/00000542-200404000-00023] [PMID: 15087628]

[62]   Norris MC, Fogel ST, Dalman H, Borrenpohl S, Hoppe W, Riley A. Labor epidural analgesia without an intravascular "test dose". Anesthesiology 1998; 88(6): 1495-501.
[http://dx.doi.org/10.1097/00000542-199806000-00012] [PMID: 9637642]

[63]   Hermanides J, Hollmann MW, Stevens MF, Lirk P. Failed epidural: causes and management. Br J Anaesth 2012; 109(2): 144-54.
[http://dx.doi.org/10.1093/bja/aes214] [PMID: 22735301]

[64]   Kasten GW, Martin ST. Resuscitation from bupivacaine-induced cardiovascular toxicity during partial inferior vena cava occlusion. Anesth Analg 1986; 65(4): 341-4.
[http://dx.doi.org/10.1213/00000539-198604000-00005] [PMID: 3954108]

[65]   Santos AC, Arthur GR, Roberts DJ, *et al.* Effect of ropivacaine and bupivacaine on uterine blood flow in pregnant ewes. Anesth Analg 1992; 74(1): 62-7.
[http://dx.doi.org/10.1213/00000539-199201000-00011] [PMID: 1734800]

[66]   Beilin Y, Guinn NR, Bernstein HH, Zahn J, Hossain S, Bodian CA. Local anesthetics and mode of delivery: bupivacaine *versus* ropivacaine *versus* levobupivacaine. Anesth Analg 2007; 105(3): 756-63.
[http://dx.doi.org/10.1213/01.ane.0000278131.73472.f4] [PMID: 17717236]

[67]   Wang LZ, Chang XY, Liu X, Hu XX, Tang BL. Comparison of bupivacaine, ropivacaine and levobupivacaine with sufentanil for patient-controlled epidural analgesia during labor: a randomized clinical trial. 2010.

[68]   Beilin Y, Halpern S. Focused review: ropivacaine *versus* bupivacaine for epidural labor analgesia. Anesth Analg. agosto de 2010; 111(2): 482-7.

[69]   Comparative Obstetric Mobile Epidural Trial (COMET) Study Group UK 2001.

[70]   Lyons GR, Kocarev MG, Wilson RC, Columb MO. A comparison of minimum local anesthetic volumes and doses of epidural bupivacaine (0.125% w/v and 0.25% w/v) for analgesia in labor. Anesth Analg 2007; 104(2): 412-5.
[http://dx.doi.org/10.1213/01.ane.0000252458.20912.ef] [PMID: 17242100]

[71]   Capogna G, Celleno D, Lyons G, *et al.* Minimum local analgesic concentration of extradural bupivacaine increases with progression of labour. Local Reg Anesth 2010; 3: 143-53.

[72]   Silva M, Halpern SH. Epidural analgesia for labor: Current techniques. Local Reg Anesth 2010; 3: 143-53.
[PMID: 23144567]

[73]   Lyons G, Columb M, Hawthorne L, Dresner M. Extradural pain relief in labour: bupivacaine sparing by extradural fentanyl is dose dependent. Br J Anaesth 1997; 78(5): 493-7.
[http://dx.doi.org/10.1093/bja/78.5.493] [PMID: 9175960]

[74]   Justins DM, Francis D, Houlton PG, Reynolds F. A controlled trial of extradural fentanyl in labour. Br J Anaesth 1982; 54(4): 409-14.
[http://dx.doi.org/10.1093/bja/54.4.409] [PMID: 7039646]

[75]   Wheelahan JM, Leslie K, Silbert BS. Epidural fentanyl reduces the shivering threshold during epidural lidocaine anesthesia. Anesth Analg 1998; 87(3): 587-90.
[http://dx.doi.org/10.1213/00000539-199809000-00017] [PMID: 9728834]

[76]   Liu WHD, Luxton MC. The effect of prophylactic fentanyl on shivering in elective Caesarean section under epidural analgesia. Anaesthesia 1991; 46(5): 344-8.
[http://dx.doi.org/10.1111/j.1365-2044.1991.tb09540.x] [PMID: 2035777]

[77]   DeBalli P, Breen TW. Intrathecal opioids for combined spinal-epidural analgesia during labour. CNS Drugs 2003; 17(12): 889-904.
[http://dx.doi.org/10.2165/00023210-200317120-00003] [PMID: 12962528]

[78]   Abboud TK, Sheik-ol-Eslam A, Yanagi T, *et al.* Safety and efficacy of epinephrine added to bupivacaine for lumbar epidural analgesia in obstetrics. Anesth Analg 1985; 64(6): 585-91.
[http://dx.doi.org/10.1213/00000539-198506000-00005] [PMID: 4003776]

[79]   Polley LS, Columb MO, Naughton NN, Wagner DS, van de Ven CJ. Effect of epidural epinephrine on the minimum local analgesic concentration of epidural bupivacaine in labor. Anesthesiology 2002; 96(5): 1123-8.
[http://dx.doi.org/10.1097/00000542-200205000-00015] [PMID: 11981152]

[80]   Skjöldebrand A, Garle M, Gustafsson LL, Johansson H, Lunell NO, Rane A. Extradural pethidine with and without adrenaline during labour: wide variation in effect. Br J Anaesth 1982; 54(4): 415-20.
[http://dx.doi.org/10.1093/bja/54.4.415] [PMID: 7066138]

[81]   Yarnell RW, Ewing DA, Tierney E, Smith MH. Sacralization of epidural block with repeated doses of 0.25% bupivacaine during labor. Reg Anesth 1990; 15(6): 275-9.
[PMID: 2291881]

[82]   Soetens FM, Soetens MA, Vercauteren MP. Levobupivacaine-sufentanil with or without epinephrine during epidural labor analgesia. Anesth Analg 2006; 103(1): 182-6.
[http://dx.doi.org/10.1213/01.ane.0000221038.46094.c0] [PMID: 16790650]

[83]   Albright GA, Jouppita R, Hollmén AI, Jouppila P, Vierola H, Koivula A. Epinephrine does not alter human intervillous blood flow during epidural anesthesia. Anesthesiology 1981; 54(2): 131-5.
[http://dx.doi.org/10.1097/00000542-198102000-00006] [PMID: 7469091]

[84]   Wang TT, Sun S, Huang SQ. Effects of Epidural Labor Analgesia With Low Concentrations of Local Anesthetics on Obstetric Outcomes: A Systematic Review and Meta-analysis of Randomized Controlled Trials. 2017.
[http://dx.doi.org/10.1213/ANE.0000000000001709]

[85]   Paech LJ. Patient-controlled epidural analgesia in obstetrics. 1996.
[http://dx.doi.org/10.1016/S0959-289X(96)80010-0]

[86]   Halpern SH, Carvalho B. Patient-controlled epidural analgesia for labor. Anesth Analg. marzo de 2009; 108(3): 921-8.

[87]   Bullingham A, Liang S, Edmonds E, Mathur S, Sharma S. Continuous epidural infusion *vs* programmed intermittent epidural bolus for labour analgesia: a prospective, controlled, before-an--after cohort study of labour outcomes. 2018.
[http://dx.doi.org/10.1016/j.bja.2018.03.038]

[88]   Viitanen H, Viitanen M, Heikkilä M. Single-shot spinal block for labour analgesia in multiparous

parturients. Acta Anaesthesiol Scand 2005; 49(7): 1023-9.
[http://dx.doi.org/10.1111/j.1399-6576.2005.00803.x] [PMID: 16045666]

[89]   http://www.rcoa.ac.uk/system/files/CSQ-NAP3-Full_1.pdf

[90]   Eisenach JC. Combined spinal-epidural analgesia in obstetrics. 1999.

[91]   Carrie LES, O'Sullivan G. Subarachnoid bupivacaine 0.5% for caesarean section. Eur J Anaesthesiol 1984; 1(3): 275-83.
[PMID: 6536516]

[92]   Norris MC, Fogel ST, Conway-Long C. 92. Norris MC, Fogel ST, Conway-Long C. Combined spinal-epidural *versus* epidural labor analgesia. Anesthesiology. octubre de 2001; 95(4): 913-20.

[93]   Wilson MJ, Cooper G, MacArthur C, Shennan A. Comparative Obstetric Mobile Epidural Trial (COMET) Study Group UK. Randomized controlled trial comparing traditional with two «mobile» epidural techniques: anesthetic and analgesic efficacy. Anesthesiology. diciembre de 2002;97 (6):1567-75. 2002; 97(6): 1567-75.

[94]   Riley ET, Hamilton CL, Ratner EF, Cohen SE. A comparison of the 24-gauge Sprotte and Gertie Marx spinal needles for combined spinal-epidural analgesia during labor. Anesthesiology 2002; 97(3): 574-7.
[http://dx.doi.org/10.1097/00000542-200209000-00009] [PMID: 12218522]

[95]   Mardirosoff C, Dumont L, Boulvain M, Tramèr MR. Fetal bradycardia due to intrathecal opioids for labour analgesia: a systematic review 2002.
[http://dx.doi.org/10.1111/j.1471-0528.2002.01380.x]

[96]   Abrão KC, Francisco RPV, Miyadahira S, Cicarelli DD, Zugaib M. Elevation of uterine basal tone and fetal heart rate abnormalities after labor analgesia: a randomized controlled trial 2009.

[97]   Norris MC, Grieco WM, Borkowski M, *et al.* Complications of labor analgesia: epidural *versus* combined spinal epidural techniques. Anesth Analg 1994; 79(3): 529-37.
[http://dx.doi.org/10.1213/00000539-199409000-00022] [PMID: 8067559]

[98]   McGrady E, Litchfield K. Epidural analgesia in labour. Contin Educ Anaesth Crit Care Pain 2004; 4(4): 114-7.
[http://dx.doi.org/10.1093/bjaceaccp/mkh030]

[99]   Shaw IC, Birks RJS. A case of extensive block with the combined spinal-epidural technique during labour. Anaesthesia 2001; 56(4): 346-9.
[http://dx.doi.org/10.1046/j.1365-2044.2001.01785.x] [PMID: 11284821]

[100]   Holmström B, Rawal N, Axelsson K, Nydahl P-A. Risk of catheter migration during combined spinal epidural block: percutaneous epiduroscopy study. Anesth Analg 1995; 80(4): 747-53.
[PMID: 7893029]

[101]   Cambic CR, Wong CA. Labour analgesia and obstetric outcomes. Br J Anaesth. diciembre de 2010;105 Suppl 1:50-60.
[http://dx.doi.org/10.1093/bja/aeq311]

[102]   Wong CA, McCarthy RJ, Sullivan JT, Scavone BM, Gerber SE, Yaghmour EA. Early compared with late neuraxial analgesia in nulliparous labor induction: a randomized controlled trial 2009.
[http://dx.doi.org/10.1097/AOG.0b013e3181a1a9a8]

[103]   Wang F, Shen X, Guo X, Peng Y, Gu X. Labor Analgesia Examining Group. Epidural analgesia in the latent phase of labor and the risk of cesarean delivery: a five-year randomized controlled trial. 111. octubre de 2009; 4: 871-0.

[104]   Zhang J, Landy HJ, Ware Branch D, *et al.* Contemporary patterns of spontaneous labor with normal neonatal outcomes. Obstet Gynecol 2010; 116(6): 1281-7.
[http://dx.doi.org/10.1097/AOG.0b013e3181fdef6e] [PMID: 21099592]

[105]   Sng BL, Leong WL, Zeng Y, *et al.* Early *versus* late initiation of epidural analgesia for labour.

Cochrane Libr 2014; (10): CD007238.
[http://dx.doi.org/10.1002/14651858.CD007238.pub2] [PMID: 25300169]

[106] Miro M, Guasch E, Gilsanz F. Comparison of epidural analgesia with combined spinal-epidural analgesia for labor: a retrospective study of 6497 cases. Int J Obstet Anesth 2008; 17(1): 15-9.
[http://dx.doi.org/10.1016/j.ijoa.2007.07.003] [PMID: 18162199]

[107] Mullington CJ, Low DA, Strutton PH, Malhotra S. A mechanistic study of the tremor associated with epidural anaesthesia for intrapartum caesarean delivery 2020.
[http://dx.doi.org/10.1016/j.ijoa.2020.02.007]

[108] Beilin Y, Zahn J, Bernstein HH, Zucker-Pinchoff B, Zenzen WJ, Andres LA. Treatment of incomplete analgesia after placement of an epidural catheter and administration of local anesthetic for women in labor. Anesthesiology 1998; 88(6): 1502-6.
[http://dx.doi.org/10.1097/00000542-199806000-00013] [PMID: 9637643]

[109] Simmons SW, Taghizadeh N, Dennis AT, Hughes D, Cyna AM. Combined spinal-epidural *versus* epidural analgesia in labour. Cochrane Libr 2012; 10(10): CD003401.
[http://dx.doi.org/10.1002/14651858.CD003401.pub3] [PMID: 23076897]

[110] Dyer RA, Reed AR, van Dyk D, *et al.* Hemodynamic effects of ephedrine, phenylephrine, and the coadministration of phenylephrine with oxytocin during spinal anesthesia for elective cesarean delivery. Anesthesiology 2009; 111(4): 753-65.
[http://dx.doi.org/10.1097/ALN.0b013e3181b437e0] [PMID: 19741494]

[111] Kinsella SM, Pirlet M, Mills MS, Tuckey JP, Thomas TA, Thomas TA. Randomized study of intravenous fluid preload before epidural analgesia during labour. Br J Anaesth 2000; 85(2): 311-3.
[http://dx.doi.org/10.1093/bja/85.2.311] [PMID: 10992845]

[112] Kubli M, Shennan AH, Seed PT, O'Sullivan G. A randomised controlled trial of fluid pre-loading before low dose epidural analgesia for labour. Int J Obstet Anesth 2003; 12(4): 256-60.
[http://dx.doi.org/10.1016/S0959-289X(03)00071-2] [PMID: 15321453]

[113] Banerjee A, Stocche RM, Angle P, Halpern SH. Preload or coload for spinal anesthesia for elective Cesarean delivery: a meta-analysis. Can J Anaesth 2010; 57(1): 24-31.
[http://dx.doi.org/10.1007/s12630-009-9206-7] [PMID: 19859776]

[114] Chooi C, Cox JJ, Lumb RS, *et al.* Techniques for preventing hypotension during spinal anaesthesia for caesarean section 2020.

[115] Mhyre JM, Greenfield MLVH, Tsen LC, Polley LS. A systematic review of randomized controlled trials that evaluate strategies to avoid epidural vein cannulation during obstetric epidural catheter placement. Anesth Analg 2009; 108(4): 1232-42.
[http://dx.doi.org/10.1213/ane.0b013e318198f85e] [PMID: 19299793]

[116] Van Zundert A, Vaes L, Soetens M, *et al.* Every dose given in epidural analgesia for vaginal delivery can be a test dose. Anesthesiology 1987; 67(3): 436-40.
[http://dx.doi.org/10.1097/00000542-198709000-00030] [PMID: 3631617]

[117] Booth JM, Pan JC, Ross VH, Russell GB, Harris LC, Pan PH. Combined spinal epidural technique for labor analgesia does not delay recognition of epidural catheter failures: a single-center retrospective cohort survival analysis. Anesthesiology 2016; 125(3): 516-24.
[http://dx.doi.org/10.1097/ALN.0000000000001222] [PMID. 27380107]

[118] Gambling DR, Huber CJ, Berkowitz J, *et al.* Patient-controlled epidural analgesia in labour: varying bolus dose and lockout interval. Can J Anaesth 1993; 40(3): 211-7.
[http://dx.doi.org/10.1007/BF03037032] [PMID: 8467542]

[119] Richardson MG, Lee AC, Wissler RN. High spinal anesthesia after epidural test dose administration in five obstetric patients. Reg Anesth 1996; 21(2): 119-23.
[PMID: 8829404]

[120] Choi PT, Galinski SE, Takeuchi L, Lucas S, Tamayo C, Jadad AR. PDPH is a common complication

of neuraxial blockade in parturients: a meta-analysis of obstetrical studies. Can J Anaesth 2003; 50(5): 460-9.
[http://dx.doi.org/10.1007/BF03021057] [PMID: 12734154]

[121] Crawford JS. Some maternal complications of epidural analgesia for labour. Anaesthesia 1985; 40(12): 1219-25.
[http://dx.doi.org/10.1111/j.1365-2044.1985.tb10664.x] [PMID: 4083452]

[122] Leighton BL, Halpern SH. Epidural analgesia and the progress of labor. In: Halpern SH, Douglas MJ, Eds. Evidence-based Obstetric Anesthesia 2005.
[http://dx.doi.org/10.1002/9780470988343.ch2]

[123] Cook TM, Counsell D, Wildsmith JAW. Royal College of Anaesthetists Third National Audit Project. Major complications of central neuraxial block: Report on the Third National Audit Project of the Royal College of Anaesthetists. Br J Anaesth 2009; 102: 179-90.
[http://dx.doi.org/10.1093/bja/aen360] [PMID: 19139027]

[124] de Orange FA, Passini R Jr, Amorim MMR, Almeida T, Barros A. Combined spinal and epidural anaesthesia and maternal intrapartum temperature during vaginal delivery: a randomized clinical trial. Br J Anaesth 2011; 107(5): 762-8.
[http://dx.doi.org/10.1093/bja/aer218] [PMID: 21743067]

[125] Dias Cicarelli D, Frerichs E, Martins Benseñor FE. Incidence of neurological complications and post-dural puncture headache after regional anesthesia in obstetric practice: A retrospective study of 2399 patients. Rev Colomb de Anestesiol 2014; 42(1): 28-32.
[http://dx.doi.org/10.1016/j.rca.2013.09.009]

[126] Ruppen W, Derry S, McQuay H, Moore RA. Incidence of epidural hematoma, infection, and neurologic injury in obstetric patients with epidural analgesia/anesthesia. Anesthesiology 2006; 105(2): 394-9.
[http://dx.doi.org/10.1097/00000542-200608000-00023] [PMID: 16871074]

[127] Birnbach DJ, Browne IM. Anesthesia for obstetrics. Churchill Livingstone 2009; 2215-5.

[128] Wong CA. Epidural and Spinal Analgesia: Anesthesia for Labor and Vaginal Delivery 2020; 474.

[129] Novikova N, Cluver C. Local anaesthetic nerve block for pain management in labour 2012.
[http://dx.doi.org/10.1002/14651858.CD009200.pub2]

[130] Lopez Timoneda F. Analgesia y Anestesia obstetrica.Tratado de la Sociedad Española de Ginecologia y Obstetricia. 2nda Ed. Ed Medica Panamericana; 2014; pp. 1191-8.

[131] Rosen MA. Paracervical block for labor analgesia: A brief historic review. Am J Obstet Gynecol 2002; 186(5) (Suppl Nature): S127-30.
[http://dx.doi.org/10.1016/S0002-9378(02)70187-7] [PMID: 12011878]

[132] Miranda L. Analgesia y anestesia obstétrica. Folia Clín Obstet Ginecol 2005; 50: 6-27.

CHAPTER 9

Uterotonic Agents

Juan José Correa Barrera[1,*], **Blanca Gómez del Pulgar Vázquez**[1], **Adriana Orozco Vinasco**[1] and **Enrique Alonso Rodríguez**[1]

[1] *Department of Anaesthesiology, University Hospital Severo Ochoa, Leganes, Madrid, Spain*

Abstract: Postpartum haemorrhage due to uterine atony is one of the major causes of maternal morbidity and mortality worldwide. Different control strategies have been postulated, especially during the third stage of labour, but the gold standard treatment is the use of uterotonic drugs. There are currently three well-defined groups of drugs: oxytocics, ergot derivatives and prostaglandins. Although the literature is heterogeneous, it is clear that oxytocin is the uterotonic of choice in both prophylaxis and treatment of postpartum haemorrhage. Detailed knowledge of protocols based on current evidence is mandatory, which vary according to the different medical societies and dictate the doses and order of administration of different drugs.

Keywords: Caesarian Section, Carbetocin, Dinoprostone, Ergot Alkaloids, Methylergometrine, Misoprostol, Obstetric Myometrium, Oxytocin, Oxytocics, Postpartum Haemorrhage, Prostaglandins, Prostaglandins Synthetic, Uterotonics, Uterine Contraction.

INTRODUCTION

Nowadays, postpartum haemorrhage (*PPH*) is still the main cause of maternal death from obstetric haemorrhage, despite great efforts to reduce its incidence, especially in developed countries [1 - 6].

Uterine atony is the leading cause of PPH, both in caesarean section and vaginal delivery [3, 4]. Active control of the third stage of labour, through the administration of uterotonic drugs, early cord clamping and controlled traction of the umbilical cord until placental prevent bleeding during this period [1, 3 - 5].

Historically, the first drugs used as uterotonics were ergot alkaloids, later oxytocin and finally modern prostaglandins [5, 7]. According to available evidence, the order of administration of these drugs has been modified based on their efficacy, tolerance and adverse effect profile [5].

* **Corresponding author Juan José Correa Barrera:** Department of Anaesthesiology. Hospital Universitario Severo Ochoa, Madrid, Spain; Email: correabarrera83@gmail.com

Eugenio Daniel Martinez-Hurtado, Monica Sanjuan-Alvarez & Marta Chacon-Castillo (Eds.)
All rights reserved-© 2022 Bentham Science Publishers

Oxytocics are currently considered the drugs of choice for the prevention of PPH, since they have a safety and efficacy profile that is superior to that of other drugs of this group [4, 5, 7, 8].

Ergotamine derivatives, despite being effective in the prevention of postpartum haemorrhage, have greater adverse effects, so they are reserved as a second therapeutic step.

Prostaglandins play an important role in the treatment of postpartum haemorrhage, but they are not considered first-line drugs, neither for prophylaxis nor for treatment [4, 5, 7, 8].

Uterine atony risk factors include uterus overdistension, oxytocin infusion during labour, chorioamnionitis, placenta previa, previous uterine atony, multiple gestations and high parity [8].

Prompt communication between the obstetrician and the anesthesiologist is very important in order to establish the patient's individual needs according to the clinical setting, which determines uterotonic requirements in each specific case.

UTEROTONIC AGENTS

Uterotonic drugs promote adequate uterine contraction by increasing uterine basal tone and activating the frequency, intensity and duration of uterine smooth muscle contractions [1, 3, 4].

The characteristics of an ideal uterotonic are shown in Table **1** [4].

The administration of uterotonic drugs, therapeutically or prophylactically, is a fundamental measure to reduce the incidence of PPH due to uterine atony [4].

Oxytocin

Oxytocin is a hormone synthesized in the hypothalamus and secreted by the posterior pituitary gland in a pulsatile fashion. It is also synthesized in the umbilical cord, chorion and decidua, and is responsible, among other actions, for uterine contractions [1, 3, 5 - 7].

Table 1. Characteristics of an ideal uterotonic.

- Highly effective
- Few adverse effects
- Thermoresistant
- Easy to administer
- Predictable and optimal pharmacokinetic profile

Oxytocin was discovered in 1906 by Sir Henry Dale [6, 7]. Since Vincent du Vigneaud first artificially synthesized it in 1954, it has become an essential drug in obstetric practice for both, induction and optimization of labour, and subsequently for the prevention and control of PPH [4 - 8]. In the postpartum period, it acts by slowing placental bed haemorrhage [6].

Oxytocin is also synthesized in peripheral tissues such as the uterus, corpus luteum, amnion, umbilical cord, placenta and testis. It is involved in various physiological and pathological actions like maternal behaviour, milk ejection, erectile dysfunction and ejaculation [1, 3, 5, 6].

Oxytocin is poorly protein bound, can be administered intravenously and it has an onset of action of 1 to 2 minutes and a half-life of 15 minutes. Therefore, it should be given as a continuous infusion. Intramuscular administration is also feasible; by this route, its onset of action is 2 to 4 minutes and its half-life is lengthened, lasting between 30 and 60 minutes [4].

The concentration of oxytocin receptors in the myometrium of non-pregnant women is low, increasing progressively during pregnancy until labour, when it is doubled [1, 6, 8]. Both oxytocin and carbetocin do not show significant uterine contraction in non-pregnant women [8].

Oxytocin and its analogues are agonists of the transmembrane oxytocin receptor (*OTR*), G-protein-coupled receptors family involved in the transmission and signalling of various intracellular pathways [1, 5, 6, 8]. Although some of these routes and mechanisms are not fully elucidated, OTR functions are clear in the physiology of pregnancy and childbirth [1]. OTR is expressed throughout the body, *e.g.* in the circulatory system, the central nervous system, as well as in the myometrium and endometrium [6, 8].

Oxytocin molecule binding to OTR leads to activation of a phospholipase that catalyses the conversion of phosphoinositide-bis-phosphate (*PIP2*) to inositol-tri-
-phosphate (*IP3*) and diacylglycerol (*DAG*) [1, 6]. IP3 enhances calcium release from the sarcoplasmic reticulum and thus, cytoplasmic calcium increases, which results in the stimulation of Ca^{2+}-dependent calmodulin. The latter activates a myosin light chain kinase (*MLCK*) that triggers the contraction-relaxation cycle of smooth muscle [1, 3, 6]. Additionally, DAG, through a series of kinase-mediated cascades, increases prostaglandin E2 synthesis, which is also involved in myometrial muscle contraction [1, 6].

The action of oxytocin has a ceiling effect. Once all the receptors are blocked, a phenomenon called oxytocin receptor desensitization, uterine contractions intensity will not increase, predisposing to increased bleeding and potentiation of drug adverse effects [1, 4, 6, 8]. Different *in vivo* and *in vitro* studies have demonstrated a decrease in uterine contractility after exposure to high concentrations of oxytocin mediated by a receptor downregulation phenomenon [1, 6]. It is important to highlight that this reduction in contractility does not limit the use of second-line agents to control PPH [1].

Despite being the most widely used uterotonic, oxytocin has a number of adverse effects to be considered (Table **2**). Those effects are more pronounced when administered as a *bolus,* hence the preference for continuous infusions [1, 8].

Table 2. Adverse effects of oxytocin

- Fetal bradycardia and hyperbilirubinemia at high doses.
- Nausea and vomiting
- Fetal desaturation
- Uterine hyperactivity
- Flushing
- Antidiuretic effect (fluid retention, hyponatremia, seizure, coma)
- Headache
- Preterm labour, placental abruption, uterine atony and postpartum haemorrhage.
- Cardiovascular effects: hypotension, tachycardia, myocardial ischemia, arrhythmias, ST alterations.

Cardiovascular sideeffects are associated to the worst outcomes; those are especially dangerous in hypovolemic patients, cardiomyopathies and preeclampsia [3, 4, 8]. The dose and infusion rate of the drug are factors that influence the occurrence of adverse effects [4, 8]. Oxytocin has been directly or indirectly involved in some maternal deaths [3, 8].

Clinical considerations

Oxytocin is considered the uterotonic of choice; however, it is a drug under continuous review. Its evidence is based on heterogeneous studies, which makes it difficult to establish an adequate and standardized dose and administration pattern [2 - 4]. Doses will be different for treatment and prophylaxis, as well as for vaginal delivery and caesarean section. Table **3** shows different recommendations for PPH prophylaxis in caesarean section according to different medical societies around the world [8]. It can be noted that, although all these guidelines have been developed for PPH prevention, the recommendations differ [1].

Table 3. Recommendations for the use of uterotonics in caesarean sections according to different official agencies.

Institution	First-line Drug for Postpartum Haemorrhage (PPH) Prophylaxis	Second-line Drug for PPH Prophylaxis
Safe Motherhood and Newborn Health Committee Prevention and treatment of postpartum haemorrhage in low-resource settings. International Federation of Gynecology and Obstetrics (FIGO)	Rule out another infant by palpating the mother's abdomen before the first minute of the infant's birth and administer oxytocin 10 IU i.m. Oxytocin has a fast action time of 2-3 minutes, few adverse effects, and can be used in all pregnant women, thus it is the recommended uterotonic. If oxytocin is not available, ergometrine or methylergometrine at a dose of 0.2 mg i.m., syntometrine i.m. (which is a combination of oxytocin 5 IU and ergometrine 0.5 mg), or misoprostol 600 µg orally can be used (which is a combination of oxytocin 5 IU and ergometrine 0.5 mg per ampoule), or misoprostol 600 µg orally.	FIGO guideline discusses the management of established haemorrhage and recommends that oxytocin be used over ergometrine or methylergometrine alone, a fixed-dose combination of ergometrine and oxytocin, carbetocin and/or prostaglandins such as misoprostol. In cases where oxytocin cannot be started, or if bleeding does not respond to oxytocin or ergometrine, a fixed-dose combination of oxytocin and ergometrine, carbetocin or misoprostol should be offered as a second-line treatment. If the second-line drugs are not available, or if bleeding remains unresponsive to treatment, the proposed third line of treatment is a prostaglandin such as carboprost tromethamine, if available.
National Institute of Health and Care Excellence (NICE), UK	It is recommended to administer Oxytocin 5 IU i.v. in slow infusion.	Not discussed
Association of Women's Health, Obstetric and Neonatal Nurses, USA	It is recommended to administer an i.v. bolus of oxytocin followed by an infusion for 4 h after delivery. In case of caesarean section, it is recommended to continue the infusion beyond 4 h, adjusting the infusion rate and duration of infusion according to uterine tone and haemorrhage.	Not discussed

(Table 3) cont.....

Institution	First-line Drug for Postpartum Haemorrhage (PPH) Prophylaxis	Second-line Drug for PPH Prophylaxis
Royal College of Obstetricians and Gynaecologists, UK, 2016	It is recommended to administer Oxytocin 5 IU i.v. in slow infusion.	Oxytocin and ergometrine reduce the risk of minor PPH (500-1000 ml), so they can be used in the absence of hypertension. If the risk of PPH is high, a combination of preventive measures should also be used together with oxytocin.
American College of Obstetricians and Gynecologists Practice Bulletin number 183 Postpartum Haemorrhage, 2017	It is recommended to use oxytocin prophylactically by bolus of 10 IU i.v. or intramuscular injection of 10 IU.	This guideline discusses the management of established haemorrhage, recommending uterotonic agents as first-line treatment for PPH secondary to uterine atony. However, they leave the choice of uterotonic to the discretion of the health care provider.
Royal Australian and New Zealand College of Obstetricians and Gynaecologists, 2017	Prophylactic oxytocics and labour management reduce the risk of PPH, as well as the need for blood transfusion, so active management of the third stage of labour is recommended. However, they do not recommend any particular agent/dose.	This guideline discusses the management of established haemorrhage by recommending uterotonic agents as first-line treatment for PPH secondary to uterine atony.
Society of Obstetrics and Gynaecologists of Canada, 2009	It is recommended to use 100 μg of Carbetocin as a slow i.v. bolus to be administered over 1 minute.	This guideline recommends as second-line treatment the infusion of oxytocin or ergonovine (ergometrine) but only in vaginal deliveries. No specific recommendation is made as second line treatment in case of caesarean section.
French College of Obstetricians and Gynaecologists in collaboration with French Society of Anaesthesiology and Intensive Care, 2015	It is recommended to administer 5-10 IU i.v. of oxytocin as a bolus, except in women with manifest cardiovascular risk, in whom the injection should last at least 5 minutes. The maintenance dose will be 10 IU.h-1, checking every 2 hours. Although carbetocin reduces risk of PPH, in the absence of a non-inferiority trial oxytocin remains the drug of choice for prophylaxis.	Management algorithms for PPH after vaginal delivery are discussed, PPH that may occur during caesarean section, and delayed PPH after caesarean section, recommending oxytocin and sulprostone infusion.
Deutsche Gesellschaft feur Gyneakologie und Geburtshilfe, 2016	It is recommended to administer Oxytocin 3–5 IU i.v. in slow infusion.	Carbetocin 100 μg *i.v.* in slow infusion.

(Table 3) cont.....

Institution	First-line Drug for Postpartum Haemorrhage (PPH) Prophylaxis	Second-line Drug for PPH Prophylaxis
World Health Organization (WHO) Recommendations for the prevention and treatment of postpartum haemorrhage, 2018	The use of one of the following uterotonics is recommended for the prevention of PPH during the third stage of labour in all deliveries: - oxytocin (10 IU, *i.m./i.v.*) - carbetocin (100 μg, *i.m. /i.v.*) - misoprostol (either 400 μg or 600 μg, oral) - ergometrine/methylergometrine (200 μg, *i.m./ i.v.*) - oxytocin and ergometrine fixed-dose combination (5 IU/ 500 μg, i.m.) When multiple uterotonic options are available, oxytocin at a dose of 10 IU i.m./i.v. is recommended as the uterotonic agent for PPH prevention.	Not reviewed.

Modification of table found in Heesen et al. Consensus statement on uterotonic agents during caesarean section Anaesthesia 2019, 74, 1305–1319 [8].

Apparently, both oxytocin's total dose and the time of drug exposure independently increase the risk of PPH. In cases of caesarean section after prolonged labour, the effective oxytocin dose is higher than the one needed for a scheduled caesarean section. The former may require a second uterotonic, which will be useful to modulate the desensitization phenomenon and the ceiling effect of oxytocin [4, 8].

Oxytocin administration after delivery eliminates the risk of drug transfer to the neonate [3, 4].

According to the latest update of the *Royal College of Obstetrics and Gynecology*, routine prophylactic administration of oxytocin is recommended during the third stage of labour in women without risk of PPH. A dose of 5 to 10 IU is given *i.m.* after fetal anterior shoulder detachment, followed by an *i.v.* infusion of 10 IU during 4 to 6 hours. In the event of caesarean section, recommendations are 3 to 5 IU in a rapid bolus followed by a continuous infusion of 10 IU in 100 ml in low-risk cases, or 40 IU in 500 ml of saline at 125 ml/h in high-risk women [2 - 4, 8].

Over the last decade, new evidence emerged that a lower dose of oxytocin is equally effective, both in elective caesarean sections (0.3 IU-1 IU *bolus*) and in those with pre-labour (3 IU *bolus*). Afterwards, a continuous infusion between 5 and 10 IU/h should be maintained [3, 4, 8]. It is unclear how long this continuous infusion should be continued, but the total dose received is a key factor in the development of PPH [4]. The use of bolus followed by infusion results in reduced blood loss, less transfusion and less use of other uterotonics than if given solely a *bolus* [8].

Classically, the most common way to administer oxytocin has been by *bolus*, especially in caesarean sections. In 2010, a novel oxytocin administration protocol, known as the *"rule of threes"*, was published. This regime consists of administering an initial loading *bolus* of 3 IU of oxytocin in 15-30 seconds, followed by a clinical assessment of the situation every 3 minutes. If the uterine tone is inadequate, 2 more boluses of 3 IU can be administered and maintenance perfusion of 3 IU/h should be administered. If uterine atony persists, uterotonics from other pharmacological families should be given [2, 4, 8]. Simultaneously, the PPH protocol must be activated when necessary.

Although protocols based on current evidence are heterogeneous, it is clear that oxytocic guidelines should be different in scheduled procedures than in those preceded by long oxytocin administration or prolonged labour and delivery [8].

Carbetocin

Carbetocin is a synthetic analogue of oxytocin, whose safety profile is similar to that of oxytocin [1, 3 - 8]. Its mechanism of action consists of oxytocin receptor binding and prostaglandin synthesis [1, 3 - 5]. Its receptor affinity is similar to that of oxytocin [7]. When oxytocin is administered beforehand, a phenomenon of attenuation of contractions occurs, indicating that carbetocin could probably also be involved in receptor desensitization phenomena [1, 6, 8].

Carbetocin half-life is 40 minutes, significantly longer than that of oxytocin, which is 10 minutes. This allows carbetocin to be administered in a single dose instead of continuous perfusion, both intramuscularly and intravenously [1, 5, 6, 8]. Its uterine effects are maintained for 60 minutes when given intravenously and 120 minutes when given intramuscularly. These pharmacokinetic features are due to its high liposolubility, its tissue distribution and its resistance to degradation by peptidases [1, 5].

Disadvantages of carbetocin include that it is more expensive and the paucity of solid evidence to support its systematic use [4]. The recommended dose is a single *bolus* of 100 µg of carbetocin, equivalent to 5 IU of oxytocin. Its prophylactic use should be individualized [1, 3 - 5, 8].

It has fewer adverse effects than ergot derivatives, and are similar to those of oxytocin, including headache, flushing, hypotension, abdominal pain, nausea, pruritus and tremor [3 - 5, 8]. Although there are studies indicating that carbetocin could be administrated safely in hypertensive patients, preeclampsia is a contraindication to its use [8].

Carbetocin transfer to breast milk is minimal, lacking clinical impact, and it is rapidly degraded by the infant's digestive tract [4, 8].

There are studies comparing carbetocin with oxytocin that show less blood loss in caesarean sections, and less need for other uterotonics and uterine massage [1, 3, 5, 6, 8].

A Cochrane study demonstrated its benefit for routine PPH prophylaxis in elective caesarean sections under regional anaesthesia and with more than one risk factor for bleeding [3, 4, 8]. However, in different systematic reviews, the evidence of this PPH reduction has been variable [3]. It has not been approved for prophylactic use in vaginal delivery, although there are studies that support its use when there is more than one risk factor for bleeding [3].

It can be kept for 1 month at temperatures over 60°, 3 months at 50°, 6 months at 40° and 3 years at 30° [1, 8]. This could be an advantage in countries where it is difficult to maintain the cold chain [1].

Ergot Alkaloids

Ergot alkaloids have been used in obstetrics since 1582, although they were discontinued because of the associated ergotism (convulsions, hallucinations, necrosis and gangrene) and very high maternal and fetal mortality [3, 7]. They were reintroduced in 1932 when Dudley and Moir synthesized methylergometrine, an alkaloid with a higher safety profile than other analogues of the group [3, 4, 7]. They are now considered second-line uterotonics.

Ergometrine (ergonovine) and methylergometrine (methylergonovine) produce an increase in uterine contractility through a non-specific mechanism on adrenergic, dopaminergic and serotonergic receptors [1, 3, 4, 8]. They behave as partial agonists and antagonists of these receptors, generating an increase in intracellular calcium concentration, which enhances uterine contraction [1, 3].

Methylergometrine has an onset of action 2-3 minutes after administration and a plasma half-life of 30-120 minutes [8]. Methylergometrine is the most commonly used alkaloid in clinical practice, administered intramuscularly or intravenously, in doses of 200 µg [1, 3, 4, 8].

Due to their effect on alpha-adrenergic and dopaminergic receptors, they produce significant vasoconstriction, which limits the use of these drugs [1, 3, 4, 7, 8].

The side effects described are: placental retention, uterine inversion, headache, hypertension, abdominal pain, skin rash, vertigo, nausea and vomiting, coronary spasm, seizures and even intracranial haemorrhage [1, 3, 4, 8]; therefore, they are contraindicated in patients with ischemic heart disease, renal or hepatic disease, sepsis, pulmonary hypertension, preeclampsia and hypertensive disorders of pregnancy [4, 8].

Several Cochrane systematic reviews regarding its prophylactic use, conclude that it reduces uterine bleeding without the need to administer other uterotonics, that when compared with oxytocin and carbetocin is not associated with less PPH but with a greater number of side effects, and that when given orally, it does not provide any advantage over placebo [1, 3, 4].

Ergometrine requires adequate storage, since its efficacy is reduced by heat, light and humidity [7].

Prostaglandins and Analogues

Prostaglandins are biological peptides derived from arachidonic acid, first isolated in 1936 by Von Euler, which play an important role in reproduction, pregnancy and childbirth [1, 7, 9]. They are third-line drugs in the treatment of PPH [4].

There are several prostaglandins with uterotonic effects. They are released and act in situ as mediators that cause multiple cellular changes, which can have stimulatory or inhibitory effects [1, 4, 9]. They carry out their activity via a G-protein-coupled receptor on target cells [1]. Unlike OTR, prostaglandin receptors are present in the uterus of non-pregnant patients and throughout pregnancy [1]. The higher the number of prostaglandin receptors, the higher the expression of OTR, which will result in an increase in cytoplasmic calcium concentration and increased uterine contractility, and maturation of the collagen matrix of the uterine cervix [1, 4, 6]. Plasma prostaglandin levels increase in late pregnancy and to a greater extent with the onset of labour [1].

Synthetic prostaglandin analogues are drugs that have been developed to obtain more stable compounds [9]. Three synthetic prostaglandin analogues are currently used in clinical practice: Prostaglandin E2 (dinoprostone), Prostaglandin F2 (carboprost) and Prostaglandin E1 (misoprostol).

Prostaglandin E2 (Dinoprostone)

Indicated for the treatment of PPH due to uterine atony [1, 3, 4, 7, 8]. Dinoprostone has a very rapid distribution and metabolism in the lung, liver, kidney and spleen. It undergoes renal elimination [3]. It has a differentiated contractility action in the upper uterine segment and relaxation in the lower uterine segment [1]. The route of administration can be intravenous, intramyometrial, rectal or vaginal [3]. Its initial dose is 2.5 µg/min intravenous [3, 4].

Side effects include nausea and vomiting, headache, diarrhoea, hypertension, bronchospasm and fever, among others [3, 4, 9]. Uterine hyperstimulation is frequent [9]. These effects mean that it should be used at the minimum dose titrated to produce adequate uterine contraction [3, 4]. It is contraindicated in patients with the cardiac, pulmonary, renal and hepatic disease [3, 4, 9].

Other indications are abortion in the second trimester of pregnancy, uterine evacuation in case of fetal death, hydatiform mole and cervical ripening in term patients with the unfavourable cervix and indication for induction of labour [9].

Prostaglandin F2α (Carboprost)

It is the prostaglandin of choice in the treatment of PPH due to uterine atony [1, 3, 4]. It is metabolized by the liver and lungs, and excreted by the kidney [10]. The chemical modifications of carboprost confer a longer half-life than natural prostaglandin [1]. It can be administered intramuscularly or intramiometrially at doses of 250 µg, which can be repeated every 10-15 minutes up to a maximum of 2 g [3, 4].

Adverse effects include fever, diarrhoea, nausea and vomiting, myalgia, flushing and hypertension [1, 8, 9]. This drug can be associated with bronchospasm even in non-asthmatic patients, so it must be used with caution in asthma [1, 8]. The most severe, but infrequent, the complication is uterine rupture [9]. It can be used for abortion induction between 13 and 20 weeks [9].

Prostaglandin E1 (Misoprostol)

This is a synthetic prostaglandin indicated for the prophylaxis and treatment of uterine atony [3, 4, 9]. It can be administered sublingually, orally or rectally [1, 3, 9]. Vaginal and sublingual routes have less absorption variation and higher plasma concentrations [3, 4, 9]. Recommended dose varies between 600 mg and 1000 mg [1, 4].

It has many advantages over other prostaglandins: lower cost, no need for refrigeration, easy administration, long half-life and its favourable safety profile [1, 3, 4, 9]. Because of its advantages, it can constitute an alternative to oxytocin in places where oxytocin is not available or when intravenous access is absent.

Nevertheless, misoprostol is not more effective than oxytocin according to current evidence. Misoprostol should not be used as initial management of the third stage of labour if first-line uterotonics are available [3, 4]. The side effects of misoprostol depend on the route of administration and dose (nausea, vomiting, diarrhoea and more frequently fever and chills) [1, 3, 4, 9].

Misoprostol can be used, with solid evidence, for pregnancy termination in the first and second trimester, for cervical ripening before surgical interruption (in the first trimester), induction of labour, treatment of incomplete miscarriage, prevention and treatment of postpartum haemorrhage, cervical ripening before hysteroscopy (non-pregnant patients); with lessen evidence it can be used for cervical ripening and intrauterine device insertion, endometrial biopsy or intrauterine insemination [9].

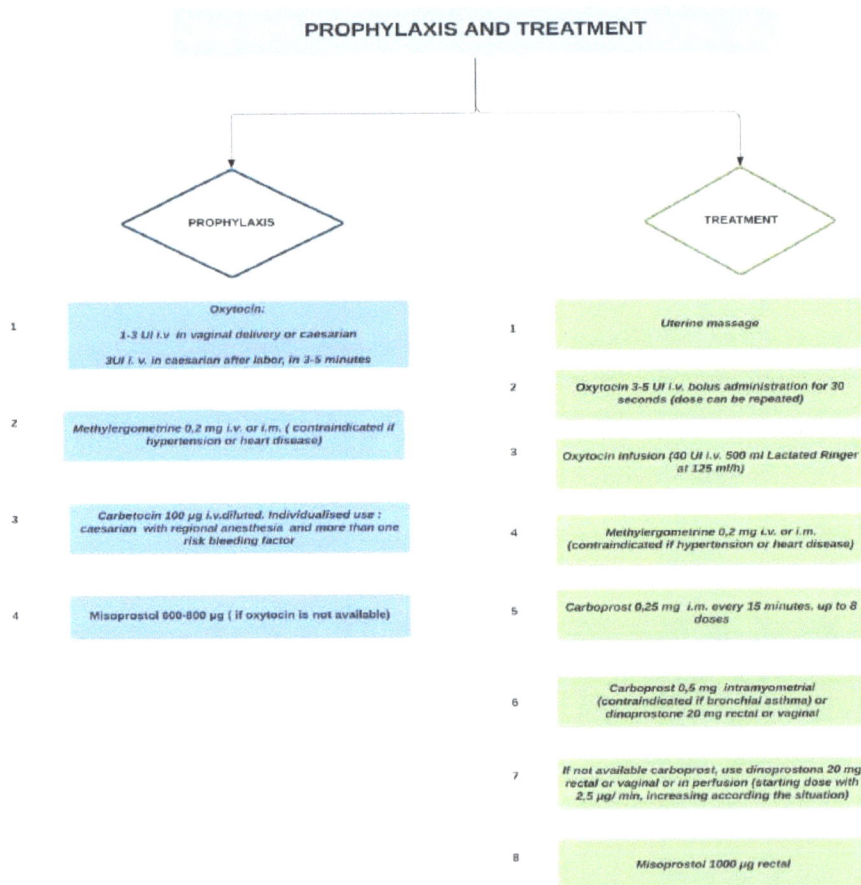

Fig. (1). Algorithm of recommendations of the Spanish Society of Anesthesiology and Resuscitation (SEDAR) for prophylaxis and treatment of PPH.

USE OF UTEROTONIC AGENTS

As mentioned before in this chapter, there are plenty of publications on PPH management, differing in routes of administration, doses and indications of uterotonic agents. Fig. (**1**) represents schematically the algorithm of recommendations of the Spanish Society of Anesthesiology and Resuscitation (*SEDAR*) for both prophylaxis and treatment of PPH [4].

CONCLUSION

Postpartum haemorrhage (*PPH*) is still the main cause of maternal death from obstetric haemorrhage. Uterine atony is the leading cause of PPH, both in caesarean section and vaginal delivery.

Oxytocics are currently considered the drugs of choice for the prevention of PPH, since they have a safety and efficacy profile that is superior to that of other drugs of this group.

Uterotonic drugs promote adequate uterine contraction by increasing uterine basal tone and activating the frequency, intensity and duration of uterine smooth muscle contractions.

Oxytocin is considered the uterotonic of choice; however it is a drug under continuous review. Its evidence is based on heterogeneous studies, which makes it difficult to establish an adequate and standardized dose and administration pattern.

Carbetocin is a synthetic analogue of oxytocin, whose safety profile is similar to that of oxytocin. Disadvantages of carbetocin include that it is more expensive and the paucity of solid evidence to support its systematic use.

Ergometrine (ergonovine) and methylergometrine (methylergonovine) produce an increase in uterine contractility through a non-specific mechanism on adrenergic, dopaminergic and serotonergic receptors. They are now considered second-line uterotonics.

Synthetic prostaglandin analogues are drugs that have been developed to obtain more stable compounds. Three synthetic prostaglandin analogues are currently used in clinical practice: Prostaglandin E2 (dinoprostone), Prostaglandin F2 (carboprost) and Prostaglandin E1 (misoprostol).

CONSENT FOR PUBLICATION

Not applicable.

CONFLICT OF INTEREST

The authors declare no conflict of interest, financial or otherwise.

ACKNOWLEDGEMENT

Declared none.

REFERENCES

[1]   Drew T, Balki M. What does basic science tell us about the use of uterotonics? Best Pract Res Clin Obstet Gynaecol 2019; 61: 3-14.
        [http://dx.doi.org/10.1016/j.bpobgyn.2019.05.017] [PMID: 31326333]

[2]   Morillas-Ramírez F, Ortiz-Gómez JR, Palacio-Abizanda FJ, Fornet-Ruiz I, Pérez-Lucas R, Bermejo-Albares L. An update of the obstetrics hemorrhage treatment protocol Rev Esp Anestesiol Reanim 2014; 61(4): 196-204.
        [PMID: 24560060]

[3]   Manrique Muñoz S, Munar Bauzà F, Francés González S, Suescun López MC, Montferrer Estruch N, Fernández López de Hierro C. Update on the use of uterotonic agents Rev Esp Anestesiol Reanim 2012; 59(2): 91-7.
        [PMID: 22480555]

[4]   Sociedad Española de Anestesiología. Reanimación y Tratamiento del dolor (SEDAR) Actualización de los protocolos asistenciales de la sección de anestesia Obstétrica de la Sedar 2a 2016; 324.

[5]   Alonso Salvador S. Estudio de la función endotelial de los fármacos oxitócicos en la prevención de la hemorragia postparto 2018.

[6]   Arrowsmith S, Wray S. Oxytocin: its mechanism of action and receptor signalling in the myometrium. J Neuroendocrinol 2014; 26(6): 356-69.
        [http://dx.doi.org/10.1111/jne.12154] [PMID: 24888645]

[7]   den Hertog CEC, de Groot ANJA, van Dongen PWJ. History and use of oxytocics. Eur J Obstet Gynecol Reprod Biol 2001; 94(1): 8-12.
        [http://dx.doi.org/10.1016/S0301-2115(00)00311-0] [PMID: 11134819]

[8]   Heesen M, Carvalho B, Carvalho JCA, Duvekot JJ, Dyer RA, Lucas DN, *et al*. International consensus statement on the use of uterotonic agents during caesarean section. Anaesthesia. 2019; 74(10): 1305-9.

[9]   Gidder B-G, Nora MM. Uso de prostaglandinas en obstetricia. RFM [Internet] 2006; 29(1): 67-73.

CHAPTER 10

Anesthesia for Non-Obstetric Surgery in Pregnancy

Irene González del Pozo[1,*], Inés Almagro Vidal[1] and **Paula Agostina Vullo[1]**

[1] *Department of Anesthesiology and Intensive Care, Hospital Central de la Defensa - Gómez Ulla, Madrid, Spain*

Abstract: The need for non-obstetric surgery during pregnancy is relatively frequent and can occur at any time during pregnancy. In this chapter, we will develop the anesthetic implications of changes in maternal physiology, and the repercussions of anesthesia on the fetus, and we will delve into the peculiarities of anesthetic management of these patients. Urgent/emergent procedures should not be postponed in these patients due to their pregnancy conditions. However, elective surgeries should be delayed whenever possible, taking into account the maternal-fetal risk-benefit.

Keywords: Anesthesia, Embryogenesis, General Anesthesia, High-Risk Pregnancy, Laparoscopy, Maternal-Fetal Risk, Monitoring, Non-Obstetric Surgery, Obstetrics Anesthesia, Obstetrics, Outcome, Positioning, Pregnancy, Preoperative Assessment, Safety, Surgical Procedures, Surgery, Spinal Anesthesia, Teratogenicity, Trimester.

INTRODUCTION

It is estimated that 1-2% of pregnant women would undergo non-obstetric surgery during pregnancy [1]. Forty-two percent of cases occur during the first trimester, 35% in the second, and 23% in the last trimester [2]. This percentage does not include patients with undetected or suspected pregnancies who undergo elective or emergency surgeries. The most frequently performed procedures are appendectomy and cholecystectomy, followed by other surgeries such as intestinal obstruction, adnexal torsions, breast pathology, and trauma interventions. Pregnancy predisposes to the development of cholelithiasis due to an increase in biliary lithogenicity and a decrease in gallbladder motility secondary to hormonal effects, and the risk of acute cholecystitis increases with advancing gestational age [3]. Some cancers are sometimes aggravated by the

---

* **Corresponding author Irene González del Pozo:** Department of Anesthesiology and Intensive Care, Hospital Central de la Defensa - Gómez Ulla, Madrid, Spain; Email: i.gonzalezdelpozo@gmail.com

Eugenio Daniel Martinez-Hurtado, Monica Sanjuan-Alvarez & Marta Chacon-Castillo (Eds.)
All rights reserved-© 2022 Bentham Science Publishers

hormonal changes in pregnancy, such as meningiomas that express estrogen or progesterone receptors and grow during this period [4].

Diagnosis of surgical processes is more complex than in non-pregnant patients due to the difficulty of the abdominal exploration and the anatomical, physiological and analytical alterations of pregnancy. This delay in diagnosis can result in diseases reaching advanced stages (*e.g.,* peritonitis) and increased maternal morbidity and mortality [5].

ANESTHETIC IMPLICATIONS OF PHYSIOLOGICAL CHANGES IN THE PREGNANT WOMAN

The physiological changes in the pregnant patient are discussed in detail in chapter **1**. In this section, we describe the implications of these changes on anesthesia and the perioperative period (Table **1**).

Table 1. Anesthetic risks of physiological changes in pregnant women.

-	Physiological changes	Risks
Respiratory	↓ functional residual capacity ↑ metabolic intake of O_2	Hypoxemia, hypercapnia, acidosis. ↓ uteroplacental blood flow Fetal hypoxemia
Airway	Edema and mucosal congestion ↑ breast and body mass	Difficult ventilation and intubation Maternal-fetal hypoxemia
Cardiovascular	*"Supine hypotensive syndrome"* Susceptibility to sympathetic blocks or vasodilator drugs	↓ cardiac output ↓ uteroplacental blood flow Fetal hypoxemia
Neuroaxial	Reduced epidural space ↑ epidural venous plexus	↑ diffusion and blockade by local anesthetics Risk of intravascular injection and local anesthetic toxicity
Gastrointestinal	↓ gastric emptying ↑ intragastric pressure ↑ intragastric acidity ↓ lower esophageal sphincter pressure	Regurgitation and aspiration Maternal-fetal hypoxemia
Hepatorenal	Hepatorenal alteration Alteration of plasma proteins	↑ drug toxicity ↑ pharmacological clearance
Hematological	Dilutional anemia Hypercoagulability	↓ symptoms of moderate bleeding ↑ thromboembolic risk

Impact of Respiratory Changes

Pregnancy is characterized by a decrease in the functional residual capacity that becomes significant around week 20 and an increase in metabolic oxygen consumption. All this predisposes to hypoxemia, hypercapnia and acidosis, which can be accentuated in the presence of hypoventilation and apnea. Pre-oxygenation with 100% oxygen, administration of supplemental oxygen in the perioperative period and the monitoring of oxygen saturation are essential. A decrease in pCO_2 can produce vasoconstriction of the uterine arteries and a decrease in uteroplacental blood flow, therefore it is mandatory to monitor CO_2 exchange, and target normocapnia. Decreased functional residual capacity and increased minute ventilation lead to an increase in the induction rate with inhalation anesthesia [5].

Impact of Changes on the Airway

The risk associated with ventilation and intubation of the pregnant patient is created by edema secondary to fluid retention, mucosal congestion, increased tongue size, reduction in the diameter of the oropharynx, and increased size of the breasts and fatty tissues. These conditions increase the risk of difficult ventilation and intubation, so it is a priority to expect problems in airway management and anticipate a failed intubation [6].

Impact of Cardiovascular Changes

In the second half of pregnancy, attention must be paid to aortocaval compression produced by the uterus, which reduces venous return, preload, and cardiac output in a condition known as *"supine hypotensive syndrome"* [7]. A drop in cardiac output of up to 25% can occur when the patient is placed supine with respect to the left lateral decubitus, while the displacement of the uterus to the left decreases compression, increasing end-diastolic volume, stroke volume, and left ventricular ejection fraction [8]. Neuroaxial or general anesthesia can accentuate cardiovascular depression in the supine position, due to sympathetic block or vasodilation.

Impact of Neuroaxial Changes

The epidural space of the pregnant woman presents distended venous plexuses and a decreased capacity for distension, increasing the risk of intravascular injection of local anesthetics, more extensive dissemination of local anesthetics, and blockage of unwanted levels.

Impact of Digestive Changes

Mechanical and hormonal factors delay gastric emptying, increase intragastric pressure and acidity, and decrease the pressure of the lower esophageal sphincter (*LEE*), increasing the risk of regurgitation and aspiration from the second trimester. Therefore, in pregnant women, over 18 to 20 weeks, prophylaxis thirty minutes prior to anesthesia induction with a non-particulate oral antacid (*e.g.*, sodium citrate), H_2 antihistamines (*e.g.*, ranitidine) and/or metoclopramide may be indicated.

The use of ranitidine is preferable to cimetidine since the latter can cause adverse effects on the mother such as hypotension, arrhythmias, decreased hepatic blood flow, and increased toxicity of local anesthetics. The latest recommendations suggest individualizing the need for aspiration prophylaxis, indicating it, for example, in case of pregnant women who do not comply with fasting, pregnant women with obesity, pregnant women with symptomatic gastroesophageal reflux or evidence of stomach content evaluated by ultrasound [5, 9].

Impact of Hepato-Renal Changes

During pregnancy, there is an increase in the metabolic demands of these organs. At the renal level, there is an increase in plasma flow, glomerular filtration and tubular reabsorption. On a practical level, there is a decrease in blood levels of creatinine, urea, uric acid and amino acids. The alteration of liver function and plasma proteins can lead to increased drug toxicity during pregnancy. However, clearance of some drugs such as cefazolin or acetaminophen (paracetamol) is increased in pregnant women [5].

Impact of Hematological Changes

Dilutional anemia leads to a better tolerance of moderate perioperative bleeding as long as it is not accompanied by other causes of anemia. Pregnancy involves a state of hypercoagulability that persists until the puerperium and therefore pregnant women undergoing non-obstetric surgery should be screened for venous thromboembolism risk and should have the appropriate perioperative prophylaxis administered [10].

IMPACT OF ANESTHESIA ON THE FETUS

Anesthesia, Embryogenesis and Fetal Outcome

Surgery and anesthesia have a direct effect on the mother and the fetus and its development. Maternal hypotension, hypovolemia, severe anemia, hypoxemia and increased sympathetic tone can severely compromise the uteroplacental circulation and promote fetal distress [11]. Fetal damage can result from the teratogenic effects of drugs administered, changes in uteroplacental blood flow and maternal hypoxemia. Outcomes of fetal distress can be the development of organ malformations, miscarriage or premature delivery.

Currently, the toxicity and teratogenicity of anesthetics in the fetus remain an unexplored field, as most of the data obtained to date are based on the results of animal experimentation studies. So far, retrospective studies on humans have not been fully conclusive and no anesthetic agent has been identified as a definitive human teratogen [5]. We know that anesthetic drugs potentially cross the placental barrier due to their properties such as low molecular weight, high lipid solubility, low degree of ionisation, and low protein binding [12].

Regarding the effect of drugs during embryogenesis and subsequent development of the fetus, three stages of susceptibility are recognized. The most critical period is from the third to the eighth week of gestation (days 18 to 58 post-conception), which corresponds to the organogenesis period, in which the influence of drugs or teratogenic insults correspond to serious fetal malformations and considerable abnormalities later development. Between conception and implantation, insults to the embryo can result in its death and miscarriage or in intact survival.

From the eighth week onwards, organogenesis is practically complete and the growth of the organs is completed. The alterations that can result from this period are usually minor, but significant physiological abnormalities and growth retardation can continue to occur.

To date, no study has so far reported a higher incidence of congenital defects in neonates of mothers who underwent general anesthesia during pregnancy, but it has been related to a slightly increased risk of miscarriage, premature delivery and low birth weight, all these outcomes being closely related to the stage of pregnancy in which it was performed [13].

Teratogenicity of Anesthetic Agents

Induction Agents

No anesthetic drug has been proven to be teratogenic, nor are propofol, etomidate, thiopental, or ketamine at clinically effective doses known to cause fetal adverse effects. While studies have been performed on rats and rabbits, there is a lack of adequate and well-controlled studies on pregnant women [11]. Ketamine can cause uterine contractions during early pregnancy and should therefore be avoided. It has been observed that there is a decrease in cortisol production in neonates less than 6 hours after using etomidate; however, the clinical significance of the finding is not known.

Inhalation Anesthesia

Volatile anesthetics are highly soluble, have a low molecular weight, and are transferred to the fetus. Fetal concentrations depend on the maternal plasma concentration and the duration of administration of the anesthetic before delivery. Sevoflurane and desflurane are considered safe products; however, there has been a lot of controversy about nitrous oxide (N_2O). Although DNA production is affected by nitrous oxide (it inhibits methionine synthetase activity through oxidation of vitamin B12, leading to interference with DNA synthesis and myelin deposition), it does not impair fetal outcome after a brief maternal exposure [11]. No teratogenic findings have been reported in humans with the worldwide use of halothane, isoflurane, and enflurane [5].

Neuromuscular Blocking Agents

Depolarizing and non-depolarizing neuromuscular relaxants in clinically significant amounts do not reach fetal circulation. After their administration, only a small amount reaches the fetus due to its high degree of ionization and low liposolubility. However, teratogenic effects have not been reported after the administration of neuromuscular blocking agents to pregnant women [5, 11].

Neuromuscular Block Reversers

The neostigmine-atropine combination has not exhibited teratogenic effects on the fetus, but its administration can cause fetal hemodynamic alterations such as an increase in the fetal heart rate (*FHR*) due to the passage of atropine into the fetal circulation. Sugammadex has low placental transfer rates due to its molecular structure and high molecular weight [5]. However, the potential effects of sugammadex on the fetus are unknown at this time, and there are not enough studies to recommend its use in pregnant women [5, 14].

Local Anesthetics

No teratogenic relationship has been found at the usual clinical doses [5]. Hence, spinal anesthesia is a safe technique since there is no maternal-fetal transfer of local anesthetics. This fact has been confirmed by animal experimentation studies [11].

Analgesics

The idea that acetaminophen is a safe drug and in fact widely used for the treatment of pain during pregnancy has been widely accepted [13]. There is no known teratogenic risk of acetaminophen so far. However, recent studies have been published linking exposure to acetaminophen before birth and an increased risk for multiple behavioral difficulties, which may be due to an intrauterine mechanism. Stergiakouli *et al* have presented that exposure during the third trimester led to more behavioral difficulties than exposure during the second trimester; the third trimester is a period of active brain development and, therefore, a sensitive fetal phase.

Another recent study published by Masarwa *et al* has linked intrauterine exposure to acetaminophen with behavioral disorders such as attention-deficit/hyperactivity disorders [13, 15, 16]. Non-steroidal anti-inflammatory drugs (*NSAIDs*) can also cause serious disorders. The use of NSAIDs and aspirin in the first trimester has increased the risk for pregnancy loss and cardiac defects, notably ventricular and atrial septum defects or a combination of both. In the third trimester, NSAIDs and aspirin are usually avoided because of risks of renal injury, oligohydramnios, gastroschisis, and intrauterine constriction of the ductus arteriosus in the fetus. There is a serious recommendation to discontinue its use during pregnancy [13].

Opioids

Despite recent studies concluding that maternal opioid use was associated with an increased risk for various cardiac birth defects, spina bifida, and gastroschisis, little data is available regarding their potential adverse effects in pregnancy to conclude teratogenicity. Studies in mice using a wide range of morphine, fentanyl, sufentanil, and alfentanil doses have not revealed an increase in the incidence of malformations although fetal growth restriction was present, and offspring mortality was increased. Excessive antepartum use can also lead to neonatal opioid withdrawal symptoms. Tramadol exposure in early pregnancy was associated with a higher number of spontaneous abortions, and it should be avoided in the first trimester [13].

Sedatives

Perinatal use of benzodiazepines by pregnant women has been associated with newborn hypotonia, hypothermia, and respiratory depression. Likewise, it has also been linked to a small increase in the risk of preterm birth and low weight at birth. Regarding the possible teratogenic effects of benzodiazepines in the first trimester of pregnancy, there is no strong evidence. As this fact has not been confirmed by other studies, there is a strong recommendation in the current bibliography not to use benzodiazepines, even though the risk is low [13].

Maternal Anesthesia and Neurocognitive Outcomes

A controversial issue in this topic is the possible influence of general anesthesia on pregnancy and its potential effects on fetal neurodevelopment and neurocognition [17]. Synaptogenesis is believed to occur primarily during the third trimester of pregnancy. From the data obtained from population cohort studies, it is suggested that repeated exposures to general anesthesia have a crucial influence and increase the risk of suffering alterations in the learning of calculation and reading, and have been specially related to alterations in memory.

Between the 5th and 25th postmenstrual weeks, neoblastic proliferation and fetal brain development are at their peak, and we know that the interaction of anesthetic agents with GABA and the NMDA-subtype of glutamate receptors causes a decrease in synaptic activity, proliferation, and even apoptotic cell degeneration.

This effect has been especially thoroughly studied in the hippocampal area in animal models and associated in the long term with alterations in spatial orientation and memory [18]. It is believed that repeated exposure of GABA and glutamatergic systems of the fetal brain to anesthetic agents may have a negative modulatory effect that can affect neurogenesis and neurocognitive modulation through damage caused in synaptogenesis. However, more studies are still needed to confirm these facts [12].

ANESTHETIC MANAGEMENT

Practical Considerations

When the need for non-obstetric surgery arises in a pregnant patient, a multidisciplinary team comprising a surgeon, anesthesiologist, obstetrician, and perinatologist must be set up to assess the right time to perform it. These surgeries should be performed in a hospital with a neonatal ICU [10]. In the case of elective surgery, it should be delayed until six weeks after delivery once maternal physiology is recovered (Fig. **1**) [19]. On the other hand, non-urgent surgery should preferably be performed in the second trimester as this is when there is less likelihood of teratogenesis, spontaneous abortion, and preterm labor [5, 20]. Urgent surgery should not be deferred as it can lead to both maternal and fetal risk [19].

The main objective of surgery during pregnancy in an urgent and serious situation is to preserve maternal life. The more advanced the cause requiring surgery, the greater the maternal and fetal morbidity and mortality [5]. It has been reported that complications in the fetus are rare; however, a higher prevalence of preterm and low birth weight babies has been observed [19, 21]. These are more frequent in those women who suffered procedures under general anesthesia; although it is difficult to define if this is due to the surgery itself or the underlying surgical condition [19].

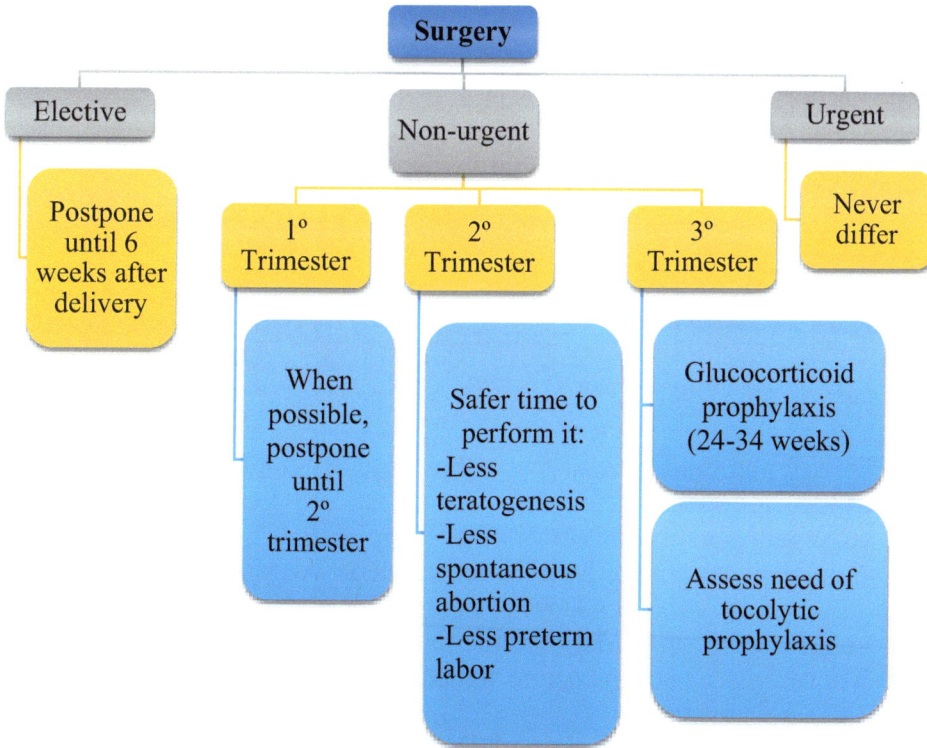

Fig. (1). Algorithm for non-obstetric surgery during pregnancy.

Regarding the surgical approach, laparoscopy is currently the most recommended technique in the three trimesters since it decreases postoperative pain and hospitalization time. Although an increase in its use has been observed in the first two periods, its use in the final stretch of pregnancy continues to be scarce. This is probably due to the technical difficulties conferred by the size of the gravid uterus [5, 20]. During this time, open access should be used to prevent uterine damage. To avoid fetal acidosis, provoked by CO_2 absorption, laparoscopy should be conducted with low pressure (< 12–15 mmHg). On the other hand, maternal cardiac output and lung compliance can be reduced, not only by high intra-abdominal pressure but also by forced Trendelenburg position. Meanwhile, reverse Trendelenburg can diminish venous return and, consequently, affect maternal hemodynamic stability and uteroplacental prefusion. However, all these changes can be controlled by using careful anesthetic techniques and adequate monitoring (Table **2**) [4, 12, 20, 21].

Table 2. Important factors in maternal laparoscopy

- Use an open technique to open abdomen - Avoid maternal hypercapnia: monitor maternal end-tidal CO_2 level or arterial blood gases - Avoid hypotension: treatment with volume or vasopressors, low pneumoperitoneum pressure (<12-15 mmHg) or gasless technique - Avoid extreme positions (Trendelenburg or reverse Trendelenburg) or rapid positioning - Monitor fetal heart rate and uterine tone when feasible - Prevent deep vein thrombosis in the lower limbs by wearing intra-operative intermittent pneumatic compression stockings
Modified from Reitman E, Flood P. Anaesthetic considerations *for* non-obstetric surgery during pregnancy. *Br J Anaesth* 2011;*107 Suppl 1:i72-8.*

Preoperative Assessment

In the case of non-emergent surgery, the patient should be assessed in the preoperative period with a complete blood test and ECG, and the risks and benefits of surgery and anesthesia should be explained [5, 19, 20]. If the fetus is viable and the patient is in the 24-34 weeks, glucocorticoids will be administered 24–48 hours before surgery. This is contraindicated in septic patients since steroids would alter the maternal immune response. In addition, informed consent for an urgent cesarean section must be signed if the fetus is viable [10, 19].

Fasting should be, as indicated in the guidelines, 6–8 hours depending on the fat content of the last food ingested. As mentioned before, acid aspiration prophylaxis with sucralfate, ranitidine (in patients with more than 16 weeks along), and metoclopramide will be performed, which will increase the pH of the gastric content and gastric emptying as well as increase the tone of the LEE [5, 19 - 21].

Antibiotic prophylaxis depends on the surgical procedure; however, the type of antibiotic selected and its safety in pregnancy should be taken into account [19]. The risk of thrombosis is also evaluated because pregnancy is a pro-coagulant state. Therefore, depending on the procedure, the surgical technique, and the patient's personal history, the need for intermittent pneumatic compression stockings and/or low molecular weight heparins should be assessed [5, 19, 21].

Regarding premedication, it should be noted that benzodiazepines cross the placenta and can lead to neonatal depression. In addition, if administered during the first trimester, they can lead to fetal malformations, such as cleft lip and palate. Its use should be restricted to specific situations where there is a contraindication for the use of other drugs and the doses used should be minimal (*e.g.*, 0.5–2 mg midazolam) to ensure the least amount of fetal depression [20].

The use of anticholinergic drugs may be necessary to decrease secretions and bradycardia associated with anesthesia induction. To this end, glycopyrrolate is safer than atropine because it does not cross the placental barrier and can be administered intramuscularly an hour before surgery or intravenously during induction. However, it should be noted that it decreases the tone of the LEE [20].

Intraoperative Assessment

While the main objective is to preserve maternal life, during the procedure, the anesthesiologist must maintain maternal hemodynamic stability that ensures good uterine perfusion to conserve the fetus' well-being [20]. Therefore, he or she must evaluate the technique and the drugs to be used in advance. Although no one technique has been demonstrated to be better than another, loco-regional anesthesia should be used whenever possible since it provides good postoperative analgesia, reduces exposure to teratogenic agents, and decreases the risk of failed intubation or bronchial aspiration [5, 19, 21]. On the contrary, special attention should be paid to the hypotension associated with the sympathetic blockade [19]. However, since most surgical pathologies in pregnancy are abdominal, most are performed under general anesthesia.

The patient's position is of vital importance from 18–20 weeks to avoid aortocaval compression [5, 19]. This can be prevented with a 15° left lateral tilt or with a wedge placed under the right hip and can be assessed by the right femoral pulse [20, 21]. Each mobilization should be done slowly to prevent sudden hemodynamic changes.

Rapid sequence general anesthesia should be used, with good pre-oxygenation, cricoid pressure, fast-acting muscle relaxants, and orotracheal intubation [5]. Anesthetic drugs are considered safe in pregnancy, as long as their particular characteristics are taken into account [21].

As previously stated, benzodiazepines are not recommended, unless maternal anxiety that could lead to decreased uterine blood flow needs to be controlled [5, 19]. Opioids are used to control pain induced by laryngoscopy, which would reduce uterine flow. However, their use should be considered if a cesarean section is planned because they diminish FHR and produce fetal depression. Hypnotics such as propofol and thiopental are reliable for anesthesia induction and are quickly eliminated from fetal circulation; however, they produce dose-dependent hypotension and can decrease uteroplacental perfusion [20]. The latter may be useful in hypertensive patients for better control of hypertension associated with airway management.

On the other hand, ketamine reaches a higher concentration in the fetus than in the maternal blood and increases uterine contractions during the first trimester [21]. However, ketamine can be used safely during late pregnancy for its analgesic and sympathomimetic properties. Volatile halogenated agents decrease uterine contractility and should be used at 0.75–1 minimal alveolar concentration since, at higher doses, they reduce maternal blood pressure and depress the fetal central nervous system and heart rate.

Nitrous oxide has been avoided because it easily diffuses into the bowel and the pneumoperitoneum, which can increase intra-abdominal pressure, and into the cuff of the endotracheal tube, which can cause lesions in the mucosa (already edematized by pregnancy) [19, 20]. In addition, its use avoids the administration of high concentrations of oxygen. Neuromuscular relaxants barely cross the placenta and it is advisable to use those that reach a peak concentration quickly (succinylcholine or rocuronium) to secure the airway rapidly [20].

Maternal monitoring should include ECG, blood pressure, pulse oximetry, and, in the case of general anesthesia, capnography, nerve stimulator, and anesthetic depth monitor [5]. The latter helps to adjust the hypnotic dose to avoid light anesthesia, which produces catecholaminergic release that impairs placental perfusion, or deep anesthesia, which causes a reduction of systemic vascular resistance [19].

It is important to control maternal homeostasis. Therefore, hypothermia, prolonged hypoxemia, and hypercapnia should be avoided since they cause uterine vasoconstriction, reduce placental perfusion, and lead to fetal hypoxemia and acidosis [19 - 21]. On the other hand, hypocapnia also reduces uterine flow; therefore, CO_2 levels should be kept within normal limits [19, 21]. Aggressive management of hypotension with drug dose adjustment, fluid therapy, patient positioning, and vasoactive drugs should be performed. No difference in efficacy has been found between ephedrine and phenylephrine in maintaining blood pressure; however, the latter significantly improves fetal acid-base balance [19, 21].

Fetal Monitoring

It is recommended that FHR be monitored before and after surgery by a skilled professional, starting at week 18 [5, 10, 19]. If surgical technique allows it, FHR may be monitored throughout the procedure to detect early fetal compromise [21]. FHR variability could also be used after 25 weeks but should be distinguished from variations produced by anesthetic drugs or maternal position, hypotension, hypoxia, or acidosis [5].

Whenever possible, intraoperative tocometry should be used to take early therapeutic measures (improve maternal hemodynamic stability, tocolytic treatment, *etc.*) [5, 19, 20]. The use of tocolytic prophylaxis is not recommended by default [21]. Its use can be considered in pelvic surgery during the third trimester [19].

Postoperative Analgesia

Special attention should be given to the management of postoperative pain since adrenergic discharge increases the risk of premature birth. Whenever possible, regional anesthesia should be administered to reduce respiratory depression associated with large doses of opioids. The latter can be used safely in association with acetaminophen. However, the use of NSAIDs for more than 48 hours should be avoided since they induce the closure of the ductus arteriosus and decrease fetal kidney function, which may cause oligohydramnios [19].

CONCLUSION

The need for non-obstetric surgery during pregnancy can occur at any time during pregnancy and urgent/emergent procedures should not be postponed due to the pregnancy condition. Diagnosis of surgical processes is more complex than in non-pregnant patients and delay in diagnosis increases maternal morbidity and mortality, Surgery and anesthesia have a direct effect on the mother and the fetus, and they can severely compromise utero-placental circulation and promote fetal distress. Fetal damage can result from the teratogenic effects of drugs administered, changes in uteroplacental blood flow, and maternal hypoxemia. The influence of general anesthesia in pregnancy and its possible effects on neurodevelopment and fetal neurocognition is, in the absence of further studies, controversial. In the case of non-obstetric surgery in a pregnant patient, multidisciplinary work between the surgeon, anesthesiologist, obstetrician and perinatologist is essential to evaluate the appropriate time and form to perform it.

CONSENT FOR PUBLICATION

Not applicable.

CONFLICT OF INTEREST

The authors declare no conflict of interest, financial or otherwise.

ACKNOWLEDGEMENT

Declared none.

REFERENCES

[1]   Balinskaite V, Bottle A, Sodhi V, *et al.* The risk of adverse pregnancy outcomes following nonobstetric surgery during pregnancy: estimates from a retrospective cohort study of 6.5 million pregnancies. Ann Surg 2017; 266(2): 260-6.
[http://dx.doi.org/10.1097/SLA.0000000000001976] [PMID: 27617856]

[2]   Mazze RI, Kallén B. Reproductive outcome after anesthesia and operation during pregnancy: A Registry study of 5405 cases. Am J Obstet Gynecol 1989; 161(5): 1178-85.
[http://dx.doi.org/10.1016/0002-9378(89)90659-5] [PMID: 2589435]

[3]   Augustin G, Majerovic M. Non-obstetrical acute abdomen during pregnancy. Eur J Obstet Gynecol Reprod Biol 2007; 131(1): 4-12.
[http://dx.doi.org/10.1016/j.ejogrb.2006.07.052] [PMID: 16982130]

[4]   Reitman E, Flood P. Anaesthetic considerations for non-obstetric surgery during pregnancy. Br J Anaesth 2011; 107 (Suppl. 1): i72-8.
[http://dx.doi.org/10.1093/bja/aer343] [PMID: 22156272]

[5]   Bauchat JR, Van De Velde M. Non-obstetric surgery in pregnancy. In: Chestnut DH, Wong C, Tsen L, Eds. Chestnut's Obstetric Anesthesia: Principles and Practice 6th ed. 2019; 368-91.

[6]   Mushambi MC, Kinsella SM, Popat M, *et al.* Obstetric Anaesthetists' Association and Difficult Airway Society guidelines for the management of difficult and failed tracheal intubation in obstetrics. Anaesthesia 2015; 70(11): 1286-306.
[http://dx.doi.org/10.1111/anae.13260] [PMID: 26449292]

[7]   Rossi A, Cornette J, Johnson MR, *et al.* Quantitative cardiovascular magnetic resonance in pregnant women: cross-sectional analysis of physiological parameters throughout pregnancy and the impact of the supine position. J Cardiovasc Magn Reson 2011; 13(1): 31.
[http://dx.doi.org/10.1186/1532-429X-13-31] [PMID: 21708015]

[8]   Higuchi H, Takagi S, Zhang K, Furui I, Ozaki M. Effect of lateral tilt angle on the volume of the abdominal aorta and inferior vena cava in pregnant and nonpregnant women determined by magnetic resonance imaging. Anesthesiology 2015; 122(2): 286-93.
[http://dx.doi.org/10.1097/ALN.0000000000000553] [PMID: 25603203]

[9]   Arzola C, Perlas A, Siddiqui NT, Downey K, Ye XY, Carvalho JCA. Gastric ultrasound in the third trimester of pregnancy: a randomised controlled trial to develop a predictive model of volume assessment. Anaesthesia 2018; 73(3): 295-303.
[http://dx.doi.org/10.1111/anae.14131] [PMID: 29265187]

[10]   ACOG Committee Opinion Number 775: non obstetric surgery during pregnancy. Obstet Gynecol 2019; 133(4): e285-6.
[http://dx.doi.org/10.1097/AOG.0000000000003174] [PMID: 30913200]

[11]   Allaert SE, Carlier SP, Weyne LP, Vertommen DJ, Dutré PE, Desmet MB. First trimester anesthesia exposure and fetal outcome. A review. Acta Anaesthesiol Belg 2007; 58(2): 119-23.
[PMID: 17710900]

[12]   Sharpe EE, Arendt KW. Anesthesia for obstetrics. In: Gropper MA, Ed. Miller's Anesthesia 9th ed. 2020; 2006-41.

[13]   Gin T. Pharmacology during Pregnancy and Lactation. In: Chestnut DH, Wong C, Tsen L, Eds. Chestnut's Obstetric Anesthesia: Principles and Practice 6th ed. 2019; 313-35.

[14]   Richardson MG, Raymond BL. Sugammadex Administration in Pregnant Women and in Women of Reproductive Potential. Anesth Analg 2020; 130(6): 1628-37.
[http://dx.doi.org/10.1213/ANE.0000000000004305] [PMID: 31283616]

[15]   Stergiakouli E, Thapar A, Davey Smith G. Association of acetaminophen use during pregnancy with behavioral problems in childhood: evidence against confounding. JAMA Pediatr 2016; 170(10): 964-70.

[http://dx.doi.org/10.1001/jamapediatrics.2016.1775] [PMID: 27533796]

[16]   Masarwa R, Levine H, Gorelik E, Reif S, Perlman A, Matok I. Prenatal Exposure to Acetaminophen and Risk for Attention Deficit Hyperactivity Disorder and Autistic Spectrum Disorder: A Systematic Review, Meta-Analysis, and Meta-Regression Analysis of Cohort Studies. Am J Epidemiol 2018; 187(8): 1817-27.
[http://dx.doi.org/10.1093/aje/kwy086] [PMID: 29688261]

[17]   Flick RP, Katusic SK, Colligan RC, *et al.* Cognitive and behavioral outcomes after early exposure to anesthesia and surgery (published correction appears at Pediatrics. 2012;129(3):595). Pediatrics 2011; 128(5): e1053-61.
[http://dx.doi.org/10.1542/peds.2011-0351] [PMID: 21969289]

[18]   Esakoff TF, Kilpatrick SJ. Fetal and neonatal neurologic injury. In: Chestnut DH, Wong C, Tsen L, Eds. Chestnut's Obstetric Anesthesia: Principles and Practice 6th ed. 2019; 199-222.

[19]   Upadya M, Saneesh PJ. Anaesthesia for non-obstetric surgery during pregnancy. Indian J Anaesth 2016; 60(4): 234-41.
[http://dx.doi.org/10.4103/0019-5049.179445] [PMID: 27141105]

[20]   Kuczkowski KM. The safety of anaesthetics in pregnant women. Expert Opin Drug Saf 2006; 5(2): 251-64.
[http://dx.doi.org/10.1517/14740338.5.2.251] [PMID: 16503746]

[21]   Van De Velde M, De Buck F. Anesthesia for non-obstetric surgery in the pregnant patient. Minerva Anestesiol 2007; 73(4): 235-40.
[PMID: 17473818]

CHAPTER 11

Anesthetic Management of the Pregnant Patient with Comorbidities

Anna Pascual Carreño[1,*], Aleix Clusella Moya[1], Mireia Pozo Albiol[1], Eva Maria Blazquez Gomez[1] and **Esperanza Martin Mateos[1]**

[1] *Department of Anesthesiology, Hospital Sant Joan de Déu, Esplugues, Barcelona, Spain*

Abstract: An increase in pregnant patients with comorbidities has been seen in the last decade. Nevertheless, these patients are able to enjoy longer and better quality lives nowadays. During pregnancy, patients can experience decompensations of their chronic disease which can be sometimes challenging for the medical team. Complexity has risen; that is why the anesthesiologist must be updated and capable of facing different scenarios both in the delivery room and before or after birth.

This chapter offers a practical and synthetical approach to the most common situations in which a general anesthesiologist can be involved, aiming to emphasize main points for safe and accurate anesthetic care.

Keywords: Anemia, Aortic Stenosis, Autoimmune, Chorioamnionitis, Cardiovascular, Comorbidity, Coagulation, Diabetes Mellitus, Epilepsy, Epidural, Fever, Hepatic, Hyperthyroidism, Lupus, Mitral Stenosis, Multiple Sclerosis, Myasthenia Gravis, Neurologic, Neuraxial, Neurofibromatosis, Obesity, Platelets, Pregnancy, Pulmonary Hypertension, Renal, Respiratory, Sepsis, Septic Shock, Spinal Cord Injury, Thromboprophylaxis.

INTRODUCTION

Neurological, neuromuscular and musculoskeletal disorders can influence the obstetric outcome during operative deliveries, and ideally all such operative interventions should be referred to tertiary care centers.

During the preanesthetic stage, cardiorespiratory evaluation should be thoroughly done. Regional anesthesia is preferred in the majority of these patients except for a few strong contraindications such as increased intracranial pressures, tethered spinal cord and others. Patients with the high risk of developing intra-operative

* **Corresponding author Anna Pascual Carreño:** Department of Anesthesiology, Hospital Sant Joan de Déu, Esplugues, Barcelona, Spain; Email: apascual@sjdhospitalbarcelona.org

Eugenio Daniel Martinez-Hurtado, Monica Sanjuan-Alvarez & Marta Chacon-Castillo (Eds.)
All rights reserved-© 2022 Bentham Science Publishers

respiratory insufficiency should preferably be administered regional anesthesia in an incremental manner.

Multiple Sclerosis

For labor analgesia with epidural, use lower concentrations of local anesthetic when possible. Neuraxial anesthesia is the preferred anesthetic technique for cesarean delivery. Anyway, the type of anesthesia selected does not influence the relapse rate. If general anesthesia is given, succinylcholine should be administered cautiously and only if strongly indicated.

Spinal Cord Injury

Epidural analgesia should be used as soon as the patient goes into labor to prevent autonomic hyperreflexia (injuries at or above T6) and mass reflex. For cesarean section, epidural anesthesia is preferable to spinal anesthesia because the chances of hypotension are less. If general anesthesia is essential, avoid succinylcholine. Also remember that pregnancy may aggravate medical complications of spinal cord injury (decreased respiratory reserve, atelectasis, pneumonia, anemia, deep venous thrombosis, renal insufficiency, decubitus ulcers, autonomic hyperreflexia).

Myasthenia Gravis

Neuraxial anesthesia is preferred for labor analgesia, and amide local anesthetics are preferable. Because of the need for a higher level of sensory anesthesia for cesarean delivery, there is a danger of impairment of the respiratory and swallowing muscles following regional anesthesia. Unless contraindicated because of respiratory insufficiency, regional anesthesia should be the technique of choice.

We should have caution with the use of opioids, and avoid magnesium sulfate, aminoglycosides, fluoroquinolones, tetracyclines, and macrolides antibiotics. Also, patients are extremely sensitive to non-depolarizing muscle relaxants and resistant to depolarizing muscle relaxants. There is a risk for postoperative ventilation if the duration of myasthenia is greater than 6 years, there is a history of chronic respiratory disease, pyridostigmine dose is higher than 750 mg/day, and female gender.

Epilepsy

There is no contraindication to the administration of neuraxial analgesia or anesthesia. If general anesthesia is necessary, we should avoid ketamine, enflurane, and meperidine, as these may lower the seizure threshold. Some antiepileptic medications induce liver enzymes, which may lead to the rapid breakdown of anesthetic agents metabolized by the liver.

Muscular and Myotonic Dystrophy

Neuraxial anesthesia is preferred due to a higher risk of apnea with opioids in these patients.

Neurocutaneous Syndromes

Severe kyphoscoliosis may be present, and lesions that involve the neck and larynx are common in neurofibromatosis type 1. Asymptomatic paraspinal and intracranial tumors may be present; clinical and radiologic evaluations may be indicated prior to neuraxial anesthesia.

Brain Tumors

Painful uterine contractions and bearing-down efforts increase intracranial pressure; hence epidural analgesia may be indicated, but bear in mind the consequences of accidental dural puncture. General anesthesia is preferred for cesarean deliveries.

Cerebrovascular Accidents

For labor and delivery, a continuous epidural block is advisable. The use of forceps is indicated to shorten the second stage. In the immediate postpartum period, one should be prepared to treat hypertension aggressively if it occurs. For cesarean delivery, an epidural block is the anesthesia of choice; however, if there is fetal distress or if general anesthesia is indicated for some other reason, be careful about the hypertensive response following endotracheal intubation.

PREGNANT PATIENT WITH CARDIOVASCULAR DISORDERS

Heart disease is the primary medical cause of non-obstetric maternal mortality. The most common cardiac condition encountered in pregnant women in developed countries is congenital heart disease followed by rheumatic heart disease.

During pregnancy, there are physiological changes in hemodynamics such as: an increase in the intravascular volume, a decrease in systemic vascular resistance (SRV), an increase in the heart rate (HR) and thus in cardiac output (CO). There is also a hypercoagulability status and a decrease in the functional residual capacity. Due to all these changes, cardiac decompensation is the main concern in pregnant patients with a heart disease.

Not only by monitoring the pregnant patient, but by monitoring the fetal status we will detect early compromise and we will be able to apply different measures to correct it. We summarize the hemodynamic parameters that can be modified by the anesthesiologist using different anesthetic techniques and drugs (Table **1**).

Table 1. Hemodynamic parameters affected by the anesthetic management.

Parameter	Increase	Decrease
PRELOAD	- Fluids - Capacitance vessel constriction (phenylephrine)	- Bleeding - Capacitance vessel dilation (nitroglicerine) - Ventilation (large tidal volumen, PEEP)
SVR	- Phenylephrine - Ketamine	- Nitroprusside - Sevoflurane - Propofol - Thiopental
PVR	- ↑ PaCO2 - Hypoventilation - ↓ PaO2 - Acidosis	- ↓ PaCO2 - Hyperventilation - ↑ PaO2 - Alcalosis
HR	- Atropine	- BBlockers - fentanyl
Contractility	- Ionotropes - Calcium - Digoxine - Milrinone	- BBlockers - Propofol - Sevoflurane

Every cardiac lesion needs an individualized management. Table **2** describes the ideal hemodynamic parameters in the most common cardiac lesions.

Table 2. Anesthetic considerations for specific cardiovascular pathological processes.

Disease	Anesthetic considerations
Mitral stenosis	- Maintain sinus rythm and prevent taquicardia. - If new onset of atrial fibrillation: control heart rate and consider cardioversion. • Increase in preload not well tolerated. • Monitor closely for fluid overload the first 24h after delivery. • Prevent pain, hipoxemia, acidosis. - If: Valve area > 1.5 cm2, without pulmonary hypertension: Neuraxial anesthesia generally well tolerated. - If: Valve area ≤ 1.5 cm2 + pulmonary hypertension: • High –risk. • Consider percutaneous valvuloplasty before labor.

(Table 2) cont.....

Disease	Anesthetic considerations
Aortic stenosis	- If transvalvular gradient<25mmHg, valve área < 1.0cm2, normal LV function: • Neuraxial anesthesia is well tolerated. • Maintain normal preload and afterload. • Monitor closely for volume overload 24h after delivery. - If transvalvular gradient > 25 mmHg, valve área ≤ 1.0 cm2, impaired LV function: • High risk group. • Consider risk/benefits of neuraxial vs general anesthesia. • Avoid abrupt decrease in SVR with sympathectomy. • Avoid myocardial depressants or vasodilators. • Maintain normal preload and afterload. • Maintain sinus rhythm and prevent tachycardia. • Monitor closely for volume overload 24h after delivery.
Pulmonary Hipertension	- Mild-Moderate: • Attention to preload. - Severe: • Very high risk. • Maintain SVR. • Maintain preload • Avoid increase in PVR (avoid hypoxemia, hypercarbia, acidosis) • Avoid myocardial depression • Prevent/treat pain - Consider pulmonary vasodilators
Fontan Repair	- Low and high preload poorly tolerated. - Positive-pressure ventilation is poorly tolerated because it increases thoracic pressure and thus impedes venous return.
Repaired Transposition of Great Arteries	- Meticulous attention to preload during labor and the early postpartum period, because there is a propensity to right ventricular dysfunction. - High incidence of arrhythmias.

Table **3** describes the optimal cardiovascular parameters for a parturient with shunt.

Table 3. Optimal cardiovascular parameters for parturient with shunt.

Shunt	- Right to Left shunt. - Cyanotic. - Tetralogy of Fallot (unrepaired).	- Left to right shunt. - Acyanotic. - Persistence of ductus arteriosus. - Atrial septal defect. - Ventricular septal defect
SVR	- ↑ - Caution with induction or central neuraxial block	- ↓ - Avoid cold, anxiety, pain.

(Table 3) cont.....

	- ↓ - Avoid hypoxia. - Hypoventilation or excessive positive pressure ventilation.	- ↑ - Avoid pulmonary artery depressants.
PVR		
HR / Rhythm	- N / Sinus	- N / Sinus
PRELOAD	- Maintain.	- Maintain.
CONTRACTILITY	- N	- N / ↑ - Avoid myocardial depressants
Other recommendations	- Risk of air embolism. Ensure avoidance of bubbles in iv lines. - Use oxytocin cautiously. - Avoid prostaglandin F2-alfa.	- Risk of air embolism. Ensure avoidance of bubbles in iv. lines. - Avoid ergometrine.
↑: Increase, ↓: decrease, N: normal, PVR: pulmonary vascular resistance, SVR: systemic vascular resistance, HR: heart rate.		

PREGNANT PATIENT WITH RESPIRATORY DISORDERS

Patients with a respiratory disease like asthma, pneumonia, smokers, cystic fibrosis or respiratory failure may have hypoxemia that can lead to loss of fetal well-being.

As anesthetists we must avoid the appearance of hypoxemia and respiratory symptoms.

The goals of analgesia for labor and delivery in women with a respiratory disease include two important outcomes, the first one is providing adequate pain relief because it could trigger respiratory symptoms like the stimulation of the airway and consequently its obstruction. The second is to prevent maternal hyperventilation and maternal stress because it increases the work of breathing and may cause decompensation of the respiratory disease.

Neuraxial anesthesia is preferred in the majority of patients with pulmonary disorders, but there is a very important consideration for neuraxial anesthesia, which is to avoid a high thoracic motor block, which may impair ventilation, and decrease vital capacity and the ability to cough. Also, a high thoracic block could cause pulmonary sympathetic denervation with an unopposed parasympathetic system causing bronchoconstriction.

Epidural anesthesia is preferred over spinal anesthesia for delivery and cesarean section because it allows titration of the local anesthetic agent to achieve the desired sensory level. Neuraxial anesthesia also avoids positive-pressure ventilation, which may enlarge a preexisting pneumothorax.

Also, if an emergency cesarean section is needed, the presence of an epidural catheter can facilitate epidural anesthesia avoiding the need for airway instrumentation because tracheal intubation has shown to evoke bronchoconstriction. For pain relief during labor, parenteral opioid analgesia may worsen pulmonary function by depressing respiratory drive and inhibiting cough.

If general anesthesia is required, a bronchodilator should be administered, but carefully because most bronchodilators also produce uterine relaxation. However, their administration by aerosol should minimize their effects on uterine tone.

Also, we have to know what drugs would provoke bronchoconstriction and should be avoided. For anaesthesia induction, propofol is better than thiopental, as it has been shown to induce less bronchoconstrictor. Another good hypnotic is ketamine for its bronchodilator properties. Inhalational anesthesia, and particularly sevoflurane, are effective bronchodilators.

Drugs that cause histamine release such as morphine, atracurium, mivacurium, and neostigmine, and H2-receptor blockers like ranitidine should be avoided. Also Beta-adrenergic receptor antagonists like labetalol, that is used to treat hypertension, should be avoided.

Finally, there are some drugs used as uterotonic agents for the treatment of postpartum hemorrhage that should be used carefully because they have been associated with episodes of bronchospasm. We are talking about 15-methyl prostaglandin F2α (carboprost, Hemabate) and ergot alkaloids (ergometrine/methylergotamine). Oxytocin is preferred and can be used safely because it does not significantly affect the airway tone.

PREGNANT PATIENT WITH INFECTIOUS DISORDERS

Clinically, temperature measurements greater than 39°C in a measure or 38°C in two measurements 30 minutes apart represent fever.

This can result from drugs, diseases or infectious processes. In pregnant women, fever can result from the infection of fetal membranes, urinary tract, respiratory tract and postpartum uterine cavity.

- *Sepsis and septic shock*: remains an important cause of maternal mortality and morbidity.
- Usually due to untreated chorioamnionitis, genitourinary infection, pneumonia.

- Several screening tools for the identification of end-organ injury like SOFA score.

- *Microorganisms*: E. coli, Staphylococcus, Streptococcus and gram-negative organisms.
- Necessary monitoring: invasive arterial pressure, oxygen saturation, temperature, respiratory rate, heart rate and urine output.
- *Antibiotic therapy*: a combination of gentamicin, clindamycin and penicillin or vancomycin and piperacillin/ tazobactam.
- To treat hypotension (target MAP: 65mmHg): in the first 3 hours, give 30 ml/kg of IV crystalloid fluid and use norepinephrine as the first line vasopressor +/- vasopressin or epinephrine.
- *Assess other therapies*: thromboembolic prophylaxis, anemia prophylaxis/ treatment, glycemic control and stressulcer prophylaxis.
- Fetal monitoring if gestational age > 28 weeks every 24h.
- In some cases, maternal sepsis may require delivery, even before the age of viability.
- Neuraxial anesthesia should be avoided in the setting of sepsis, although it can be assessed individually taking into account the risk/benefit of regional anesthesia, anesthetic alternatives and the risk of infection of the central nervous system (*CNS*).
- Many anesthesiologists will administer neuraxial anesthesia to patients with systemic infection if appropriate antibiotic therapy has begun.

VHS

Neuraxial anesthesia is safe for both labor and cesarean in the presence of recurrent infections, as long as the lesions are far from the needle insertion site. Reactivations of the virus have been observed after neuraxial opioid administration. No guidelines have been given for neuraxial opioid administration in patients in labor with cold sores or a history of exacerbation.

VIH

After the studies were carried out, there is no evidence of accelerated disease progression after neuraxial anesthesia, and there were no neurologic or infectious complications immediately after delivery and at 4 to 6 months postpartum. The prevention of infectious complications of neuraxial anesthesia depends on a strict aseptic technique.

General anesthesia is not contraindicated but it is necessary to ask for the patients with a high risk to develop infectious complications.

CONCLUSION

There should be a thorough pre-anesthetic evaluation of patients with fever and infection. In the case of fever and infection, the etiology of the same should be determined, in order to administer antimicrobial therapy early and appropriately before performing neuraxial anesthesia, which can be performed safely for most patients with established infection, as long as sepsis is not established.

PREGNANT PATIENT WITH ENDOCRINE DISORDERS

Diabetes Mellitus

One of the most challenging aspects in diabetic parturient involves the adequate control of blood sugar so as to prevent the occurrence of neonatal hypoglycemia. There exists a high association of diabetes mellitus with other comorbid diseases. The presence of autonomic neuropathy makes a diabetic parturient vulnerable to hemodynamic instability [1].

For labor and vaginal delivery, a lumbar epidural block can provide excellent pain relief. Spinal anesthesia can also be used if required at the time of delivery. It is important to realize that the fetus of a diabetic mother might be quite susceptible to hypoxia secondary to maternal hypotension.

For cesarean section, regional anesthesia is much safer. It can be used safely if maternal diabetes is well controlled, if dextrose-containing solutions are not used for maternal intravascular volume expansion before delivery, and if maternal hypotension is avoided [1].

General anesthesia is more hazardous due to the high probability of difficult airway management, unpredictable response to stress during intubation and impaired counter-regulatory responses to fluctuating blood sugar levels. Also metoclopramide should be used preoperatively because of the high incidence of gastric stasis.

Finally, remember the significant decrease in insulin requirement after delivery. As such, perioperative status has to be optimized with an appropriate insulin regimen taking care not to induce hypoglycemia.

Therefore, monitoring should be intense in patients with comorbidities and ideally they should be taken up in tertiary care centers with intensive care unit back-up facilities.

Hyperthyroidism

Thyrotoxicosis needs special attention during operative or vaginal delivery besides a good control during the antenatal period. The evaluation of cardiac status is mandatory during the preanesthetic examination. Spinal anesthesia may be avoided, especially for cesarean delivery, if the mother is taking high doses of propranolol due to exaggerated post-spinal hypotension. Epidural anesthesia is a reasonable alternative.

Obesity

There are numerous alterations in obese parturients. The associated comorbidities make them prone to develop complications during anesthetic management.

For labor and vagnal delivery, epidural analgesia is preferable and should be used if technically possible. Continuous spinal analgesia has also been used with success.

Regional anesthesia should be a preferred choice for an elective cesarean section. Single-shot spinal anesthesia should be used cautiously, if at all, because of a high incidence of hypotension and also because it can reach higher levels and cause further compromise of the already abnormal pulmonary function.

General anesthesia is associated with a higher incidence of perioperative mortality and morbidity. The major goals during anesthetic management of obese parturients include: titration of anesthetic drugs, aspiration prophylaxis, difficult airway management and maintenance of stable hemodynamics.

Postoperative analgesia should be adequate to prevent any obstruction or limitation of breathing movements due to pain.

PREGNANT PATIENT WITH AUTOIMMUNE DISORDERS

- Pregnancy does not worsen the long-term course of autoimmune disorders, which can lead to renal, cardiac, and pulmonary dysfunction.
- Systemic lupus erythematosus (*SLE*) can result in maternal thrombocytopenia. Patients with lupus anticoagulants do not have a bleeding tendency in the absence of an underlying coagulation disorder and can safely receive neuraxial anesthesia because it has no clinical anticoagulant activity. It can also result in false elevations of aPTT.
- A history of dyspnea on exertion or unexplained tachycardia may suggest pericarditis or myocarditis in patients with SLE. Cardiac tamponade and myocardial infarction in young women have been reported.
- Central and peripheral sensorimotor and autonomic neuropathies are observed in 25% of patients with SLE, and vocal cord palsy has been reported. These deficits should be documented before the administration of either neuraxial or general anesthesia.

- Migraine headache and cerebral vasculitis resulting from SLE must be considered in the differential diagnosis of a postpartum headache.
- Patients with scleroderma are at increased risk for difficult airway management. This disease can also prolong the duration of neuraxial anesthesia. Due to vasoconstriction usually seen in scleroderma, patients are usually volume contracted and neuraxial analgesia may contribute to refractory hypotension. Radial artery catheterization is contraindicated in patients with Raynaud's phenomenon because of the risk for hand ischemia.
- Patients with polymyositis/dermatomyositis may have an atypical response to muscle relaxants. Also, neuraxial anesthesia must be administered cautiously because of intercostal weakness. If muscle weakness is present, spirometry should be performed, as well as cardiovascular evaluation. Some investigators have advocated the avoidance of agents known to trigger malignant hyperthermia in patients with polymyositis/dermatomyositis and elevated creatine kinase levels, but the association is speculative and is not supported by published clinical experience.
- Women receiving long-term corticosteroid therapy should receive a peripartum stress dose of a corticosteroid.

PREGNANT PATIENT WITH COAGULATION DISORDERS

- A number of at least 70-80.000 platelets/mm^3 is considered safe for an epidural technique, between 50-70.000/mm^3 should be analyzed in each patient. Under 50.000/mm^3, the risk is higher than the benefit [2].
- Antiphospholipid syndrome, which is usually associated with autoimmune thrombocytopenia, is the most common acquired thrombophilia. Thromboprophylaxis is indicated if the patient has documented thrombotic events [3].
- APCR/Factor V Leyden, Antithrombin III deficiency and protein C or S deficiency are the most common congenital thrombophilia disorders. Patients affected may receive thromboprophylaxis.
- Disseminated intravascular coagulation is due to systemic activation of blood coagulation secondary to an underlying disorder, which leads to a lack of coagulation factors and platelets resulting in a bleeding diathesis. The main goal of the treatment is the removal of the underlying cause as well as supportive care and replacement of blood products.
- The main goals to avoid complications in patients with sickle cell disease are: warm, good oxygenation and hydration, and movement. Hemoglobin should be above 8-9 g/dl.
- Bernard-Soulier sd. and Glanzmann thrombasthenia are congenital thrombophilia. Bleeding episodes may require tranexamic acid, desmopressin, rFVIIa and platelet transfusion.

- Coagulation status should be checked both before performing a neuraxial technique and prior to removal of the peridural catheter in women with congenital disease. Then, if it is in its normal range, there would be no contraindication to its placement.

- Von Willebrand disease is the most common bleeding disorder in the general population and the commonest form (type 1) should improve during pregnancy even if coagulation may rapidly deteriorate after delivery in both Von Willebrand disease and Hemophilia.

- Epidural anesthesia may be used in hemophilias if coagulation defects have been corrected and the relevant factor level is above 50% or has been raised to more than 50%. Hemophilia B carriers do not respond to DDAVP and should receive prophylactic FIX concentrate for factor levels less than 40–50 IU/dL or in the setting of acute bleeding.

- After 4 days of receiving heparin, a platelet count should be checked to exclude heparin induced thrombocytopenia. Neuraxial anesthesia should be placed after 12 or 24h of the last LMWH injection depending on the administration of prophylactic or therapeutic doses. LMHW administration should be delayed 4 hours after catheter removal.

- There is a controversy between NACO and neuraxial techniques. In general, they should be avoided in an emergency and delayed by 24-48h for scheduled procedures [4].

PREGNANT PATIENT WITH RENAL DISEASE

Women with renal disease require special attention during pregnancy. If the kidney disease is stable with well-controlled hypertension, euvolemia and without dialysis, therapy requires fewer considerations, and routinary controls are enough. We have to differentiate between if the parturient has an acute renal failure, a chronic renal failure, if she is on dialysis treatment or has renal transplantation.

Preeclampsia, hemorrhage and sepsis are the most common causes of acute renal failure during pregnancy [5, 6]. In that cases, our priority is to prevent renal damage, we should maintain an adequate intravascular volume and a good control of the blood pressure to ensure renal perfusion and treat the main cause.

Patients with chronic renal failure have an incresed risk for maternal complications like hypertension or preeclampsia and fetal complications like intrauterine growth restriction or preterm births according to the degree of impairment in renal function. We must know that most parturients with chronic kidney disease have anemia, platelet defects, dyselectrolytemia, vitamin deficiency and also gastric emptying is reduced.

Dialysis treatment should be started if Glomerular Filtration Rate (*GFR*) is < 20ml/min or the serum creatinine level is >3.5 mg/dl. It is important to avoid hypotension because it may cause fetal distress, so fetal monitoring should be performed during hemodialysis. If instead of hemodialysis therapy, a peritoneal dialysis is being performed, we should know that the uterus may reduce peritoneal blood flow and make ineffective this therapy. If it is possible they should undergo dialysis before delivery or cesarean surgery.

Parturients with renal transplantation are immunosuppressed patients, so we have to extent the asepxia for anaesthetic procedures. Also if they are receiving corticosteroids, we should give an additional dose during delivery or cesarean section.

Neuraxial anaesthesia is the best choice for labor and cesarean delivery if there is no thrombocytopenia or no coagulopathy. Epidural technic is preferred to spinal anaesthesia because spinal anaesthesia may lead to a profound sympathetic blockade and consequently greater hypotension and decreased renal perfusion. Invasive hemodynamic monitoring is a good option to avoid hypotension and for the management of fluid therapy and vasopressors always in order not to decrease the renal perfusion pressure.

If general anesthesia ir required, we are going to use drugs that have less kidney metabolism, with a short duration of action and being non-toxic to the kidney. The standard induction agents like propofol or etomidate are safe. The best opioid option is remifentanil because of its rapid metabolism by plasma esterases also alfentanilsufentanil or fentanyl because they are short duration acting drugs and minimally excreted by the kidney. Meperidine and morphine have active metabolites and may accumulate, both are neurotoxic. Atracurium and cisatracurium are the safest nondepolarizing muscle relaxants (*NMBAs*) because they are metabolized by Hoffman elimination. We recommend neuromuscular monitoring, and being careful with patients treated with magnesium sulfate, for example to treat hypertension because hypermagnesemia and metabolic acidosis could prolong the time of action of the NMBAs. If rocuronium or vecuronium is used, the duration of action is prolonged; sugammadex could be used safely. Succinylcholine should also be avoided because it can increase serum potassium levels.

Finally, other drugs used in anaesthesia that may worsen the renal function should be avoided like nonsteroidal antiinflammatory drugs or fluids containing potassium like plasmalyte or lactated ringer.

PREGNANT PATIENT WITH HEPATIC DISEASE

Liver diseases may already be present before pregnancy and complicate it, or they may be specific to pregnancy. We have to think about liver disorders if: alanine and aspartate aminotransferases (*ALT* and *AST*), gamma-glutamyl transferase (*GGT*), Bilirubin, Lactate, Prothrombin time/international normalized ratio (*PT/INR*) or ammonia increased. Also, thrombocytopenia, hypoglycemia, hypoalbuminemia and metabolic acidosis must be checked [5, 6].

Liver diseases can alter the normal pharmacokinetics of anesthetics and other drugs, because the drug clearance and the synthesis of plasma proteins may be decreased (Table **4**).

Neuraxial anaesthesia is the best choice for labor and cesarean delivery but before performing it, we must be sure of the absence of: intravascular volume depletion, coagulopathy, encephalopathy, ascites, respiratory compromise or any other contraindication [7].

In the case of general anesthesia, we can use the standard induction agents without reducing their dose. If we perform a rapid sequence induction we can use succinylcholine in the same dose as in healthy patients, taking into account that its metabolism may be delayed. However, as an alternative we can use rocuronium and sugammadex to reverse its effect. For anesthetic maintenance, it is recommended to administer agents that do not have hepatic metabolism like desflurane, cisatracurium, and remifentanil [8].

Table 4. Drugs in pregnancy.

Drugs to Avoid/Use with Caution	Safe Drugs
- Opioids: Morphine, meperidine and alfentanil. (decreased clearance) - Fentanyl and sufentanil (continuous dosing may be problematic). - Codeine and tramadol. - Hypnotics: etomidate and benzodiazepines. - Neuromuscular blocking agents: vecuronium, rocuronium, succinylcholine, pancuronium (longer duration of action). - Local anesthetics: amide and ester (half lives may be prolonged). - Analgesics: nonsteroidal anti-inflammatory drugs.	- Opioid: Remifentanil, methadone. - Hypnotics: Propofol, methohexital and thiopental. - Neuromuscular blocking agents: atracurium and cisatracurium. - Analgesics: Acetaminophen for acute pain (chronic administration can produce hepatic injury), ketorolac.

CONCLUSION

The planning of anesthesia is mandatory in obstetric patients with comorbidities. During the perioperative period, multidisciplinary teamwork, specific precautions and pre-anesthetic optimization can certainly contribute to an improved outcome in patients during the peripartum period.

CONSENT FOR PUBLICATION

Not applicable.

CONFLICT OF INTEREST

The authors declare no conflict of interest, financial or otherwise.

ACKNOWLEDGEMENT

Declared none.

REFERENCES

[1]   Bajwa SJ, Kalra S. Diabeto-anaesthesia: A subspecialty needing endocrine introspection. Indian J Anaesth 2012; 56(6): 513-7.
[http://dx.doi.org/10.4103/0019-5049.104564] [PMID: 23325933]

[2]   Sociedad Española de Anestesiología, Reanimación y Tratamiento del dolor (SEDAR). Actualización de los protocolos asistenciales de la sección de anestesia Obstétrica de la Sedar. 2a. Madrid: SEDAR 2016.

[3]   Gunaydin B, Ismail S. Obstetric anesthesia for co-morbid conditions. Springer International Publishing AG. 1st Ed: Switzerland. 2018.
[http://dx.doi.org/10.1007/978-3-319-93163-0]

[4]   Sacks D, Baxter B, Campbell BCV, Carpenter JS, Cognard C, Dippel D, *et al.* Multisociety Consensus Quality Improvement Revised Consensus Statement for Endovascular Therapy of Acute Ischemic Stroke. Int J Stroke. 2018; 13(6): 612-32.

[5]   Bajwa SJ, Bajwa S, Ghuman G. Pregnancy with co-morbidities: Anesthetic aspects during operative intervention. Anesth Essays Res 2013; 7(3): 294-301.
[http://dx.doi.org/10.4103/0259-1162.123207] [PMID: 25885972]

[6]   Datta S, *et al.* High-Risk Pregnancy: Maternal Comorbidity. In Obstetric Anesthesia Handbook. 2016; 251-258-94-296.

[7]   Reide PJW, Yentis SM. Anaesthesia for the obstetric patient with (non-obstetric) systemic disease. Best Pract Res Clin Obstet Gynaecol 2010; 24(3): 313-26.
[http://dx.doi.org/10.1016/j.bpobgyn.2009.11.012] [PMID: 20335074]

[8]   Chestnut DH, Wong CA, Tsen LC, *et al.* Chestnut's obstetric anesthesia: principles and practice 6th ed., 2019.

CHAPTER 12

Anesthetic Management of Pregnant Patients with Infectious Disease

Serafín Alonso Vila[1,*], Elena Suárez Edo[1], Elena Sánchez Royo[1], Anna Conesa Marieges[1] and Susana Manrique Muñoz[1]

[1] *Department of Anesthesiology and Intensive Care, Hospital Universitario Vall d'Hebron, Barcelona, Spain*

Abstract: Fever is often the result of an infection. The most common sites for infection during pregnancy are fetal membranes, urinary and respiratory tracts, and the postpartum uterine cavity. The most frequent etiologies of intrapartum fever are chorioamnionitis and neuraxial anesthesia. Maternal and fetal exposure to hyperthermia and inflammation is associated with adverse consequences for the mother and the neonate. In pregnant women with fever, anesthesiologists are not only involved in providing analgesia, but also in the correct anesthetic management for the surgical treatment of the infectious region. Thus, as pyrexia may change both obstetric and anesthetic management, preventing maternal fever is imperative. Emerging and challenging infectious diseases, as COVID-19, remind us of the susceptible nature of pregnant and early postpartum women to severe respiratory infections, reinforcing the importance of vaccines and therapeutic measures during pregnancy.

Keywords: Anesthetic Management, Chorioamnionitis, COVID-19, Epidural Analgesia, Epidural Abscess, Febrile Pregnant, Fever, Fetal Membranes, Inflammation, Infection, Intrapartum Fever, Intraamniotic Infection, Labor, Maternal Fever, Neuraxial Procedures, Neuraxial Anesthesia, Postpartum Infection, Pregnancy, Pyrexia, Sepsis.

INTRODUCTION

Fever is defined as an elevation of body temperature above normal daily variation, occurring when the hypothalamic thermoregulation centre is reset at a higher temperature by the systemic release of endogenous pyrogens, including cytokines, interleukin (*IL*)-1, IL-6, tumor necrosis factor (*TNF*) and interferon-alpha (*IFN-α*), produced in response to infection, inflammation, injury or antigenic challenge. This cascade is chiefly commanded by IL-6 and IL-1B and is inhibited by the

* **Corresponding author Serafín Alonso Vila:** Department of Anesthesiology and Intensive Care, Hospital Universitario Vall d'Hebron, Barcelona, Spain; Email: egomin@yahoo.es

Eugenio Daniel Martinez-Hurtado, Monica Sanjuan-Alvarez & Marta Chacon-Castillo (Eds.)
All rights reserved-© 2022 Bentham Science Publishers

anti-pyrogenic cytokine IL-1 receptor antagonist (*IL-1ra*) [1]. High circulating levels of inflammatory biomarkers, such as IL-6 and IL-10, have been demonstrated in patients with active labor [2].

Intrapartum fever refers to maternal oral temperature $\geq$ 38°C, as axillar measurements (1-2°C lower), are susceptible to user error. The vaginal temperature might be affected by epidural analgesia-induced sympathectomy and vaginal mucosal vasodilation. Fetal/intrauterine temperature is 0.2-0.9°C higher. A progressive increase of temperature with each contraction over time (from 1.5 °C to 0.5°C depending on parity) has been known since the XIX century, attributed to the muscular work of the uterus. Some studies have shown that it is more likely to occur in women with placental inflammation.

A prospective cohort study among 6057 deliveries suggested that the incidence of maternal intrapartum fever was approximately 6.8%, even though its incidence has been reported to be higher in long labors (> 18h) compared to shorter ones (< 6h) (36% *vs.* 7%) [3].

Burgess *et al.* showed that its development is associated with: nulligravidity, length of first stage $\geq$ 720 minutes (min), length of second stage $\geq$ 120 min, membrane rupture $\geq$ 240 min, increasing number of vaginal exams, oxytocin, and meperidine. Other related factors are induced labor, use of epidural analgesia, method of how analgesia is administered, duration of exposure to epidural analgesia, higher birthweight and prolonged gestation.

Maternal and fetal exposure to hyperthermia and inflammation causes both significant maternal effects (increased maternal heart rate, cardiac output, oxygen consumption, and catecholamine production) and adverse neonatal outcomes. Associated morbidity includes caesarean delivery (C-section), Apgar score < 7 at 5 min, and neonatal intensive care unit admission due to hypotonia, assisted ventilation and seizures in the newborn [4, 5].

Different treatments have been tested, with diverse results: high-dose methylprednisolone resulted in lower levels of IL-6 and less fever, but it is associated with increased risk of neonatal bacteremia [6]. Prophylactic acetaminophen and preventive antibiotics are not useful. Intrapartum magnesium-sulfate reduced temperature during labor, either by inhibiting the expression of IL-6 [7], or inducing peripheral vasodilation [8]. And dexmedetomidine can reduce both intrapartum fever and pain during labor, with no increased adverse events, by inhibiting cytokines and alleviating inflammation.

ETIOLOGY OF MATERNAL FEVER

Infectious Causes

Intraamniotic Infection (Chorioamnionitis)

Chorioamnionitis refers to infection of the amniotic fluid, membranes, placenta, and/or decidua, and is one of the most common infections in pregnancy. Independent risk factors include low parity, a history of prior chorioamnionitis, the number of vaginal examinations, both duration of total labor and ruptured membranes, and use of internal monitors [9].

The diagnosis of chorioamnionitis has been based upon the presence of maternal fever ($\geq 38°C$) and at least two of the following: maternal tachycardia (> 100 beats per minute [bpm]), fetal tachycardia (> 160 bpm), uterine tenderness, foul odor of the amniotic fluid, and maternal leukocytosis (> 15.000 cells/mm^3) [10].

Since intrapartum fever is the key clinical sign of a chorioamnionitis, and as there are no findings either sensitive nor specific, antibiotics are usually administered in the presence of maternal fever when other infection sources have been excluded. Once chorioamnionitis is suspected, prompt treatment with broad-spectrum antibiotics with coverage for group B *Streptococcus* must be initiated (*i.e.* Ampicillin plus gentamicin) as this reduces maternal and neonatal morbidity.

The most common isolated organisms from the amniotic fluid in chorioamnionitis are *Bacteroides* species (sp.), group B *Streptococcus*, *Mycoplasma* and *Ureaplasma sp.*, and *E. coli*. Additionally, general supportive measures (acetaminophen, rehydration…) are very important.

Maternal complications of this infection include preterm labor, placental abruption, postpartum infection, uterine atony, postpartum hemorrhage, peripartum hysterectomy, sepsis, and death [9].

The cornerstone of obstetric management of these patients is prompt delivery. Several studies suggest that early, antepartum, treatment results in decreased maternal and neonatal morbidity. The early use of antibiotics may also affect the anesthesiologist's decision regarding the performance of neuraxial technique [9].

Urologic Infections

Urinary tract infections are common in pregnancy due to increased concentrations of progesterone (which causes ureteral dilatation that facilitates bacterial ascent from the bladder) and the partial ureteral obstruction caused by the gravid uterus (provoking urinary stasis) [9].

Signs and symptoms of upper or complicated urinary tract infections include fever, flank pain, nausea, vomiting, and costovertebral angle tenderness with or without lower urinary tract symptoms (dysuria, frequency, urgency, suprapubic pain, hematuria) and 14% to 17% of pregnant women with pyelonephritis will develop bacteremia. Simple cystitis is not associated with fever. The most common causative organisms are *E. coli*, gram-positive organisms (including group B *Streptococcus*), *Klebsiella*, *Enterobacter* and *Proteus sp* [9].

An 18-year retrospective study concluded that preterm birth was higher in women who have had pyelonephritis during pregnancy [11], nevertheless its incidence is less than 5%, similar to the general pregnant population [9].

Asymptomatic bacteriuria (*AB*) occurs in 2% to 7% of pregnant women, and, if left untreated, up to a 30% will eventually develop a symptomatic urinary tract infection, so its screening and treatment is important, as this is associated with a reduced incidence of pyelonephritis and low-birth-weight infants, although not with a decreased incidence of preterm delivery [9].

Treatment should be performed with a tailored antibiotic regimen, taking into account its safety during pregnancy, which can include beta-lactams, nitrofurantoin, and fosfomycin. The optimal duration of antibiotics is uncertain, traditional 7-day regimens are likely more effective but short courses are preferred to minimize the antimicrobial exposure to the fetus, as they are also effective; nevertheless, single-dose regimens may not be as effective as slightly longer regimens [12 - 14]. An exception is single-dose fosfomycin, which successfully treats bacteriuria.

It is generally accepted that penicillins, cephalosporins, aztreonam and some carbapenems (meropenem, ertapenem, and doripenem) are safe in pregnancy, as well as fosfomycin.

Respiratory Tract Infection

Most respiratory tract infections during pregnancy are harmless upper respiratory tract viral infections, with common clinical manifestations (nasal congestion, rhinorrhea, sore throat, cough). Fever, if present, tends to be low grade. Supportive treatment is indicated.

Many lower respiratory tract infections are also viral and self-limited, and may intensify characteristic hyperemia and hypersecretion of the gestational respiratory tract mucosa. These excess secretions may predispose to a bacterial superinfection.

Pregnant patients are an especially vulnerable population for community-acquired pneumonias, most of which are bacterial in origin, as they are more susceptible to respiratory pathogens due to physiological changes (such as increased oxygen consumption, elevation of the diaphragm, edema in respiratory tract mucosa and decreased functional residual capacity) and immune adaptations (such as altered T lymphocyte immunity), that may increase maternal hypoxemia [9, 15].

Pneumonia incidence during pregnancy is similar to general population, and is associated with significant maternal and fetal morbidities. Risk factors include anemia, asthma, smoking, illicit drug use, and immunosuppressive illness or therapy.

Classic symptoms are fever, pleuritic chest pain, shortness of breath, and productive cough of purulent sputum. In order, the most common pathogens are *Streptococcus pneumoniae*, *Mycoplasma pneumoniae* and influenza. *Legionella pneumophila*, *Chlamydia*, *Staphylococcus aureus*, and varicella are less common. Varicella pneumonia has been associated with up to 40% of maternal mortality and maternal-fetal morbidity, so it is very important to establish the immune status prior to a planned pregnancy, vaccinating those who are not yet immune.

Both acyclovir and valacyclovir have been successfully used to treat gestational varicella pneumonia and have warranted to reduce the risk of respiratory failure and maternal death.

For pregnant women with mild community-acquired pneumonia, a combination of amoxicillin or amoxicillin/clavulanate plus azithromycin is suggested as outpatient treatment. Clindamycin could be an alternative in those allergic to beta-lactams.

If hospitalization is required, combination therapy with an antipneumococcal beta-lactam plus azithromycin, will be the first option; with clindamycin plus aztreonam used in case of allergy. In cases of severe pneumonia, vancomycin should be added (for MRSA coverage and drug-resistant *S. pneumoniae*). Some antibiotics to be avoided in pregnancy include tetracyclines, clarithromycin, and fluoroquinolones.

Influenza pandemics of 1918, 1957, and 2009 showed increased morbidity (risk of fetal death) and mortality in pregnant and puerperal women, so as immunization is safe, inactivated influenza vaccine is strongly recommended regardless of trimester of pregnancy. Passive protection to the newborn can last up to 20 weeks after birth [9]. Prompt empiric treatment should be given if suspected or confirmed acute influenza in pregnant and two weeks postpartum women, due to the seriousness of infection in these patients.

This virus is usually susceptible to neuraminidase inhibitors, oseltamivir, zanamivir, and peramivir, with benefits outweighing the potential risks during pregnancy [16, 17]. Oseltamivir is the drug of choice because of its systemic absorption and the greater clinical experience in pregnancy. The usual duration of treatment is five days, but longer treatment courses can be considered in severely ill patients. No data are available on the use of baloxavir in pregnancy.

Genital Herpes Infection

The typical presentation includes painful vesicular or papular lesions on the skin or mucous membranes of the genital tract. Primary maternal herpes simplex virus (*HSV*) type 2 infection is either asymptomatic or associated with transient viremia (fever, headache, lymphadenopathy) and causes locally recurring disease characterized by asymptomatic periods alternated with episodes of reactivation from sites in the sensory ganglia. Up to 2% of pregnant women will be primarily infected during gestation.

HSV type 1 (*HSV-1*) is now the predominant cause of new genital herpes infections in some populations. Maternal antibodies prevent the recurrence of viremia in recurrent infection, even though the site of lesions on the external genitalia may present severe symptoms [9].

The major obstetric concern is the potential transmission to the infant at birth, by one of two ways: direct contact during vaginal delivery or secondary to an intrauterine infection (by ascent after membranes rupture). Neonatal HSV infection is a life-threatening condition with potential for permanent central nervous system sequelae, with an increased risk for infection in the setting of a primary maternal infection. Its severity may be reduced by early initiation of antiviral therapy (acyclovir or valacyclovir). Passive transfer of HSV-antibodies from the mother to the fetus is protective in recurrent herpes infection. C-section reduces the risk for HSV labor-related transmission when cervix/external genitalia cultures to HSV are positive. Safety of neuraxial anesthesia in primary HSV infection remains unclear [9].

Postpartum Infection

Bacteria colonizing genital tract (cervix and vagina) gain access to the amniotic fluid during labor, and may invade devitalized uterine tissue postpartum. Postpartum endometritis is a common cause of postpartum fever and uterine tenderness, and is 10-to-30-fold more common after C-section than vaginal delivery. Prolonged rupture of membranes and/or duration of labor increase its incidence. Both vaginal preparation before elective or emergent C-section and prophylactic administration of antibiotics, decrease the incidence of postpartum uterine infection and post-surgical wound infection. Likewise, prophylactic antibiotics should be given in the setting of complex perineal repairs [9].

Treatment is indicated for symptom relief and to prevent sequelae (peritonitis, salpingitis, oophoritis, phlegmon or abscess, and septic pelvic thrombophlebitis), with broad spectrum parenteral antibiotics that include coverage for beta-lactamase-producing anaerobes, given the microbiology of these infections: Their prompt initiation is critical in septic patients [18]. Oral antibiotics are an option for mild endometritis diagnosed after the patient has been discharged, especially those post-vaginal birth.

As a previous endometritis increases risk for uterine rupture, anesthesiologists and obstetricians must be aware of this serious complication in future pregnancies [19].

Non-Infectious Causes

Non-infectious causes of maternal fever include medications (such as prostaglandin E2 agents), elevated ambient temperature and administration of neuraxial analgesia [20].

Neuraxial Analgesia

It has been described an association between the use of epidural analgesia and an increase in maternal core temperature (mean increase of 0.18°C/hour), with non-statistically significant differences found between the different techniques (epidural *vs.* combined spinal-epidural [*CSE*]) or with the use of opioids.

The etiology is not clearly known yet, but the most reasonable mechanism is a non-infectious inflammatory process due to the direct effect of local anesthetics (impairing the release of the anti-pyrogenic IL-1ra, by reducing caspase-1 activity and reducing plasma IL-1ra/IL-1β ratio) on endothelial tissue, with studies showing less febrile rate in lower concentrations of local anesthetics. Around 20-30% of patients who receive this analgesia have fever during labor, observing increasing IL-6 concentrations associated with its duration (and especially after the 4th hour of exposure) [21, 22]. As per all these data, fever appears to have an inflammatory etiology more than being secondary to the alteration of thermoregulation related to the epidural technique [23 - 25].

The use of low doses of epidural dexamethasone leads to a decrease in both maternal fever and IL-6 levels. Antibiotics have no effect in reducing temperature.

ANESTHETIC MANAGEMENT FOR THE FEBRILE OR INFECTED PARTURIENT

This management will depend on the characteristics of the patient and the situation.

Neuraxial Anesthesia

The greatest concern on the use of neuraxial anesthesia [26] in the febrile or infected pregnant patient is the development of meningitis or an epidural abscess. It is difficult to stablish a proper incidence of these complications due to the great variability in the reported incidence in the literature.

Multiple theories explain the association between performing a dural puncture in patients with bacteremia and the appearance of meningitis, from direct inoculation when the venous plexus that surrounds the spinal cord is broken, to the rupture of the dural barrier itself. The introduction of a catheter into the epidural space is a source of infection in these patients involving a greater risk of complications than spinal techniques.

A full clinical evaluation and the review of blood studies is recommended to identify patients with high risk of complications and to balance the risks/benefits of performing a neuraxial technique. Leukocytes, C-reactive protein (*CRP*) and erythrocyte sedimentation rate are elevated during pregnancy, so these parameters are not reliable to determine the severity of infection in these patients.

Notwithstanding the low incidence of infectious complications, the choice to go on neuraxial procedures in pregnant patients with fever or infection should be carefully individualized.

- Spinal or epidural anesthesia can be safely performed to healthy patients at low-grade risk for bacteremia.
- If treatment with antibiotics is started before the procedure and there is evidence of a clinical improvement, parturients with systemic infection may safely receive spinal anesthesia. The security of placing an epidural catheter is still under discussion in these cases.
- It appears to be wise not to perform neuraxial anesthesia in untreated pregnant women with evident signs of sepsis.

General Anesthesia

Pregnant patients with systemic infection own some peculiarities that every anesthesiologist should consider before performing a general anesthesia [27]:

- Risk of pulmonary aspiration due to delayed gastric emptying. Premedication and a rapid sequence induction are recommended in these patients.
- Adequate pre-oxygenation before induction should be performed because of the reduction of functional residual capacity. The increased oxygen consumption, characteristic of both pregnancy and infection, also contributes to this situation.
- Prevention of aortocaval compression by displacing the uterus to the left. Prompt hypotension treatment with adequate fluid resuscitation and inotropic drugs should be performed.

ANESTHETIC CONSIDERATIONS OF THE MOST COMMON INFECTIONS DURING PREGNANCY [13, 32]

Herpes Simplex Virus (*HSV*)

• HSV-1: Spinal or epidural administration of morphine has been associated with the reactivation of thoracic and perioral lesions.

• HSV-2: The presence of an active lesion at the puncture site contraindicates regional anesthesia in both groups of patients.

    • Primary infection (genital lesions with systemic symptoms): Safety of regional anesthesia remains unclear (risk of central nervous system infection due to viremia).

    • Secondary/recurrent infection: neuraxial anesthesia is secure.

Hepatitis

Early correction of dehydration and electrolyte abnormalities should be performed in parturients with acute viral hepatitis.

Likewise, avoid those factors associated with an hepatic blood flow reduction (hypotension, high sympathetic stimulation, *etc.*).

- *General anesthesia*: use drugs with extrahepatic metabolism.
- *Regional anesthesia*: check for platelet or coagulation abnormalities before performing neuraxial procedures.

Human Inmunodeficiency Virus (*HIV*)

- *Regional anesthesia*: neuraxial procedures are safe. If a dural puncture occurs, a blood patch using autologous blood is a secure treatment.
- *General anesthesia*: there is a high risk of difficult intubation and aspiration because of oropharyngeal/esophagical problems. Adjust anesthestic doses due

to compromised hepatic and renal functions, and loss of muscle mass. If there is

respiratory compromise, higher fraction of inspired oxygen concentration may be needed.

Urinary Tract Infections

Early correction of dehydration and electrolyte abnormalities should be performed in parturients with acute pyelonephritis. Special care on the pulmonary monitoring must be provided to prevent a respiratory failure. Aspiration prophylaxis should be administered. There is no contraindication for regional anesthesia previous antibiotic therapy.

Chorioamnionitis

There is no evidence that regional anesthesia is contraindicated previous antibiotic therapy. So, its administeration before treatment has not been proven harmful.

It is associated with an increased risk of postpartum hemorrhage, uterine atony and sepsis.

Pneumonia

- *Regional anesthesia*: there is no contraindication previous antibiotic therapy. It may contribute to control the increased oxygen consumption characteristic of both pregnancy and infection.
- *General anesthesia*: indicated if there is a severe respiratory failure (oxygen arrival to fetus must be ensured due to rapid desaturation).

Septic Shock

- *Regional anesthesia*: the combination of low cardiac ouput, dehydratation, hypotension and coagulation abnormalities contraindicates it.
- *General anesthesia*: choice of drugs should be focused on the maintenance of uteroplacental flow and maternal hemodynamia.

COVID-19 & PREGNANCY

Coronavirus disease of 2019 (*COVID-19*) is a multi-system disease caused by the Severe Acute Respiratory Syndrome Coronavirus-2 (*SARS-CoV-2*) first identified in December 2019 in Wuhan, China, with symptoms ranging from asymptomatic to fatal. The overall mortality rate ranges from 3% to 4%, with a high rate of patients requiring intensive care [15, 28, 29].

COVID-19 during pregnancy is more likely to develop a severe illness with increased rate of admission to the intensive care unit, need for supplemental oxygen, ventilation, and mortality than in general population. Also, Dubey et al. found that up to 27% of patients had increased risk of preterm birth, fetal vascular malperfusion, and premature fetal membrane rupture [15, 30].

Predominant symptoms on pregnancy are fever, cough, and dyspnea, followed by anosmia, ageusia, myalgia, fatigue, sore throat, malaise, rigor, headache, and anorexia [15, 31]. The most reported laboratory abnormalities are leukocytosis (with lymphopenia and increased neutrophil ratio), leukopenia, elevated CRP, D-dimer, and lactate dehydrogenase (*LDH*). Commonest CT findings in pneumonia in pregnant patients include ground glass opacities and bilateral infiltrates [15].

Treatments on pregnancy are limited, including, currently, dexamethasone, convalescent plasma, and remdesivir [15]. It is unclear whether uterine decompression improves maternal respiratory status, but prolonged maternal hypoxemia may ultimately cause fetal acidemia, which should be avoided [32, 33].

Anesthetic Management

Recommendations are based on data on viral transmission risks combined with the shared experience from maternity units caring for these patients and applied to women with confirmed or suspected COVID-19 [34].

Evaluation and monitoring for an appropriate level of care and planning for potential deterioration should include history, assessment of respiratory symptoms, physical examination, frequent vital signs (with the addition of continuous pulse oximetry [SpO_2 goal $\geq$ 95%]), review of laboratory tests and strict fluid balance to assure proper restriction [32, 34]. High-flow nasal oxygen (*HFNO*) or non-invasive ventilation may be considered. If acute distress respiratory syndrome (*ADRS*) is diagnosed, the patient should undergo endotracheal intubation and intensive care support [32]. Awake patients should wear a surgical facemask at all times to avoid droplet transmission [34, 35].

Labor Analgesia

Neuraxial analgesia is recommended, all types of procedures are acceptable and they should be considered as a mean to avoid general anesthesia [36]. There is no evidence that these procedures are contraindicated in the presence of coronaviruses and the risk of causing meningitis or encephalitis is extremely low even in infected patients [32, 34, 36].

Mild thrombocytopenia appears to be common in non-pregnant patients with

COVID-19, the more moderate with the more severe illness. Therefore, platelet count should be checked before initiation of technique [34]. A platelet count of 70,000 E106/L has a low risk for spinal epidural hematoma, and lower levels should be considered safe in cases with a high risk for respiratory compromise with general anesthesia [36].

As labor ventilation is non-aerosol-generating procedure (*AGP*), a hat, eye protection, a surgical mask, sterile fluid-resistant long-sleeved gown and sterile gloves should be worn for neuraxial placement. Closed-loop communication is always recommended to the staff. All personal protective equipment (*PPE*) should be donned outside the labor room.

Use of a NO_2 breathing system neither constitutes an AGP, so, same measures should apply. However, the equipment circuit must contain an anti-viral filter [32, 37].

There are no current data about the use of remifentanil PCA in these patients, but it should be used with caution and avoided if SpO_2 < 95% due to the risk of respiratory depression [34].

Caesarean Section

Neuraxial anesthesia is recommended, as is standard in obstetric anesthesia, to minimize the risk of aerosolization associated with general anesthesia. To reduce complications, the block should be performed by the most appropriate anesthetist available [34]. Donning PPE for AGP should be considered for emergency cases because of the risk of failed block and the consequent need for mid-procedural conversion to general anesthesia [37].

As the more severe cases of COVID-19 are more prone to hypotension, the use of a prophylactic intravenous infusion of a vasopressor is recommended in these patients to prevent hypotension associated with neuraxial anesthesia [32, 34]. Refractory secondary hypotension is more observed in patients having an epidural top-up or CSE [38]. Antiemetic medication should also be administered. Uterotonics can be associated with cardiovascular disturbance and should be administered by slow bolus or infusion [32, 34, 39].

General Anesthesia

The same operating theatre, with the essential and -if possible- disposable equipment to minimize its contamination, and the same anesthetic machine should be used and restricted for COVID-19 cases. A heat and moisture exchanger with viral filtration should be present within the anesthesia circuit [34].

The major concerns are both the risk of infection spreading and the impact of tracheal intubation on a patient with acute respiratory compromise. Intubation and extubation are AGP and the risk of viral transmission is greater than with non-AGP procedures. Minimizing staff in theatre, use of PPE that include protection against aerosol exposure and two pairs of gloves to the intubating clinician are recommended [34, 35, 40]. Antacid prophylaxis and positioning adjuncts should be added as in routine obstetric practice.

As there is an increased risk of difficult and failed airway management in obstetric practice, the most skilled anesthetist should make the first intubation attempt, using a videolaryngoscope, to maximize the first-pass success. Respiratory impairment due to COVID-19 together with pregnancy-related lung changes, provokes a rapid desaturation following induction: preoxygenation is mandatory (tight-fitting face mask with two-hand technique) with standard flow-rate oxygen.

Avoid increased risk of aerosolization using HFNO or face mask oxygen. Low-pressure manual ventilation may be necessary if desaturation occurs. Cardiovascular collapse following induction may happen and vasopressors should be immediately available for its management. Decontamination of work surfaces around the anesthetic machine and patient's head should be performed at all times.

A variety of effective agents have been evaluated to avoid coughing on extubation, being dexmedetomidine ranked as the most effective [34, 35, 41]. Their use should be careful because of the respiratory and hemodynamic effects on the mother [34].

As the real risk of general anesthesia outweighs the theoretical risk of causing meningitis/encephalitis, performing neuraxial procedures in parturients with COVID-19, unless otherwise contraindicated, is recommended [36].

Postoperative/Postpartum Care

Postoperative location and usual postpartum issues (postpartum hemorrhage, pain, hemodynamic status), judicious fluid management, surveillance for respiratory decompensation, and early involvement of subspecialty care as needed [32] should be discussed prior to intervention.

The use of NSAIDs in patients with COVID-19 is not related to worse outcomes [32, 35].

Precautionary separation of the mother and neonate may minimize transmission, but there is insufficient evidence to guide management [37, 42, 43]. If done, breastfeeding must involve strict adherence to hand hygiene and droplet precautions to limit viral spread.

Patients with COVID-19 are hypercoagulable (usual prolonged aPTT and increased D-Dimer) and as pregnancy is a prothrombotic state, infected patients are more vulnerable to thromboembolism. Recommendations on anticoagulation should be performed in all pregnant women admitted with COVID-19, unless birth is expected within 12 h [34, 35, 37].

SPECIAL SITUATIONS

- Uterine atony (postpartum hemorrhage): oxytocin is the first-line treament, followed by methylergonovine. Carboprost has increased potential for bronchospasm [32].
- Postdural Puncture Headache: usual conservative care followed by epidural blood patch, applying usual contraindications (fever, thrombocytopenia or other coagulation issues). In actively ill women postponing the blood patch is recommended, even though individual assessment should be performed [32, 35].
- Peripartum fever should be treated with usual protocols (as previously seen).
- Gestational hypertension/preeclampsia: pharmacological control should be performed with labetalol or urapidil, as nicardipine has undesirable effects in pulmonary function. ACE inhibitors for postpartum hypertension can be started or continued [44].
- Magnesium sulfate: benefits of its use exceed risk of central respiratory depression [35].

CONCLUSION

Vertical transmission to the fetus is uncommon.

Fever is an alarming symptom, especially during pregnancy. Although it usually has an infectious etiology, there are other causes of fever, and a correct differential diagnosis and adequate treatment are particularly important.

Diagnosis of infection in pregnancy raises questions about neuraxial anesthesia safety. Infection does not always contraindicate regional anesthesia, and decision should be based on an individual risk-to-benefit ratio.

Pregnant women are particularly susceptible to respiratory pathogens and severe pneumonia due to their immunosuppressive state and the physiological adaptations secondary to pregnancy.

COVID-19 clinical manifestations do not differ form general population, but is more likely to develop severe illness during pregnancy.

Avoid general anaesthesia unless absolutely necessary. Early epidural analgesia should be recommended to women in labour with suspected or confirmed coronavirus disease 2019. Due to increased risk of thrombocytopenia, platelet count must be checked.

CONSENT FOR PUBLICATION

Not applicable.

CONFLICT OF INTEREST

The authors declare no conflict of interest, financial or otherwise.

ACKNOWLEDGEMENT

Declared none.

REFERENCES

[1]   Evans SS, Repasky EA, Fisher DT. Fever and the thermal regulation of immunity: the immune system feels the heat. Nat Rev Immunol 2015; 15(6): 335-49.
[http://dx.doi.org/10.1038/nri3843] [PMID: 25976513]

[2]   Neal JL, Lamp JM, Lowe NK, Gillespie SL, Sinnott LT, McCarthy DO. Differences in inflammatory markers between nulliparous women admitted to hospitals in preactive vs active labor. Am J Obstet Gynecol 2015; 212(1): 68.e1-8.
[http://dx.doi.org/10.1016/j.ajog.2014.07.050] [PMID: 25086275]

[3]   Towers CV, Yates A, Zite N, Smith C, Chernicky L, Howard B. Incidence of fever in labor and risk of neonatal sepsis. Am J Obstet Gynecol. 2017; 216(6): e1-5.

[4]   Burgess APH, Katz JE, Moretti M, Lakhi N. risk factors for intrapartum fever in term gestations and associated maternal and neonatal sequelae. gynecol obstet invest 2017; 82(5): 508-16.
[http://dx.doi.org/10.1159/000453611] [PMID: 28103590]

[5]   Greenwell EA, Wyshak G, Ringer SA, Johnson LC, Rivkin MJ, Lieberman E. Intrapartum temperature elevation, epidural use, and adverse outcome in term infants. Pediatrics 2012; 129(2): e447-54.
[http://dx.doi.org/10.1542/peds.2010-2301] [PMID: 22291120]

[6]   Goetzl L, Zighelboim I, Dadell M, *et al.* Maternal corticosteroids to prevent intrauterine exposure to hyperthermia and inflammation: A randomized, double-blind, placebo-controlled trial. Am J Obstet Gynecol 2006; 195(4): 1031-7.
[http://dx.doi.org/10.1016/j.ajog.2006.06.012] [PMID: 16875647]

[7]   Lange EMS, Segal S, Pancaro C, *et al.* association between intrapartum magnesium administration and the incidence of maternal fever. anesthesiology 2017; 127(6): 942-52.
[http://dx.doi.org/10.1097/ALN.0000000000001872] [PMID: 28863031]

[8]   Zweifler RM, Voorhees ME, Mahmood MA, Parnell M. Magnesium sulfate increases the rate of hypothermia *via* surface cooling and improves comfort. Stroke 2004; 35(10): 2331-4.
[http://dx.doi.org/10.1161/01.STR.0000141161.63181.f1] [PMID: 15322301]

[9]   Bauer ME, Albright CM, Scott S, Wlody DJ. Fever. In: Chest, editor. Chestnut's Obstetric Anesthesia: Principles and Practice. 6 ed: Elsevier 2019; 878-96.

[10]   Newton ER. Chorioamnionitis and intraamniotic infection. Clin Obstet Gynecol 1993; 36(4): 795-808.
       [http://dx.doi.org/10.1097/00003081-199312000-00004] [PMID: 8293582]

[11]   Wing DA, Fassett MJ, Getahun D. Acute pyelonephritis in pregnancy: an 18-year retrospective analysis. Am J Obstet Gynecol 2014; 210(3): 219.e1-6.
       [http://dx.doi.org/10.1016/j.ajog.2013.10.006] [PMID: 24100227]

[12]   Tan JS, File TM Jr. Treatment of bacteriuria in pregnancy. Drugs 1992; 44(6): 972-80.
       [http://dx.doi.org/10.2165/00003495-199244060-00006] [PMID: 1282867]

[13]   Vercaigne LM, Zhanel GG. Recommended treatment for urinary tract infection in pregnancy. Ann Pharmacother 1994; 28(2): 248-51.
       [http://dx.doi.org/10.1177/106002809402800218] [PMID: 8173146]

[14]   Widmer M, Lopez I, Gülmezoglu AM, Mignini L, Roganti A. Duration of treatment for asymptomatic bacteriuria during pregnancy. Cochrane Database Syst Rev. 2015; (11).

[15]   Boushra MN, Koyfman A, Long B. COVID-19 in pregnancy and the puerperium: A review for emergency physicians. Am J Emerg Med 2020.
       [PMID: 33162266]

[16]   Van Bennekom CM, Kerr SM, Mitchell AA. Oseltamivir exposure in pregnancy and the risk of specific birth defects. Birth Defects Res 2019; 111(19): 1479-86.
       [http://dx.doi.org/10.1002/bdr2.1563] [PMID: 31397115]

[17]   Chambers CD, Johnson D, Xu R, Luo Y, Jones KL, Group OCR. Oseltamivir use in pregnancy: Risk of birth defects, preterm delivery, and small for gestational age infants. Birth Defects Res 2019; 111(19): 1487-93.
       [http://dx.doi.org/10.1002/bdr2.1566] [PMID: 31397112]

[18]   Bauer ME, Lorenz RP, Bauer ST, Rao K, Anderson FWJ. Maternal Deaths Due to Sepsis in the State of Michigan, 1999–2006. Obstet Gynecol 2015; 126(4): 747-52.
       [http://dx.doi.org/10.1097/AOG.0000000000001028] [PMID: 26348189]

[19]   Shipp TD, Zelop C, Cohen A, Repke JT, Lieberman E. Post-cesarean delivery fever and uterine rupture in a subsequent trial of labor. Obstet Gynecol 2003; 101(1): 136-9.
       [PMID: 12517658]

[20]   Higgins RD, Saade G, Polin RA, *et al.* Evaluation and Management of Women and Newborns With a Maternal Diagnosis of Chorioamnionitis. Obstet Gynecol 2016; 127(3): 426-36.
       [http://dx.doi.org/10.1097/AOG.0000000000001246] [PMID: 26855098]

[21]   del Arroyo AG, Sanchez J, Patel S, *et al.* Role of leucocyte caspase-1 activity in epidural-related maternal fever: a single-centre, observational, mechanistic cohort study. Br J Anaesth 2019; 122(1): 92-102.
       [http://dx.doi.org/10.1016/j.bja.2018.09.024] [PMID: 30579413]

[22]   Anim-Somuah M, Smyth RMD, Cyna AM, Cuthbert A. Epidural versus non-epidural or no analgesia for pain management in labour. Cochrane Libr 2018; 2018(5)CD000331
       [http://dx.doi.org/10.1002/14651858.CD000331.pub4] [PMID: 29781504]

[23]   Li CJ, Xia F, Xu SQ, Shen XF. Concerned topics of epidural labor analgesia: labor elongation and maternal pyrexia: a systematic review. Chin Med J (Engl) 2020; 133(5): 597-605.
       [http://dx.doi.org/10.1097/CM9.0000000000000646] [PMID: 32032081]

[24]   Sultan P, David AL, Fernando R, Ackland GL. inflammation and epidural-related maternal fever. anesth analg 2016; 122(5): 1546-53.
       [http://dx.doi.org/10.1213/ANE.0000000000001195] [PMID: 27101499]

[25]   Zhou X, Li J, Deng S, Xu Z, Liu Z. Ropivacaine at different concentrations on intrapartum fever, IL-6

and TNF-α in parturient with epidural labor analgesia. Exp Ther Med 2019; 17(3): 1631-6.
[PMID: 30783430]

[26]   Practice Advisory for the Prevention, Diagnosis, and Management of Infectious Complications
Associated with Neuraxial Techniques: An Updated Report by the American Society of
Anesthesiologists Task Force on Infectious Complications Associated with Neuraxial Techniques and
the American Society of Regional Anesthesia and Pain Medicine. Anesthesiology. 2017; 126(4): 585-
601.

[27]   Bowyer L, Robinson HL, Barrett H, *et al.* SOMANZ guidelines for the investigation and management
sepsis in pregnancy. Aust N Z J Obstet Gynaecol 2017; 57(5): 540-51.
[http://dx.doi.org/10.1111/ajo.12646] [PMID: 28670748]

[28]   Wang D, Hu B, Hu C, *et al.* clinical characteristics of 138 hospitalized patients with 2019 novel
coronavirus–infected pneumonia in wuhan, china. jama 2020; 323(11): 1061-9.
[http://dx.doi.org/10.1001/jama.2020.1585] [PMID: 32031570]

[29]   Di Mascio D, Khalil A, Saccone G, *et al.* Outcome of coronavirus spectrum infections (SARS, MERS,
COVID-19) during pregnancy: a systematic review and meta-analysis. Am J Obstet Gynecol MFM
2020; 2(2)100107
[http://dx.doi.org/10.1016/j.ajogmf.2020.100107] [PMID: 32292902]

[30]   Moore KM, Suthar MS. Comprehensive analysis of COVID-19 during pregnancy. Biochem Biophys
Res Commun 2021; 538: 180-6.
[http://dx.doi.org/10.1016/j.bbrc.2020.12.064] [PMID: 33384142]

[31]   Di Toro F, Gjoka M, Di Lorenzo G, De Seta F, Maso G, Risso FM, *et al.* Impact of COVID-19 on
maternal and neonatal outcomes: a systematic review and meta-analysis. Clin Microbiol Infect 2020.
[PMID: 33148440]

[32]   Bauer ME, Bernstein K, Dinges E, *et al.* Obstetric Anesthesia During the COVID-19 Pandemic.
Anesth Analg 2020; 131(1): 7-15.
[http://dx.doi.org/10.1213/ANE.0000000000004856] [PMID: 32265365]

[33]   Society for Maternal Fetal Medicine, Perinatology. Labor and Delivery COVID-19 Considerations.
2020.

[34]   Bampoe S, Odor PM, Lucas DN. Novel coronavirus SARS-CoV-2 and COVID-19. Practice
recommendations for obstetric anaesthesia: what we have learned thus far. Int J Obstet Anesth 2020;
43: 1-8.
[http://dx.doi.org/10.1016/j.ijoa.2020.04.006] [PMID: 32437912]

[35]   Ung N, Bonnet MP. Obstetric anaesthesia during the COVID-19 pandemic Prat Anesth Reanim 2020;
24(4): 196-201.
[http://dx.doi.org/10.1016/j.pratan.2020.07.005] [PMID: 32837210]

[36]   Bauer ME, Chiware R, Pancaro C. Neuraxial Procedures in COVID-19–Positive Parturients: A
Review of Current Reports. Anesth Analg 2020; 131(1): e22-4.
[http://dx.doi.org/10.1213/ANE.0000000000004831] [PMID: 32221171]

[37]   RCOG.   Coronavirus   (COVID-19)   infection   in   pregnancy..
https://www.rcog.org.uk/globalassets/documents/guidelines/2020-10-14-coronavirus-covid-19-infectio
n-in-pregnancy-v12.pdf Ed2020; 26-35.

[38]   Chen R, Zhang Y, Huang L, Cheng B, Xia Z, Meng Q. Safety and efficacy of different anesthetic
regimens for parturients with COVID-19 undergoing Cesarean delivery: a case series of 17 patients.
Can J Anaesth 2020; 67(6): 655-63.
[http://dx.doi.org/10.1007/s12630-020-01630-7] [PMID: 32180175]

[39]   Kinsella SM, Carvalho B, Dyer RA, *et al.* International consensus statement on the management of
hypotension with vasopressors during caesarean section under spinal anaesthesia. Anaesthesia 2018;
73(1): 71-92.

[http://dx.doi.org/10.1111/anae.14080] [PMID: 29090733]

[40]　Wittenberg MD, Vaughan DJA, Lucas DN. A novel airway checklist for obstetric general anaesthesia. Int J Obstet Anesth 2013; 22(3): 264-5.
[http://dx.doi.org/10.1016/j.ijoa.2013.03.001] [PMID: 23669487]

[41]　Tung A, Fergusson NA, Ng N, Hu V, Dormuth C, Griesdale DEG. Medications to reduce emergence coughing after general anaesthesia with tracheal intubation: a systematic review and network meta-analysis. Br J Anaesth 2020; 124(4): 480-95.
[http://dx.doi.org/10.1016/j.bja.2019.12.041] [PMID: 32098647]

[42]　Favre G, Pomar L, Qi X, Nielsen-Saines K, Musso D, Baud D. Guidelines for pregnant women with suspected SARS-CoV-2 infection. Lancet Infect Dis 2020; 20(6): 652-3.
[http://dx.doi.org/10.1016/S1473-3099(20)30157-2] [PMID: 32142639]

[43]　Rasmussen SA, Smulian JC, Lednicky JA, Wen TS, Jamieson DJ. Coronavirus Disease 2019 (COVID-19) and pregnancy: what obstetricians need to know. Am J Obstet Gynecol 2020; 222(5): 415-26.
[http://dx.doi.org/10.1016/j.ajog.2020.02.017] [PMID: 32105680]

[44]　Vogel JP, Tendal B, Giles M, *et al.* Clinical care of pregnant and postpartum women with COVID-19: Living recommendations from the National COVID-19 Clinical Evidence Taskforce. Aust N Z J Obstet Gynaecol 2020; 60(6): 840-51.
[http://dx.doi.org/10.1111/ajo.13270] [PMID: 33119139]

CHAPTER 13

Obstetric Hemorrhage

María de la Flor Robledo[1,*] and **Pablo Solís Muñoz**[2]

[1] *Department of Anesthesia, University Hospital Severo Ochoa, Leganes, Madrid, Spain*

[2] *University Hospital Infanta Elena, Valdemoro, Madrid, Spain*

Abstract: Postpartum hemorrhage (*PPH*) is the most common cause of obstetric hemorrhage (*OH*) and the first cause of maternal death worldwide. However, its mortality has decreased in the United States in recent decades due to the implementation of certain measures. Several factors are significantly associated with the onset of PPH. Identifying them early will help us to establish an appropriate strategy for the management of these patients. One of the most useful prevention measures is the active management of the third stage of labor, especially the routine administration of oxytocin. The existence of acting algorithms will also contribute to a rapid and orderly response to the presence of expected or unplanned bleeding.

Keywords: Artery Embolization, Bleeding, Blood Bank, Cesarean Birth, Clamping Umbilical Cord, Coagulopathy, Disseminated Intravascular Coagulation, Hemorrhage, Hysterectomy, Intrauterine Tamponade Balloon, Labor, Massive Transfusion, Massive Obstetric Hemorrhage, Oxytocin, Postpartum Period, Postpartum Hemorrhage, Placental Disorders, Rotational Thromboelastography, Thromboelastography, Trauma, Uterotonic Drug, Uterine Atony, Uterine Massage, Vaginal Delivery.

INTRODUCTION

Postpartum hemorrhage (*PPH*) is the most common cause of obstetric hemorrhage (*OH*) and the first cause of maternal death worldwide. When the bleeding occurs within the first 24 hours after delivery, PPH is called early PPH, and it will be the subject of this chapter. Hemorrhage between 24 hours and 6-12 weeks after delivery is called late PPH [1].

Definitions vary depending on the author or organization, with the World Health Organization's (*WHO*) definition being one of the most frequently used. According to it, PPH is a blood loss greater than 500 mL within the first 24 hours

* **Corresponding author María de la Flor Robledo:** Department of Anesthesia, University Hospital Severo Ochoa, Leganes, Madrid, Spain; Email: mfr16382@hotmail.com

Eugenio Daniel Martinez-Hurtado, Monica Sanjuan-Alvarez & Marta Chacon-Castillo (Eds.)
All rights reserved-© 2022 Bentham Science Publishers

postpartum. When the blood loss is larger than 1000 mL within the same time frame, it is considered a severe PPH, and if the blood loss is greater than 40% of the patient's total blood volume, which during pregnancy is increased by 100 mL/kg, it is named massive obstetric hemorrhage (*MOH*).

The American College of Obstetricians and Gynecologists defines PPH as bleeding associated with the process of childbirth that either has an accumulated blood volume loss greater than 1000 mL or any blood loss accompanied by signs or symptoms of hypovolemia, regardless of the type of delivery (vaginal or cesarean section) [2].

The incidence of PPH depends on the diagnostic criteria used. When the diagnostic criteria are met by quantified blood loss, PPH incidence is higher than when the losses are estimated. Its mortality has decreased steadily in the United States since the late 1980s, due to increased transfusions and hysterectomy rates.

CAUSES OF POSTPARTUM HEMORRHAGE

The mnemonic rule of the "*4Ts*" summarizes the most frequent causes of PPH [3]:

- *Tone*: This includes abnormalities in uterine contractions. Uterine atony is the most common cause of PPH and is responsible for at least 80% of cases, mainly in its diffuse type. Uterine atony occurs when the uterus cannot contract after delivery, and it can happen with or without tissue retention. A soft, poorly contracted uterus suggests this diagnosis.

In diffuse atony, blood loss can be significantly greater than clinically estimated as a substantial amount of blood can remain inside a flaccid and dilated uterus. When the atony is focal, only the lower segment of the uterus tends to be the most affected, and it is difficult to detect during physical examination.

- *Tissue*: This includes causes of PPH related to retained products of conception.
- *Trauma*: When the bleeding is due to any type genital trauma during childbirth. The most frequent are secondary to genital tract lacerations (in this case, diagnosis can be delayed until excessive vaginal bleeding ensues), uterine body lacerations, surgical incisions in cesarean deliveries (generally due to lateral extension of the incisions), or uterine rupture.
- *Thrombin*: Postpartum hemorrhage due to clotting disorders. Both acquired and hereditary coagulopathies are responsible for at least 7% of PPH cases. Also, coagulopathies can result from PPH when significant and persistent bleeding induces a severe reduction of the clotting factors.

Risk Factors

Several factors are significantly associated with the onset of PPH. However, many patients without any risk factor also develop OH.

The following tables list the main risk factors according to the moment of onset (Tables **1** and **2**) [3].

Table 1. Main risk factors according to the moment of onset. Presentation before delivery: significant risk of PPH.

RISK FACTOR	4T	Odds ratio (CI 95%)
Placental abruption	Thrombin	13 (7,61-12,9)
Placenta previa	Tone	12 (7,17-23)
Multiple pregnancy	Tone	5 (3,0-6,6)
Preeclampsia	Thrombin	4
Previous PPH	Tone	3
Asian ethnicity	Tone	2 (1,48-2,12)
BMI>35 kg/m2	Tone	2 (1,24-2,17)
Hemoglobin<9g/dl		2 (1,63-3,15)

Table 2. Main risk factors according to the moment of onset. Presentation during or after delivery.

RISK FACTOR	4T	Odds ratio (CI 95%)
Urgent cesarean section	Trauma	4 (3,28-3,95)
Programmed cesarean section	Trauma	2 (2,18-2,80)
Induction of labor		2 (1,67-2,96)
Retained placenta	Tissue	5 (3,36-7,87)
Mid-lateral episiotomy	Trauma	5
Instrumental delivery	Trauma	
Prolonged delivery (> 12h)	Tone	2
Large for gestational age newborn (> 4 kg)	Tone/Trauma	2 (1,38-2,60)
Fever during labor	Thrombin	2
Mother age> 40	Tone	1,4 (1,16-1,74)

The California Risk Classification subdivides risk factors according to the intensity of the risk [1]:

- *Low risk*: factors with a low risk of inducing PPH are single gestation and less than four previous vaginal deliveries.
- *Moderate risk*: this includes multiple gestations, previous uterine surgeries, multiparous women (> 4 births), presence of large myomas, previous PPH, macrosomia (> 4000 g), body mass index (*BMI*) higher than 40, anemia, chorioamnionitis, oxytocin administration for more than 24 hours, magnesium sulfide administration and a prolonged second stage of childbirth.
- *High risk*: the factors with the highest risk are the presence of placenta previa, placenta accreta, a platelet count lower than 100,000/microL, known coagulopathy, active bleeding at hospital admission, hematocrit lower than 30% and the presence of two or more moderate PPH risk factors.

MANIFESTATIONS AND DIAGNOSIS

Amount of Bleeding

The clinical manifestations of hemorrhage directly depend on the volume of blood lost.

Bleeding classifications, such as that offered by Advanced Trauma Life Support manuals, may help determine the severity of bleeding in PPH. However, many of these classifications are derived from the non-pregnant population. Therefore, there could be some differences in the postpartum period.

A specific classification for obstetric hemorrhage is outlined in The California Maternal Quality Care Collaborative OB Hemorrhage Emergency Management Plan. It distinguishes four degrees of PPH based on blood loss [1]:

- *Level 0*: this level includes all women in labor.
- *Level 1*: when there is a blood loss > 500 mL in vaginal delivery or > 1000 mL in cesarean section, or there are clinical changes (oxygen saturation < 95%, heart rate [*HR*] equal to or greater than 110 beats per minute [*bpm*], blood pressure [*BP*] less than 85/45 mmHg, or changes greater than 15% from baseline).
- *Level 2*: if the bleeding is persistent and with a total blood loss less than 1500 mL.
- *Level 3*: if the total blood loss is more than 1500 mL, hemodynamic instability, administration of more than two red blood cell (*RBC*) units, or suspected disseminated intravascular coagulation (*DIC*).

Clinical Changes

In pregnant women, hemodynamic changes and signs or symptoms of hypovolemia are usually a late PPH sign. The decrease in blood pressure and the increase in heart rate typically occur when blood loss exceeds 25% of the patient's blood volume, which can mean more than 1500 mL in these patients [4].

Laboratory Evaluation

From a laboratory point of view, hemoglobin and hematocrit values are not good indicators of acute blood loss, as the changes are often delayed. However, fibrinogen values do correlate better with the amount of bleeding. A fibrinogen level below 200 mg/dL is a predictor of the need to transfuse multiple units of blood and other blood products, the need for surgical or radiological intervention to control bleeding, and points to a higher risk of maternal death. It is recommended to maintain fibrinogen levels above 300 mg/dL.

Coagulopathy that appears in the context of OH can be due to different mechanisms (dilutional coagulopathy, consumption coagulopathy, or hyperfibrinolysis) and generally evolves rapidly. Coagulopathy is frequent in MOH secondary to tissue retention or due to coagulopathies, and hyperfibrinolysis appears particularly associated with MOH.

As indicated above, certain specific scenarios may delay the identification of PPH:

- In asymptomatic patients without evident external bleeding (for example, intra-abdominal bleeding in vaginal births).
- In patients who remain asymptomatic until blood loss exceeds 25% of their blood volume.

Thus, close monitoring and surveillance of all patients is essential to establish the diagnosis of PPH.

POSTPARTUM HEMORRHAGE PREVENTION

It is vital to identify women with risk factors for PPH and thus be able to establish an approach to delivery and a follow-up appropriate to their level of risk. In these cases, ensuring the existence of the necessary resources, both human and material, is a priority, and sometimes it may be necessary to refer these patients to specialized centers to achieve this.

The existence of PPH kits and the development of protocols for action (specific protocols for PPH and massive transfusion), with which the personnel involved in the management of the pregnant woman and her postpartum period are familiar, are some of the recommended measures.

There should be close communication with the blood bank, especially given the presence of risk factors for developing PPH. In that case, and according to the level of risk, blood should be typed and screened or crossed.

In patients at high risk of PPH, the use of intraoperative blood salvage systems could be considered, especially in the case of cesarean section, although their routine use is not cost-effective [5].

Active management of the third stage of labor is one of the most endorsed preventive measures. This could be done by administration of oxytocin, uterine massage, and umbilical cord traction. The routine use of oxytocin (dilute intravenous (*IV*) infusion or intramuscular injection) reduces the risk of PPH by at least 30% in the general obstetric population. Its combination with misoprostol or methylergonovine does not appear to be more effective than its use alone for prophylaxis. The evidence regarding uterine massage or early clamping of the umbilical cord does not appear to show significant differences in the amount of postpartum hemorrhage.

Prophylactic administration of tranexamic acid is still under study, although some authors already recommend it (Table 3) [4].

Table 3. Preventive measures for PPH [4].

Measure	Effect	Evidence level
Active management of the third stage of labor	Reduces bleeding and risk of PPH	Grade A
Routine prophylactic uterotonic drugs	Decreases the incidence and severity of PPH by 30%	Grade A
Oxytocin IV if cesarean delivery	Oxytocin IV infusion or bolus to favor uterine contraction and decrease bleeding. *Avoid bolus in women with severe heart disease.	Grade C
Multidisciplinary approach	Expert staff, blood availability, access to critical care units...	Grade C

In the postpartum period, it is advisable to perform regular complete blood count and coagulation studies in any woman at risk of developing coagulopathy or symptomatic anemia [5].

Certain entities, such as placental disorders or certain coagulopathies, require specific preventive actions that are outside the scope of this chapter.

On a final note, determining risk factors for PPH is not always clinically useful.

Most women at high risk do not experience significant postpartum bleeding, and many women who are not a priori at risk develop PPH. Thus, obstetric bleeding is unpredictable to a large extent, and we must always keep that in mind.

MANAGEMENT OF POSTPARTUM HEMORRHAGE

Objectives

The objectives of the PPH management could be summarized in the following three points:

- Identify and correct the obstetric cause of the bleeding.
- Reestablish an adequate circulatory volume to avoid hypoperfusion of vital organs and to get adequate tissue oxygenation.
- Correct the coagulopathy if it develops.

There is evidence that indicates that the use of tranexamic acid can be useful in the prevention and treatment of PPH-associated hyperfibrinolysis. Its early administration may reduce the mortality associated with bleeding when PPH occurs secondary to trauma or atony. Some studies recommend administering an initial intravenous bolus of 2g, others recommend using 4g instead, and even some authors advocate its prophylactic use in high-risk patients.

The management of uterine atony, the most frequent cause of PPH, will depend on the type of delivery and the amount of bleeding. The administration of uterotonic drugs is the initial step, with the application of progressively more invasive procedures until the bleeding is completely controlled. These procedures go from placing an intrauterine tamponade balloon initially, moving then to interventional radiology procedures such as uterine artery embolization, and finally the need for surgery (uterine artery ligation, utero-ovarian artery ligation, hysterectomy), although after a cesarean section, the invasive measures are usually considered earlier.

Bleeding secondary to trauma generally requires surgical control, either transvaginally or abdominally.

The retention of placental tissue must be quickly identified and removed as soon as possible, while the spectrum of placenta accreta will usually end in a hysterectomy.

The management of coagulopathy as the cause of the bleeding is medical, based on the transfusion of blood products or administration of deficient coagulation factors.

Specific Measures

Once the presence of PPH has been diagnosed, the rapid and simultaneous implementation of certain specific measures is crucial for the control of bleeding:

- *Multidisciplinary approach*: the joint, rapid, and coordinated action of the different specialists involved in childbirth is vital to implement effective measures to control bleeding. In this specific context of stress and seriousness, accessible protocols and diagrams of action can facilitate PPH management.
- *Routine quantification of blood loss*: determining the amount of bleeding in both vaginal and cesarean deliveries, and doing so systematically, regardless of the presence of risk factors for PPH, will allow early identification of this entity, early initiation of bleeding control measures, and avoid significant and irreversible deterioration of the patient status. Although there is not enough evidence to support the use of either method to estimate blood loss after vaginal delivery, the American College of Obstetricians and Gynecologists considers quantitative methods more accurate than visual methods since the latter may overestimate small bleeds and underestimate losses when they are high.
- *Early response*: once PPH has been diagnosed, and its cause determined, initiating adequate treatment as soon as possible is crucial, since almost 90% of PPH deaths occur in the first four hours after childbirth. This early management, to which the two above mentioned measures will contribute, would prevent poor perfusion and oxygenation of tissues and the subsequent development of acidosis, hypothermia, and coagulopathy.
- *Appropriate clinical and laboratory monitoring*: laboratory tests should at least include a complete blood count (*CBC*), coagulation studies, and calcium and potassium levels. The patient's hemodynamic status is a very important factor to consider in order to establish a strategy to control the bleeding. Thus, for example, arterial embolization procedures should not be considered for the emergency control of a PPH of an unstable patient (Table **4**).

Table 4. Acting Algorithm [1, 3, 4].

HOSPITAL ADMISSION	- Assess risk factors for PPH. - Blood Bank: • Type and screen in patients with medium risk. • Type and crossmatch 2 Units in patients with high risk.
PREVENTION	- Active management of the third stage of labor • Oxytocin (dilute IV infusión or 10 U intramuscular (IM)) • Uterine massage • Umbilical cord traction - Determine quantitative blood loss in all cases

(Table 4) cont....

BLOOD LOSS (> 500 mL vaginal or > 1000 mL cesarean) **Or** **CLINICAL CHANGES** (HR >= 110 bpm, BP < 85/45 mmHg, O2 saturation < 95%, or changes > 15% from patient baseline) (*patient could show confusion, sweatiness, oliguria*)	- Initiate PPH protocol - Notify rest of the team. - Inspection: vaginal walls, cervix, uterine cavity, placenta. - Monitorization: HR, BP, O_2 saturation. Urinary catheter. - Active patient warm-up - Ensure intravenous access: at least 18G - Increase IV fluids. Fluid heating systems - Increase oxytocin rate - Fundal massage again. - Add another uterotonic: methylergonovine 0.2mg IM (not if arterial hypertension or preeclampsia). Repeat if good response, if not, move on to 2nd level uterotonic drugs. - Type and crossmatch 2U (if not done before)
CONTINUED BLEEDING **TOTAL BLOOD LOSS < 1500 mL**	- Intensify monitoring - Intensify quantitative measurement of blood loss - Laboratory: fibrinogen, CBC, prothrombin time (*PT*)/partial thromboplastin time (*PTT*), International normalized ratio (*INR*). - Move to operating room if not already done - 2nd intravenous access (14-16G) - Next level uterotonic drugs: • Hemabate 250 mcg IM or • Misoprostol 800 mcg sublingual - Bimanual massage **Vaginal birth:** / **Cesarean birth:** *(see below)*

Vaginal birth:	**Cesarean birth:**
- Move to operating room - Repair any tears - Place intrauterine balloon - Selective embolization if haemodynamic stability	- Assess broad ligament, retained placenta and posterior part of uterus - B-Lynch suture - Place intrauterine balloon

BLOOD LOSS (> 1500 mL or > 2 units RBCs given **Or** **HAEMODYNAMIC INSTABILITY** **SUSPICION OF DI** (*patient could show lethargy or loss of consciousness*)	- Repeat labs: CBC, PT/PTT, INR, fibrinogen, blood gas, electrolytes (ionized calcium) - Monitor thromboelastography (*TEG*) or rotational thromboelastography (*ROTEM*). - Central venous access - Activate Massive Hemorrhage Protocol. • Transfuse aggressively. • 1:1 RBC:FFP • 1 platelet pack per 4-6 units RBCs • Unresponsive coagulopathy. after 8-10 units RBCs and full coagulation factor replacement: consider rFactor VIIa risk/benefit. • Administer tranexamic acid (1g IV over 10 minutes); a second dose can be given if bleeding continues • Administer fibrinogen if <2g/dL - Re-dose antibiotics. Aggressively treat acidosis, hypocalcaemia and hyperkalaemia. - Laparotomy (B-Lynch suture; uterine artery ligation, hysterectomy).

CONCLUSION

PPH is the leading cause of obstetric hemorrhage and the first cause of maternal death worldwide. However, its mortality has decreased in recent decades.

The *"4Ts"* summarizes the most frequent causes of PPH: tone, tissue, trauma, and thrombin.

Some of the factors with the highest risk of developing PPH are the presence of placenta previa, placenta accreta, a platelet count lower than 100,000/microL, or known coagulopathy.

Active management of the third stage of labor, early identification of the factors significantly related to this entity, and the existence of action protocols have undoubtedly contributed to improving its prognosis.

Many women without risk factors develop PPH. Therefore, exhaustive monitoring and follow-up of all these patients are key for the accurate diagnosis and management of this condition.

CONSENT FOR PUBLICATION

Not applicable.

CONFLICT OF INTEREST

The authors declare no conflict of interest, financial or otherwise.

ACKNOWLEDGEMENT

Declared none.

REFERENCES

[1]   Belfort MA. Overview of postpartum hemorrhage. UpToDate. [Internet]. 2020. Disponible en: www.uptodate.com

[2]   Guasch E, Gilsanz F. Hemorragia masiva obstétrica: enfoque terapéutico actual. Med Intensiva 2016; 40(5): 298-310.
[http://dx.doi.org/10.1016/j.medin.2016.02.010] [PMID: 27184441]

[3]   Guasch E, Gilsanz F. Hemorragia obstétrica: actuaciones recomendadas y protocolo de actuación. 2016.

[4]   Mavrides E, Allard S, Chandraharan E, *et al.* Prevention and management of postpartum haemorrhage. BJOG 2017; 124(5): e106-49.
[http://dx.doi.org/10.1111/1471-0528.14178] [PMID: 27981719]

[5]   Practice Bulletin No. 183: Postpartum Hemorrhage. Obstet Gynecol 2017; 130(4): e168-86.
[http://dx.doi.org/10.1097/AOG.0000000000002351] [PMID: 28937571]

Hypertensive Disorders in Pregnancy

Eugenio D. Martinez Hurtado[1,*] and **Míriam Sánchez Merchante**[2]

[1] *Department of Anesthesiology and Intensive Care, Hospital Universitario Infanta Leonor, Madrid, Spain*

[2] *Hospital Universitario Fundación Alcorcón, Madrid, Spain*

Abstract: Due to the high risk of morbidity and mortality in pregnant women with unrecognised and untreated preeclampsia, a high index of suspicion for signs of preeclampsia should be used to evaluate, treat and monitor patients. Early blood pressure control and seizure prophylaxis during labour are essential to ensure maternal safety. However, a limited proportion of pregnancies and deliveries may present a wide range of complications that may require admission to a critical care unit (*CCU*). Hypertensive disorders of pregnancy and massive hemorrhage are among the most common causes of admission to the CCU in pregnant and post-partum women.

Keywords: Blood Pressure, Biomarkers, Cardiovascular Disease, Eclampsia, Fetal Outcome, Foetus, HELLP Syndrome, Hypertension, Hypertensive Disorders, Labetalol, Maternal Morbidity, Maternal Health, Nifedipine, Pathogenesis, Placental Dysfunction, Preeclampsia, Pregnancy.

INTRODUCTION

Hypertensive pregnancy disorders (*HRD*) are a complication in about 5% to 10% of pregnancies, with a 25% increase over the past 20 years [1, 2]. Hypertensive disorders, associated with delayed or inappropriate treatment of severe systolic hypertension, remain the leading cause of maternal death. Thus, in the United States (US), there is a death/day, and worldwide there are up to 50-60,000 deaths/year [3 - 6]. The vast majority of these deaths result from hemorrhagic strokes and complications related to seizures [7 - 10]. Furthermore, for every maternal death associated with HRD, there are between 50 and 100 complications [11 - 15]. Therefore, the goal of treatment of pregnant women with HRD is to prevent morbi-mortality, which is achieved through aggressive blood pressure

---

[*] **Corresponding author Eugenio D. Martínez Hurtado:** Department of Anesthesiology and Intensive Care, Hospital Universitario Infanta Leonor, Madrid, Spain; Email: emartinez@anestesiar.org

Eugenio Daniel Martinez-Hurtado, Monica Sanjuan-Alvarez & Marta Chacon-Castillo (Eds.)
All rights reserved-© 2022 Bentham Science Publishers

(*BP*) treatment, seizure prophylaxis with magnesium, timely delivery, and post-partum surveillance.

PATHOPHYSIOLOGY OF PREECLAMPSIA

The pathophysiology of preeclampsia remains unclear. It is triggered by a marked vasoconstriction state, secondary to vascular endothelial dysfunction, when adequate vasodilation typical of normal pregnancy is not carried out.

Preeclampsia is a complex disease whose aetiology seems multifactorial. Placental disturbance plays a central role, although other genetic and immunologic factors must also be considered, as well as various predisposing factors of the fetus and the mother.

All these elements, taken together, condition a pathology that, although it begins at the placenta level, leads to multi-systemic damage, with a particular renal, hepatic and neurological impact.

There are a number of pathophysiological mechanisms which may be regarded as responsible for preeclampsia.

Uterine Artery Remodelling

The formation of the placenta is a key process in gestation, as this organ is responsible for adequate blood perfusion from the mother to the foetus, which is essential for normal fetal development. The placenta is formed from fetal cytotrophoblastic tissue, which forms the trophoblastic villi, structures that support the blood vessels of the fetus. Spiral arteries, branches of the maternal uterine artery, direct oxygenated blood and nutrients from the maternal circulation to the fetal circulation.

In some patients, it has been shown that interstitial invasion by cytotrophoblasts cannot penetrate the myometrium [16]. Trophoblast differentiation towards the endothelial phenotype characteristic of normal placentation is not effectively completed [17]. As a result, the spiral arteries remain reduced in calibre, limiting blood flow to the foetus and leading to placental ischemia.

Immunological Factors

Natural killer (*NK*) cells and macrophages are involved in the placentation process. Uterine NK cells migrate to the decidua and secrete cytokines, interferon-γ (*IFN-γ*), vascular endothelial growth factor (*VEGF*), placental growth factor (*PlGF*), among others, all of which are involved in spiral artery remodelling [18].

A predominance of uterine NK cells with an aberrant phenotype has been demonstrated in pregnant women with preeclampsia. It contributes to the disruption of placentation through the production of unusual amounts of cytokines that prevent proper interactions with cytotrophoblasts [19, 20].

On the other hand, during normal gestation, the immune system provides a privileged state for the foetus to avoid maternal reaction to fetal tissues, favouring the proliferation of Th2 lymphocytes and the action of regulatory T lymphocytes.

In contrast, a decrease in the number and activity of these lymphocyte populations has been observed in preeclampsia, at the expense of increased production of Th1 and Th17 lymphocytes, involved in the production of cytokines, such as interleukin-2, IFN-γ or tumour growth factor beta (*TGF-β*), which limit immunotolerance and induce a proinflammatory state [21 - 24].

Immune component may also contribute to the increased risk of preeclampsia in primigravid women. It has been postulated that, during early pregnancy, maternal immune system develops tolerance to paternally derived fetal antigens. And, in subsequent pregnancies, memory T cells induce immunotolerance to these antigens more rapidly, reducing the risk of developing preeclampsia [25, 26].

Genetic Factors

Preeclampsia development has a genetic component, as evidenced by the increased risk of women who have first or second-degree relatives. She present preeclampsia 5 and 2 times more, respectively, than those with no family history of preeclampsia [27 - 30].

Some family segregation studies claim that individual susceptibility to develop the disease is genetically conditioned by more than 50%.

DIAGNOSIS OF HYPERTENSIVE DISORDERS OF PREGNANCY

The most frequent manifestations of preeclampsia, hypertension and proteinuria, remain for many professionals a pre-requisite for diagnosis. However, preeclampsia is a multi-organ disorder with highly variable forms of presentation (Fig. **1**).

Preeclampsia may in some cases manifest as increased capillary permeability (proteinuria, ascites, pulmonary oedema) or as impaired haemostasis with hepatic dysfunction, but without hypertension.

Patients who do not have proteinuria are the most common, as proteinuria may not be relevant even when signs and symptoms of severe preeclampsia have already been established, such as up to 10-15% of cases of haemolysis-elevation of transaminases-plaketopenia syndrome (*HELLP*) and 35-40% of cases of eclampsia occur in the absence of hypertension or proteinuria [31 - 36]. Preeclampsia is therefore not currently conceived as a disease, but rather as a complex and heterogeneous obstetric syndrome with a broad clinical spectrum.

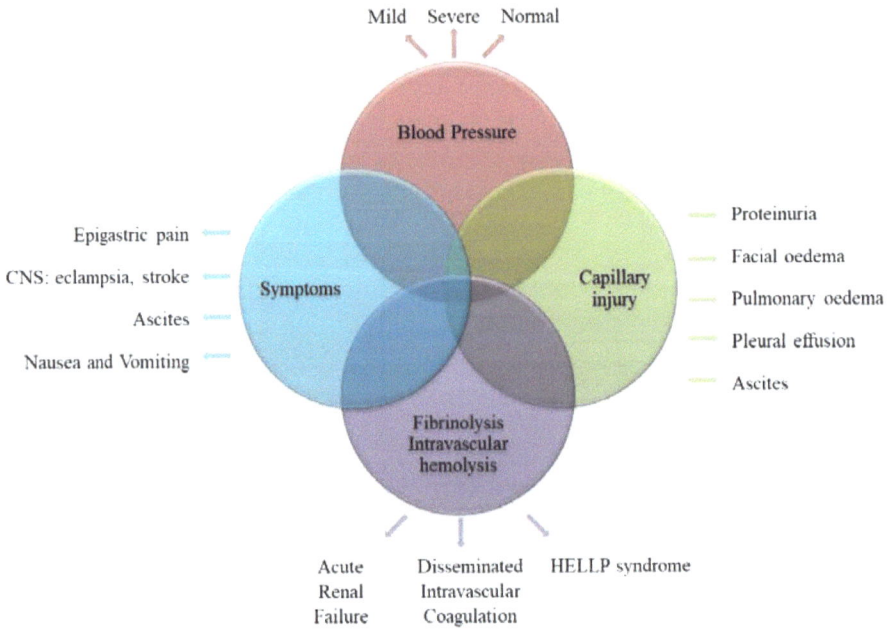

Fig 1. Clinical spectrum of preeclampsia.

In 2013, ACOG published a widespread task force review on hypertensive disorders of pregnancy [37]. In this one, Preeclampsia was defined by 2 resting blood pressure at least separated by four hours, with a result >140/90 mmHg (Table **1**).

Severe preeclampsia was defined as systolic blood pressure of 160 mmHg or diastolic blood pressure of 110 mmHg on at least 2 occasions with an interval of at least 4 hours between measurements, and/or having additional clinical or laboratory criteria (Table **1**). A hypertensive emergency is defined as a medical situation in which two elevated blood pressure values, which need not be consecutive, are taken 15-60 minutes apart.

Considering the syndromic nature of preeclampsia and its association with other

HRD related disorders, since 2013, the American College of Obstetricians and Gynaecologists (*ACOG*) has modified the diagnostic criteria for preeclampsia, becoming them more inclusive, in order to avoid scenarios in which unsuspected complications may arise due to diagnostic failure [37, 38].

ACOG admits some situations in which preeclampsia can be diagnosed without presenting proteinuria. In addition, it defines a series of clinical and laboratory findings that make preeclampsia more prone to complications and are considered criteria for severity (Table **1**).

Table 1. Diagnostic criteria of preeclampsia according to the American College of Obstetricians and Gynaecologists [37].

Blood pressure	- After 20 weeks of gestation in a woman with a previously normal blood pressure, ≥ 140 mmHg systolic blood pressure (*SBP*) or ≥ 90 mmHg diastolic blood pressure (*DBP*) on 2 occasions at least separated by 4 hours. - ≥ 160 mmHg SBP or ≥ 110 mmHg DBP, hypertension can be confirmed within a short interval (minutes) to facilitate timely antihypertensive therapy
Proteinuria	- ≥ 300 mg in 24-hour urine (or this amount extrapolated from a timed collection) or - Protein/creatinine ratio greater than or equal to 0.3 mg/dl - Dipstick reading of 1+ (used only if other quantitative methods not available)
Or, in the absence of proteinuria, new-onset hypertension with any of the following	
Thrombocytopenia	- Platelet count < 100.000/µL
Renal insufficiency	- Serum creatinine concentrations > 1.1 mg/dL or - Doubling of the serum creatinine concentration without other renal disease
Impaired liver function (*LFTs*)	- Twice-normal or greater concentration of liver transaminases.
Pulmonary oedema	- Dyspnoea and saturation 02 (SatO$_2$) < 95% or - Radiological ratification
Cerebral or visual symptoms	- Severe headache - Photopsias, blurred vision

Massive proteinuria (> 5g), previously considered a criterion of severity but not clearly associated with worse outcomes in recent studies, has been eliminated [39] (Table **2**).

Classification of Hypertensive Disorders of Pregnancy

Fig. **2** depicts the progression from gestational hypertension to preeclampsia. Transition from one to the other occurs dynamically and gradually and can be diagnosed by frequent monitoring and reassessment of maternal outcomes.

Table 2. Preeclampsia with severe features.

- Two highest BP values (SBP $\geq$ 160 or DBP $\geq$ 110) achieved within 15-60 minutes of each other - Persistent oliguria <500 ml/24 hours - Progressive renal insufficiency - Unremitting headache/visual disturbances - Pulmonary oedema - Epigastric/ Right Upper Quadrant Pain (*RUQ*) pain - Liver function tests > 2 x normal - Platelets < 100,000 - Haemolysis, elevated liver enzymes and low platelet, or red blood cell, count (HELLP) syndrome
* 5 gr of proteinuria is no longer criteria for severe preeclampsia

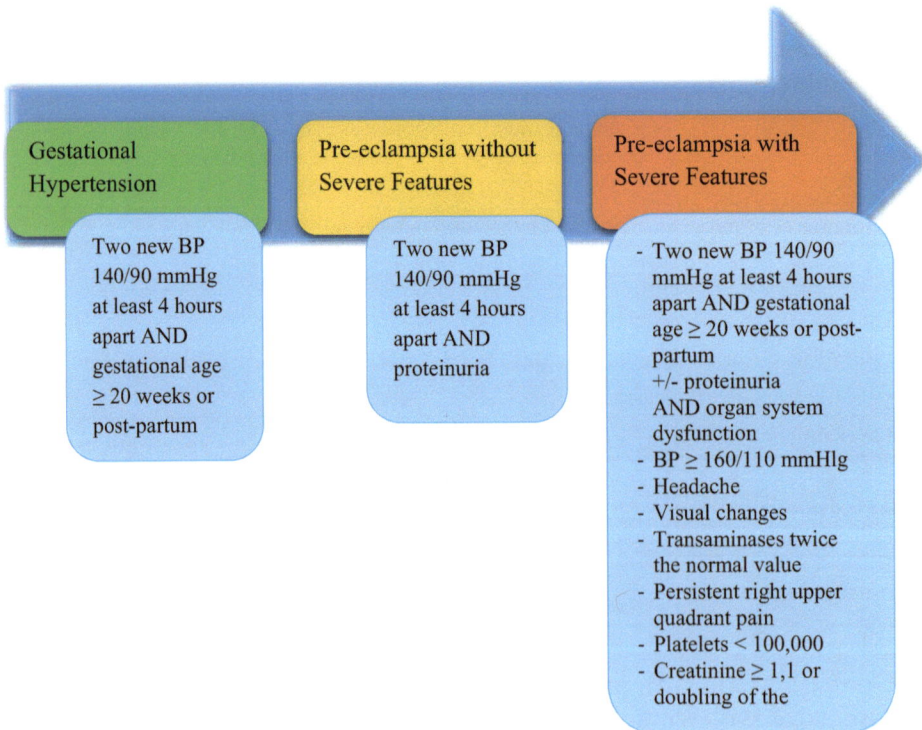

Fig. (2). Continuum of gestational hypertension and pre-eclampsia.

Thus, depending on its severity, preeclampsia can be distinguished as follows:

- *Non-severe forms*: these are the most frequent (1/20-50 pregnancies). It usually happens late in pregnancy (around 34 weeks) and has no effect on the foetus-maternal prognosis. They are usually not accompanied by fetal growth restriction.
- *Less common severe forms* (1/200-300 pregnancies) are usually of earlier onset and may present with complications such as renal failure, liver failure, coagulation disorders, hepatic hemorrhage, pulmonary oedema, maternal seizures (eclampsia) and stroke, as well as fetal growth restriction (*FGR*) and abruptio placentae.

Early-onset preeclampsia is associated with FGR in 40% of cases [40, 41] and progresses to severe and complicated forms in up to 15% [42 - 44]. It is important to remark that late-onset preeclampsia, although often more benign in course, can also progress to severe forms. Thus, FGR occurs in 15-20% of late preeclampsia, and all other complications also occur in 3-5% of late preeclampsia [45]. In fact, although early forms of preeclampsia are generally more severe, since late forms of preeclampsia are 10 times more frequent than early forms, the most severe complications of preeclampsia occur beyond 34 weeks of gestation.

In summary, the main factors conditioning the maternal and perinatal prognosis of preeclampsia are:

- Gestational age at diagnosis.
- Presence or absence of severity criteria.
- Presence or absence of associated FGR (mainly for perinatal prognosis).
- Presence or absence of predisposing conditions.
- Quality of medical care.

RISK FACTORS FOR DEVELOPING PREECLAMPSIA

If the pregnant woman has a personal history of preeclampsia in previous pregnancies, the risk of re-development of preeclampsia is seven times higher. The same happens when a first-degree parent has preeclampsia, with up to three times the risk. Other risk factors include multiple pregnancies, a mother's age of more than 40 years, diabetes, obesity, and chronic hypertension [46, 47].

Pregnancy weight gain is considered to be a risk factor for preeclampsia [48 - 50], with the risk doubling for every 5-7 kg/m^2 increase in body mass index (*BMI*) [51, 52]. However, the majority of preeclampsia cases are diagnosed in healthy pregnant women with no obvious risk factors [1, 2].

OBSTETRIC MANAGEMENT OF PREECLAMPSIA

Primary prevention of preeclampsia can be initiated with daily aspirin therapy at the end of the first trimester in pregnant women who had a history of severe preeclampsia in a previous pregnancy before 34 weeks' gestation [53 - 55]. Up to 60% reduction in preeclampsia in women at high risk of early preeclampsia has been shown with low-dose prophylactic aspirin between 11 and 14 weeks' gestation [56, 57]. Secondary prevention of crises and reduction of maternal morbidity due to preeclampsia is carried out through close surveillance, trying to detect deterioration of the maternal condition affecting, among others, cardiovascular, neurological, pulmonary or renal systems, or the development of haemolysis, elevated liver enzymes, and low platelet, or red blood cell, count (*HELLP syndrome*).

Management of Antihypertensive Drugs

Systolic hypertension untreated or inadequately treated is highly implicated in deaths related to stroke and preeclampsia [7, 58, 59]. Up to 60% of deaths are due to women not recognising the danger signs or symptoms, or there is too late or even inappropriate response by health workers [60, 61]. Pregnant women who suffer a stroke have been found to have higher mortality rates during hospitalisation and suffer complications such as the need for mechanical ventilation, pneumonia, convulsions, and prolonged hospital stay [58, 62, 63]. In preeclampsia, cerebral autoregulation is impaired, so preeclamptic pregnant women are at increased risk of intracranial hemorrhage with much lower blood pressures (> 155 mmHg) [7, 63 - 65]. The overall prevalence and mortality of stroke in older adults in the US have been declining over the past decade.

However, the rate of pregnancy-related stroke has increased by 61.5% [62, 66]. Therefore, if a blood pressure > 160/110 mmHg (severe hypertension) is monitored, repeat the measurement every 5 minutes for 15 minutes and inform the physician. If two high blood pressures are obtained within 15 minutes, treatment can be initiated. But if it persists at elevated levels for 15 minutes or more, treatment should be initiated immediately.

This treatment is with first-line agents, and should be initiated within 30-60 minutes of confirmation of severe hypertension to reduce the risk of maternal stroke [7, 63, 67 - 69].

First-line treatments are based on the use of short-acting drugs, such as intravenous labetalol or hydralazine, and oral nifedipine [70 - 73]. The use of these antihypertensive agents has comparable efficacy according to Cochrane reviews [73, 74], and oral nifedipine has been shown to be as effective as intravenous labetalol in the treatment of severe hypertension [71, 72, 75, 76].

The objective of the treatment is to obtain a blood pressure of between 140-150/90-100 mmHg, but try to make tension correction gradual and non-aggressive so as not to compromise utero-placental blood flow [37].

If an hypertension is resistant to first-line treatments, ACOG Committee Opinion recommends the continuous infusion of nicardipine or esmolol as a second line of treatment [71, 77 - 79]. If antihypertensive infusion is initiated, the Committee's advice is to consult a specialist in anaesthesiology, maternal-fetal medicine or intensive care to monitor second-line therapy.

In those cases of extreme emergency, the use of intravenous sodium nitroprusside is accepted, but with caution and for a short time due to the risk of increased maternal intracranial pressure and maternal and fetal toxicity from cyanide and thiocyanate [71, 78, 80, 81].

ACOG and the Safe Motherhood Initiative have developed a checklist for hypertensive emergencies, describing treatment with intravenous labetalol, or hydralazine, or short-acting oral nifedipine, which can be easily adapted to any clinical setting and does not require cardiac monitorization (Table 3) [82].

Table 3. Antihypertensive treatment, recommended dosing for SBP >160 or DBP >110.

- Labetalol (20, 40, 80 mg. IV* over 2 min, escalating doses, repeat at 10 minutes)   - Avoid in asthma or heart failure.
- Hydralazine (5-10 mg. IV* over 2 minutes, repeat at 20 minutes until target BP reached)
- Oral Nifedipine (10, 20, 40 mg. capsules, repeat BP at 20 minutes until target BP reached)   - Capsules should be administered orally, **not punctured** or otherwise administered sublingually
* Maximum cumulative iv-administered doses should not exceed 220 mg. labetalol or 25 mg. hydralazine in 24 hours

Note: if first line agents unsuccessful, emergency consult with specialist is recommended.

MANAGEMENT OF ECLAMPSIA

The incidence of eclampsia is between 1/2000 - 1/3500 pregnancies, and more than 90% of cases occur after 28 weeks of gestation [31, 83 - 85].

In the US, up to 20% of maternal deaths are due to HRD, and 50% are due to eclampsia [37, 86 - 88].

Severe acute hypertension causes vasogenic edema and leads to encephalopathy and seizures in pregnant women, as seen on brain imaging in most pregnant women with eclampsia [89 - 92].

The most common symptom preceding an eclampsia attack is headache [31, 93], and persistent occipital or frontal headache, blurred vision, photophobia, right upper quadrant/epigastric pain, or altered mental status are present in up to 75% of preeclampsia [31, 94, 95]. Eclampsia can be complicated by placental abruption, disseminated intravascular coagulation, acute renal failure, pulmonary edema, aspiration pneumonia, and cardiopulmonary arrest, and is therefore associated with high rates of maternal morbidity and mortality [83, 84].

The goals of eclampsia treatment are the prevention of recurrent attacks, prevention of maternal injury and aspiration, support of cardiopulmonary function, and avoidance of urgent delivery due to risk of fetal distress. Magnesium sulphate has been shown to be the most effective agent to prevent eclampsia and recurrent eclampsia [96 - 99].

Magnesium sulphate reduces the risk of eclampsia by more than 50% and probably reduces maternal death. However, there is no clear effect after hospital discharge. On the other hand, up to 25% of pregnant women report side effects from magnesium sulphate. The seizure rate with magnesium is 9.4%, compared with 23.1% with diazepam or phenytoin [96, 97, 100, 101]. A loading dose of 4g is administered over 15-20 minutes, followed by an infusion of 2 g./h. During this perfusion, up to 10% of patients will have a second seizure, and in these cases, an additional bolus of 2 g. can be given over 3-5 minutes.

Although magnesium administration is not recommended as prophylaxis for preeclampsia without severe features, its use is recommended as prophylaxis for eclampsia with severe features. In the case of the former, ongoing clinical evaluation to determine whether such severe features develop should guide the initiation of magnesium treatment [37].

For the following reasons, it will continue to be administered intraoperatively during the cesarean section despite the potential risk of exacerbation of uterine atony due [37, 102 - 108]:

- Half-life of magnesium is approximately 5 hours, and suspension is doubtful to have an immediate effect on uterine tone.
- Discontinuation of magnesium perfusion may result in sub-therapeutic levels in the post-partum period, increasing the risk of eclampsia.

Since magnesium excretion is renal, in the case of acute kidney injury secondary to preeclampsia and prophylactic magnesium treatment, serial deep tendon reflexes and serum magnesium levels should be assessed to monitor magnesium toxicity. Only if serum magnesium levels are toxic will admission to a critical care unit (ICU) and initiation of dialysis for magnesium removal be necessary, although this is rare [109 - 111].

RECOMMENDATIONS FOR DELIVERY

In case of preeclampsia with severe features, delivery at 34 weeks of gestation, at 37 weeks of gestation in the absence of severe features, and as an emergency in case of eclampsia, is usually recommended as a general rule.

Nevertheless, in the event of deterioration of the maternal or fetal condition, preparation for delivery at an earlier stage of gestation may be necessary. Despite the fact that the majority of women with preeclampsia have a successful vaginal delivery, the likelihood of a cesarean section is higher in these patients, regardless of gestational age or previous delivery history [112, 113].

Preterm preeclamptic women are more likely to have a cesarean section than non-preeclamptic women, whether they are nulliparous (29% *vs*. 7%) or multiparous (18% *vs*. 8%) [112 - 116]. Furthermore, those who have a prolonged labour lasting more than 24 hours followed by a cesarean section have a tenfold increased risk of adverse outcomes compared to those who have a cesarean section or planned vaginal delivery [112, 117, 118]. However, in patients with severe preeclampsia there is no strong evidence for physicians to indicate a scheduled cesarean section instead of vaginal delivery [119].

ANAESTHETIC MANAGEMENT OF PREECLAMPSIA

If the patient is admitted to a delivery room and the obstetric team is planning a delivery, the anesthesiologist should discuss her labour and delivery analgesic options with the labouring woman as soon as possible. And possibly the recommendation will be early neuraxial analgesia. Because of the increased risk of difficult airway in these patients, the presence of a functional epidural catheter for labour analgesia will offer the possibility of avoiding general anesthesia.

The approach to the patient with preeclampsia begins with the pre-anaesthesia assessment, which should be carried out in the latent phase of labour if possible. The idea of performing it at this stage is to establish the patient's baseline conditions and determine the severity of the hypertensive disorder, the baseline airway status, the hemodynamic condition, and the status of coagulation parameters. Preeclampsia is a dynamic disorder, the variables of which often change over time [120, 121].

Severe Preeclampsia, Preeclampsia without Criteria for Severity, and HELLP Syndrome

Severe preeclampsia is considered when blood pressure is ≥ 160 mmHg systolic pressure or ≥ 110 mmHg diastolic pressure, or ≥ 160 mmHg systolic or ≥110 mmHg diastolic pressure, or systolic blood pressure ≥ 140 mmHg or diastolic blood pressure ≥90 mmHg associated with severity criteria. The latter are symptoms that indicate target organ involvement, such as persistent tinnitus, global headache, persistent tinnitus, global headache, epigastralgia, scotomas, *etc* [122 - 126].

Pressure > 140/90 mmHg in the absence of the above are diagnostic of non-severe preeclampsia or without severity criteria.

HELLP syndrome, an entity inherent to preeclampsia, is considered a severe form of the pathology; it presents with impaired liver function, hemorrhagic function, haemolysis, and decreased platelet counts [32, 33, 127, 128].

In any case, once preeclampsia has been identified, a toxaemic profile is mandatory in order to guide treatment, both obstetric and anaesthetic.

This includes transaminases, serum bilirubin, creatinaemia, blood count, serum lactate dehydrogenase levels, and serum electrolytes [129 - 131].

Airway Assessment

Oedema and the tendency to bleed easily make the airway in the patient with preeclampsia into an anticipated difficult airway [33, 120, 132 - 134] and its management is beyond the scope of this review. However, equipment necessary for treatment must be available and, where possible, care should be carried out by personnel trained in this context [135].

Assessment of Hemodynamic Disturbances

The spectrum of hemodynamic disturbances in patients with preeclampsia includes hypertension, myocardial dysfunction due to a sudden increase in afterload in severe preeclampsia, myocardial damage, secondary pulmonary oedema, *etc*. The administration of fluids, antihypertensives and magnesium sulphate, among others, contributes to hemodynamic lability in these patients, modifying the severity of the pathology [136 - 139].

Coagulation

Coagulation disorders occur mainly in the context of HELLP syndrome, in which haemolysis (*LDH* > 600 U/L), thrombocytopenia (platelets < 150x109/L), and elevated hepatic transaminases (*AST* ≥ 70 U/L) occur.

HELLP patients with platelet counts < 75,000 represent a contraindication for neuraxial anaesthesia, as do other coagulation disorders, as well as other related coagulation disorders. These include consumption coagulopathy and changes in prothrombin times, thromboplastin and fibrinogen times, which may be found in severe forms of HELLP syndrome [128, 136, 140 - 143].

Hemodynamic Monitoring

Non-invasive hemodynamic monitoring is generally sufficient for the management of most patients with preeclampsia or even severe forms of HELLP syndrome [126, 128, 137, 144].

Nonetheless, there are some specific indications in which invasive monitoring using an arterial catheter, central venous line, or both is indicated [7, 145].

There is no evidence to support their use in pregnant women with preeclampsia, and the indications for placement of a central venous catheter and pulmonary artery catheter are usually quite nonspecific and similar to those in patients without hypertensive disorders. In general, the specific indications for placement of an arterial and/or central venous line are described in Table **4** [7, 145 - 147].

Table 4. Indications for invasive monitoring in patients with preeclampsia.

Arterial line indications	- Severe persistent hypertension (SBP > 160 mmHg, DBP > 110 mmHg) that is refractory to treatment - Need for vasoactive infusion - Need for frequent sampling* - Minimally invasive monitoring of hemodynamic parameters (volumeview®, FloTrac/Vigileo®, PiCCO®, *etc.*)
Indications for central venous catheter	- Difficulty of peripheral venous access - Administration of vasoactive agents - Cardiac function or preload measurement

* Particularly in patients in whom it is difficult to establish peripheral vascular access and in patients with impaired or with impaired metabolic or pulmonary function requiring frequent monitoring with arterial blood gases.

Transthoracic Echocardiography

Ultrasound is an ideal imaging method in terms of its safety for the pregnant patient and the foetus. It can be used to assess the cardiac impact of hypertensive disorder, especially in cases of severe preeclampsia with hemodynamic instability [148 - 152].

Blood Pressure Goals

Guidelines for the management of the patient with preeclampsia aim at achieve trans-operative blood pressure values < 160/110 mmHg, always with monitoring of fetal well-being for risk of uteroplacental hypoperfusion. In the post-partum period, the goal decreases to 150/100 mmHg, as the risk of intracranial hemorrhage and eclampsia is lower.

The different oral antihypertensives to be used are described in Table **5** with recommendations [73, 75, 124, 153 - 169].

Table 5. Oral antihypertensives in post-partum hypertension.

Diuretics (use to be only indicated in severe preeclampsia with water overload and with water overload and pulmonary oedema)	Hydrochlorothiazide	Thiazide diuretic. Very low risk to infants. Prolonged use may inhibit lactation, so it should be used at the lowest possible dose, especially in the first month post-partum*
	Furosemide	Loop diuretic. Low risk to the infant. May inhibit lactation*
	Spironolactone	Potassium-sparing diuretic Contraindicated during lactation due to anti-androgenic properties demonstrated in animals
Calcium receptor antagonists - Dihydropyridines. Choice in volume overload. Increase renal perfusion and diuresis. - Non-dihydropyridines. No evidence to recommend.	Nifedipine	Very low risk for infants Drug of choice in volume overload
	Nicardipine	Not recommended in lactation
	Amlodipine	Low risk to infant Not enough safety studies Prefer other antihypertensives.
Angiotensin type II receptor antagonists.	Theoretical risk in infants under two months of cerebral and renal hypoperfusion	
	Losartan	Insufficient evidence to recommend their use during lactation
Alpha-2-adrenergic agonists	May inhibit prolactin	
	Clonidine	Insufficient evidence to recommend its use during lactation
	Methyl-dopa	

(Table 5) cont.....

Angiotensin-converting enzyme inhibitors (ACE inhibitors)	Of choice in mothers with pregestational diabetes or chronic kidney disease	
	Enalapril	Very low risk to the infant
	Captopril	
Beta-adrenergic receptor blockers	Metoprolol	Very low risk to the infant
	Carvedilol	No evidence to recommend use during lactation
Alpha-1 adrenergic receptor blockers	Prazosin	Intermediate risk to the infant Not recommended during this period

Intravenous Fluid Management

There is no evidence to recommend the administration of colloids in the obstetric population, including patients with preeclampsia, so management guidelines recommend that only crystalloid solutions be used. The recommended rate of perfusion will be 80 - 100 mL/h, which is sufficient to meet the requirements of patients who do not have significant losses from active bleeding. This rate includes the contributions provided by magnesium sulphate or oxytocin infusions when required [170 - 177].

Although the pregnant woman with preeclampsia has a lower effective circulating volume, volume expansion has not been shown to improve maternal or foetal outcomes [177]. In contrast, excessive fluid administration, in addition to compromising hemodynamic lability, may trigger pulmonary oedema. Although the aetiology is usually multifactorial, iatrogenic volume overload is an important risk factor for the development of pulmonary edema. Diuretics should be reserved for cases of preeclampsia with pulmonary oedema, as they may inhibit lactation, especially when used in the first month post-partum [153, 158, 174, 178].

Obstetric Analgesia

The technique for neuraxial anaesthesia or analgesia is similar to that used in patients without hypertensive disorder. Epidural catheter insertion should ideally be done in the latent phase of labour, especially in patients with severe preeclampsia, in whom coagulation disturbances may appear abruptly [120, 121, 126, 133, 179, 180].

Neuraxial analgesia has demonstrated the best efficacy for pain control and for prevention of increased blood pressure, a phenomenon that could be related to a lower activation of the autonomic nervous system with less activation of the autonomic-bulbar-nociceptive circuit [181, 182]. The epidural technique does not increase the incidence of instrumental vaginal delivery, but it can induce a hypotensive response. Nonetheless, it is not recommended to administer fluids as a co-load in order to prevent it [37, 133, 174, 181, 183 - 185].

Different studies that have compared the neuraxial technique with intravenous analgesia have shown no statistically significant difference in major adverse events such as sustained hypotension, cesarean section rate, or decrease in neonatal Apgar score with either technique [186 - 189].

Vasopressors should be used with caution in cases of hypotension, but always using low doses in a titrated manner.

Patients with preeclampsia are more responsive to the action of catecholamines, and the hypertensive response to vasoactive drugs may be exaggerated, so lower doses of phenylephrine or ephedrine are recommended [26, 190 - 193].

ANAESTHETIC CONSIDERATIONS

Neuraxial anaesthesia is preferred over general anaesthesia as it avoids the need for anaesthetic induction, avoiding severe hypotension that can result from anaesthetic induction. The need for airway manipulation, with risk of unexpected difficult airway, sympathetic hypertensive discharge from laryngoscopy and intubation. And the use of muscle relaxants, the effects of which may be potentiated by the coadministration of magnesium sulphate. So far, studies have found no significant statistical differences with respect to maternal-fetal outcomes, so that either technique can be used [133, 179, 182, 194, 195].

Prevention of Post-Partum Hemorrhage

Although oxytocin represents the uterotonic of choice in the obstetric patient, whether or not she has a hypertensive disorder, it is not the only one [196].

Methylergonovine is contraindicated because it may induce severe hypertension and should be avoided in patients with preeclampsia [196 - 199].

Regarding carbetocin, despite the fact that it is often discouraged in preeclampsia, there is much scientific evidence addressing the safety of its use in preeclampsia and eclampsia [200 - 202]. So it could be concluded that carbetocin can be used in patients with preeclampsia and eclampsia, but they should be carefully monitored [203 - 205].

Misoprostol is an alternative that can be used in these patients with no major impact on the course of the disease or increase in blood pressure [206 - 209].

General Anaesthesia

General anaesthesia is reserved as an alternative in cases where cesarean section with neuraxial anaesthesia is contraindicated.

Contraindications for this type of anaesthesia are described in Table **6** [194, 195, 210, 211].

Table 6. Contraindications for neuraxial anaesthesia.

Absolute	- Patient refusal - Infection of the puncture site - Hypovolaemia - Blood clotting disorders - coagulation - Endocranial hypertension - Anatomical abnormalities - Sepsis
Related	- Cognitive or sensory deficits - Diseases of the central nervous - central nervous system - Aortic and subaortic stenosis - Use of low molecular weight heparin - Pre-existing neurological problems - including neuropathies

The different techniques for induction and maintenance of general anaesthesia are beyond the scope of this chapter. However, the implications of the drugs used on the foetus must always be considered along with the implications of the drugs used on the fetus, based on the half-life and the feto-maternal of the drug [212 - 218].

About 1% of pregnant women will have a gastric residual in excess than basal gastric secretion, even under adequate fasting guidelines. This value can be as high as 5% in pregnant women with obesity, so obstetric patients are considered to be at high risk for *"full stomach"*. For these reasons, the rapid intubation sequence is recommended for obstetric patients requiring termination of pregnancy by cesarean section under general anaesthesia [219 - 224].

Anaesthetic Management of Preeclampsia

When the patient is admitted to a delivery room and the obstetric team decides that she will deliver vaginally, it is prudent to explain labour analgesic options as early as possible. Neuraxial analgesia will be recommended if possible. Because of the increased difficulty of airway management secondary to pregnancy, which is also increased by preeclampsia, the presence of a functional neuraxial catheter will allow avoidance of general anesthesia [225].

The incidence of eclampsia has been shown to decrease from 42.6% to 0.62% with a standardised treatment of the PPH approach in which magnesium sulphate is administered. Maternal severe morbidity incidence also decreases from 16.7% to 2.4% [226]. Clinical and nursing staff in the labour and delivery unit should know how to mobilise local resources and promptly initiate treatment for preeclampsia since treatment should not be delayed while transport to an intensive care unit is arranged. In the event of failure to monitor blood pressure and vital organ perfusion (diuresis, mental status, lactate level) in the labour and delivery unit, early attention by an intensivist should be sought so that the patient can be rapidly transferred to a critical care unit.

Use of Magnesium Sulphate

Magnesium sulphate is an essential drug for pregnant neuroprotection in severe preeclampsia and for fetal neuroprotection in gestations below 32 weeks.

Its continuation in the postoperative period is recommended up to 24-48 hours post-partum [37, 227]. This drug potentiates the action of non-depolarising muscle relaxants, demonstrated in particular with rocuronium, vecuronium and cisatracurium [228 - 230]. So when using these muscle relaxants, it is advisable to use sugammadex to reverse them at the appropriate doses [231 - 233]. However, in most cases the administration of succinylcholine, which is exclusively necessary for intubation purposes, is sufficient in most cases [234, 235].

In any patient infused with magnesium sulphate, suggestive signs of magnesium sulphate toxicity should be monitored, especially if renal function is compromised. Signs of toxicity attributed to magnesium sulphate include loss of deep tendon reflexes (8-12 mg/dL), respiratory depression (12-16 mg/dL), cardiac conduction disturbances (>18 mg/dL), and cardiac arrest (>30 mg/dL) [236 - 238].

Treatment of Hypertensive Crisis

For emergency treatment of preeclampsia may be used IV hydralazine, IV labetalol and oral nifedipine [75, 161, 239 - 243].

Hydralazine selectively relaxes arteriolar smooth muscle, and its adverse effects include headache, nausea, hot flashes, and palpitations. The dose of hydralazine ranges from 50 to 300 mg/day, which can be divided into 2-4 doses. It is considered compatible with breast-feeding.

Labetalol is a non-selective β-blocking agent with the ability to block vascular α-1 receptors, and has demonstrated equivalent efficacy and better tolerability compared to hydralazine. Side effects include fatigue, lethargy, exercise intolerance, sleep disturbances, and bronchoconstriction. Dosage is variable, and can be used in boluses of 20 mg. to 40 mg., up to a maximum of 220 mg. It is usually considered compatible with breast-feeding.

Post-Operative Pain Management

Pain management usually requires non-opioid analgesics or minor opioids and must consider the impact of hypertensive disorders on various organ systems. The Nonsteroidal anti-inflammatory drugs (*NSAIDs*) may induce an increase in blood pressure, and are per se considered drugs with a hypertensive effect and with the potential to interfere with antihypertensive drugs' actions. For this reason, NSAIDs are not recommended for patients with preeclampsia, especially for those with severe preeclampsia and those who remain with elevated blood pressure after 24 hours post-partum [37]. Acetaminophen should be administered with caution, as it may be contraindicated in patients with impaired liver function such as in HELLP syndrome.

Role of Ultrasound and Echocardiography in Treatment

Echocardiography has proven to be a useful diagnostic tool in the management of patients with HRD. Its interpretation must take into account the structural anatomical changes that occur during pregnancy. For example, as normal pregnancy progresses, mild dilatation of the four chambers, increased thickness of the left ventricular wall, and increased mass of the left and right ventricles are common findings. All these changes are secondary to the increase in stroke volume and cardiac output that occurs during pregnancy [244, 245].

Mild valvular regurgitation of the mitral, tricuspid, and pulmonary valves is another common finding in pregnancy [244, 246]. Transient pericardial effusions that resolve in the post-partum period may be observed in up to 40% of pregnant women [247 - 250]. Nevertheless, aortic valvular regurgitation is not a normal finding and justifies further investigation [251].

Due to the elevated afterload of preeclampsia, all normal changes of pregnancy may be more pronounced, especially in preterm preeclampsia [252, 253]. In general, although women with HRD do not have impaired left ventricular ejection fraction, subclinical myocardial dysfunction, defined by worsening longitudinal, circumferential, and radial deformation, may be present [254, 255]. Moreover, there is a risk of diastolic dysfunction in these patients [256 - 260]. Echocardiography may even be a useful tool for predicting the development of preterm preeclampsia.

Echocardiography can also be used to predict the development of premature preeclampsia since women with placental insufficiency and impaired left ventricular function are more likely to develop preeclampsia [252]. Nevertheless, more studies will be needed to evaluate the predictive utility of echocardiography.

In addition to echocardiography, physicians have incorporated ultrasounds into a multitude of other assessments to guide medical management.

Ultrasounds has an important role in obstetric anaesthesia, and its correct use allows us to assess [258, 261 - 265]:

1. *Airway*: identifying women with an expected difficult airway can be used to avoid general anesthesia and to prescribe early analgesia in delivery.
2. *Gastric volume*: to identify women at increased risk of aspiration (*"full stomach"*).
3. *Intracranial hypertension*: to detect changes in optic nerve sheath diameter that occurs in preeclampsia.
4. *Vascular access*.
5. *Neuraxial and transverse abdominal blocks*.
6. *Pulmonary oedema*, as a way to guide fluid management [259]. Lung ultrasound can detect interstitial oedema in preeclampsia patients. B-lines indicate an increase in left ventricular pressure at the end of diastole [266, 267]. This is important because interstitial edema has been recognised as a phase that gives hardly any symptoms and precedes alveolar edema [268 - 271]. Early detection of interstitial fluid, as B-lines in the ultrasound image, will indicate the need for conservative fluid management.

Immediate and Long-Term Morbidity

Despite normalisation of blood pressure in the post-partum period, a small proportion of women with HRD remain at risk of adverse effects immediately after delivery [272 - 275]. These include hemorrhagic stroke, eclampsia, and peripartum cardiomyopathy [276 - 278].

It is assumed that HRD is a marker, rather than a cause, of the development of cardiovascular disease [63, 279]. Interestingly, the factors that predispose a woman to developing severe placental vascular disease are the same factors that predispose her to developing premature coronary heart disease and myocardial dysfunction [280].

The two most common cardiovascular morbidities in women with HRD are type 2 diabetes mellitus and hypertension [281, 282]. Women with a history of HRD have a five times greater risk of developing hypertension later in life than those without [283 - 285]. Similarly, when compared to uncomplicated pregnant women, women with a history of preeclampsia have twice the risk of developing ischemic heart disease, stroke, and venous thromboembolic events five to 15 years after pregnancy [272, 286]. Therefore, the American Heart Association and the European Society of Cardiology consider HRD to be a risk factor for cardiovascular disease in women [287, 288].

The ACOG Task Force on Hypertension in Pregnancy suggests measurement of blood pressure, lipids, fasting glucose and BMI in women with recurrent preeclampsia or who have given birth before 37 weeks gestation, but recommends that physicians, using their scientific judgment, weigh the interventions to be performed against the cost and discomfort to the patient [37].

After hospital discharge of women with HRD, cardiovascular follow-up should be performed to avoid the risk of future cardiovascular disease [289, 290].

Another complication that can occur immediately after delivery is an attack of eclampsia. Although most cases of eclampsia occur during delivery or within the first 48 hours, up to 25% of eclampsia attacks occur later, sometimes up to six weeks after delivery [277]. This necessitates informing patients of the risk of preeclampsia progression and/or eclampsia attack after discharge from the hospital.

Women with preeclampsia are up to 80% more likely to have an ischemic stroke [63, 279], and those with eclampsia may be at increased risk of developing a seizure disorder [291, 292]. Those with a history of preeclampsia have an altered metabolic phenotype years after delivery, with increased fasting glucose, low- and high-density lipoprotein levels, BMI, and blood pressure compared to women with uncomplicated pregnancies [242, 293].

The time between hospital discharge and the first post-partum visit, usually 6 weeks, is critical. Due to fluid shift and altered cerebral autoregulation following delivery, women may experience secondary silent hypertension that can lead to hemorrhagic stroke. With a maximum risk within 10 days of discharge [63, 276]. In some cases, readmission due to pregnancy-associated stroke in the post-partum period is sometimes the first time the patient is diagnosed with PPH.

Therefore, all post-partum women seen in the emergency department with discomfort should be evaluated and vigilant. Women with PPH typically have a transient drop in blood pressure for 48 hours after delivery, followed by a rise for 3 to 6 days [37, 294 - 296]. ACOG therefore recommends careful blood pressure monitoring until the third day after delivery and again 7 to 10 days later [37], emphasising education about post-partum preeclampsia and identification of danger signs/symptoms at discharge.

The maternal mortality ratio (*MMR*) is defined as the number of mothers who die per 100,000 births [297 - 301]. It serves as a meaningful indicator of the quality of care provided by health services to the mother and child [302, 303]. The annual MMR in the United States in 2013 was 28 maternal deaths / 100,000 births, which doubled from 12 per 100,000 in 1990 [304, 305]. This can potentially be attributed to significant increases in cesarean section rates and increasing age at conception, which, combined with the increased use of assisted reproductive technologies, may result in higher-risk pregnancies in patients of advanced reproductive age who are more likely to have comorbidities [306]. In 2008, the MMR in developing countries was 15 times higher than in developed countries [302, 303, 307, 308]. This discrepancy can be attributed to inadequate follow-up, lack of appropriate health services, and significantly worse living conditions in these countries [307].

In 2009, the World Health Organisation (*WHO*) introduced the terms *"near misses"*, *"Severe Maternal Morbidity"* (*SMM*) and *"Severe Associated Maternal Morbidity"* (*SAMM*) to indicate the advanced level of care required for critically ill patients [309 - 311]. The prevalence of these cases was estimated at 12.9 cases per 1,000 deliveries and 2.9 cases per 1,000 post-partum hospitalisations [312, 313]. The number of admissions to the Critical Care Unit (*CCU*) has been proposed as an indicator of maternal health quality [306, 313]. The respective admissions have been reported to range from 0.5 to 4.2 per 1,000 deliveries in developed countries [306, 314 - 316].

INTENSIVE CARE MANAGEMENT

The vast majority of pregnancies do not present major complications upon completion. Advances in global medical care and increased access to health systems have resulted in a significant decrease in maternal mortality around the world [317 - 319]. However, a limited proportion of pregnancies and deliveries present a wide range of complications that may require admission to a critical care unit (*CCU*), including post-surgery reanimation units, intensive care units (*ICU*), and high dependency units (*HDU*). The altered physiology during pregnancy, the potentially dangerous effects of certain drugs, and the limitations of certain interventions due to the need to take into account the effects on the foetus [314, 315, 320 - 322]. Hemorrhagic conditions, hypertensive disease, and sepsis are considered to be the predominant complications that can result in death [317, 319].

A key factor to consider for patients who end up in a CCU is the relative lack of experience in the management of these unique conditions on the part of the professionals involved. For this reason, the creation of specialised obstetric critical care units and the training of a multidisciplinary team that is aware of the need to manage critically ill pregnant and post-partum patients with complications has been suggested [323]. Critical care during pregnancy and post-partum is mainly based on recommendations derived from the critical care of non-pregnant patients, due to the limited data available on critically ill obstetric patients [312 - 314, 324].

Most patients admitted to CCU for obstetric complications require non-invasive monitoring and recovery support. Therefore, the provision of a dedicated intermediate care unit for obstetric cases may be beneficial for these patients to alleviate or reduce stress [319, 325]. An experienced and specialised obstetrician should lead the unit and be responsible for final decisions on patient management, based on consultation with other specialists, including anaesthesiologists and intensivists.

Family medicine specialists and neonatologists should also be part of the multidisciplinary team whenever possible. Diagnostic and care algorithms based on underlying pathology and admission indications require the contribution of such a multidisciplinary team. This is of utmost importance to improving early identification of at-risk patients in the CCU, and may help to decide the type of CCU to which each critically ill patient is admitted [312, 326]. The above modalities can not only improve the level of care for all patients, but also mitigate healthcare costs by reducing unnecessary admissions [318, 319, 325].

The proportion of pregnant patients admitted to the CCU ranged from 3.3% to 14%, with the lowest rates observed in developed countries with well-organised healthcare systems [327]. From 63 to 92% of the patients admitted to the CCU were in the post-partum period, and the mean length of stay in the CCU for women admitted before and after delivery was 2 and 1.1 days, respectively [324]. Finally, it has been shown that approximately 50% of maternal deaths can be prevented by early recognition and intervention in critically ill patients requiring admission to a CCU [10, 319].

In order to reduce maternal morbi-mortality, levels of maternal care are constantly being improved to ensure that women are provided with the necessary care during the peripartum period. According to the levels of maternity care proposed by the UK Department of Health, the care that pregnant receive in the delivery room is stratified into 4 levels according to the support and interventions required [318, 328]:

- *Level 0*: care for low-risk women in the general ward.
- *Level 1*: care requiring observation and non-invasive monitoring of the patient.
- *Level 2*: a single organ support is required, including cardiovascular, respiratory, neurological or hepatic support.
- *Level 3*: refers to women requiring mechanical ventilation for respiratory support or support of two or more organs.

The above levels can be used to decide which ward a woman with complications is admitted to, as follows [318, 328]:

- *Level 0*: patients are admitted to the general ward.
- *Levels 1 and 2*: patients are admitted to the HDU.
- *Level 3*: patients should be cared for in the ICU.

Excluding gynaecologists and obstetricians, specialists from other areas of medicine may not be as familiar with the physiological changes inherent to pregnancy, and therefore the degree of severity may be underestimated. It is therefore essential that the HDU include obstetricians, anaesthetists, specialists in maternal-fetal medicine, neonatologists, midwives, and physiotherapists. For the ICU, a multidisciplinary team is also of utmost importance for an integrated and precise approach [312, 313, 329]. In particular, the management of the obstetric patient requires knowledge of the physiology of two patients (mother and foetus [274, 314 - 316, 320, 321], because Preeclampsia is the main cause of perinatal morbi-mortality [319, 330] and, in the case of critically ill patients, the collaboration of different specialists is necessary, including anaesthesiologists, intensivists, obstetricians/gynecologists, maternal-fetal medicine (*MFM*) specialists, and neonatologists [133, 306, 312].

Patients admitted to the CCU may have obstetric and non-obstetric conditions that require continuous monitoring (invasive and non-invasive) and additional interventions (Table **7**).

Table 7. Primary indications for admission to an intensive care unit in obstetric patients.

Obstetric indication		Non-obstetric indications				
		Pre-existing diseases potentially worsened in pregnancy		High risk conditions due to pregnancy		Unrelated to pregnancy coincidental conditions
Hypertensive related pregnancy diseases	Preeclampsia Eclampsia HELLP syndrome	Autoimmune diseases Myasthenia Gravis	Systemic lupus erythematosus Autoimmune thyroiditis	Infections	Pyelonephritis Pneumonia	Trauma/car accident

(Table 7) cont.....

Obstetric indication		Non-obstetric indications					
Hemorrhagic conditions	Antepartum Post-partum Ectopic pregnancy	Cardiovascular diseases	Hypertension Vascular heart diseases Pulmonary hypertension Cardiomyopathies Arrhythmias (AF/flutter) Congenital heart disease Cardiogenic pulmonary edema/shock	Thromboembolic disease	Pulmonary embolism Deep vein thrombosis	Appendicitis
Genitourinary Infection/ sepsis	Embolism of amniotic fluid Cardiomyopathy of peripartum period Acute fatty liver of pregnancy	Neurological diseases Systemic diseases	Endometritis Chorioamnionitis	Pulmonary diseases	Asthma	Cholecystitis
Other conditions			Epilepsy Diabetes mellitus			Rupture of intracranial aneurysm

HELLP, haemolysis, elevated liver enzymes, and low platelet.

Non-obstetric conditions that may be complicated and worsen during pregnancy include immunological diseases (systemic lupus erythematosus, myasthenia gravis, and autoimmune thyroiditis), cardiovascular diseases (hypertension, valvular heart disease, pulmonary arterial hypertension, cardiomyopathies, arrhythmias, and congenital heart disease), respiratory and neurological conditions (such as asthma and epilepsy) and systemic diseases (such as diabetes mellitus).

In contrast, non-obstetric conditions associated with pregnancy can be attributed to the physiological and anatomical changes that accompany pregnancy, infectious diseases (pyelonephritis and pneumonia), thromboembolic diseases (deep vein thrombosis and pulmonary embolism), and pulmonary oedema. Finally, some additional diseases that may occur during pregnancy but are coincidental causes of admission to the CCU are trauma, appendicitis, cholecystitis, and viral infections, such as H1N1 or SARS-CoV-2 virus infection [326, 327, 331].

Obstetric indications for admission to a CCU are hypertensive disorders of pregnancy, which include preeclampsia and eclampsia, and haemolysis, elevated liver enzymes and low platelet count (HELLP syndrome), which are considered the most frequent causes of admission to a CCU in pregnant women [332 - 336]. Both represent severe conditions that can have adverse effects on maternal and foetal health, and are associated with significantly high morbidity and mortality rates. HELLP syndrome can mimic a host of non-obstetric disorders [337, 338]. Diagnosis is based on clinical symptoms, such as hypertension (up to 15% of patients with HELLP syndrome have normal blood pressure), discomfort, nausea, and epigastric pain [127, 339], and laboratory findings of microangiopathic haemolysis (schistocytes, peripheral swear, low serum hemoglobin, and elevated lactate dehydrogenase), elevated levels of serum glutamic-oxalacetic transaminase/serum glutamic-pyruvic transaminase (up to 70 IU/l) and low platelets (<100,000/μl) [127, 337, 338].

In addition, eclampsia is the most severe manifestation of pregnancy hypertensive disorders and is defined as the occurrence of tonic-clonic, focal or multifocal seizures in the absence of other causative conditions such as epilepsy, cerebral arterial ischaemia and infarction, intracranial hemorrhage or drug use [340 - 342]. Injectable magnesium sulphate is used to prevent eclampsia due to neuromuscular blockade or central action. The use of magnesium requires monitoring for potential toxicity, including observation of urine output, vital signs, and respiratory rate, as well as patellar reflex response and monitoring of serum magnesium levels, which physiologically range between 4 and 7 mEq/l [333]. Magnesium toxicity, which can occur with high magnesium levels, is another indication for admission to the CCU, and dialysis may be necessary to remove magnesium [109, 237, 343, 344]. For critically ill patients with preeclampsia, fluid management plays a key role [171, 173, 314, 316, 321].

A strict fluid balance must be maintained to simultaneously limit the risk of pulmonary oedema, potentially caused by fluid overload, and renal failure, which may be caused by volume restriction [120, 133]. Some studies have proposed a rate of 80 ml/h of intravenous fluid administration, although there is insufficient evidence for this [133]. The final treatment for the above conditions is to deliver the baby as soon as possible, taking into account the viability of the foetus and the possibility of administering corticosteroids to ensure lung maturation [319, 337].

Massive hemorrhage and subsequent hypovolemic shock are also considered a major cause of admission to the CCU in the obstetric population. Massive hemorrhage can occur both during the antepartum period, mainly due to rupture of an ectopic pregnancy, placental abruption or pathological invasion of the placenta (placenta accreta), and during the post-partum period [337]. Post-partum hemorrhage (*PPH*), described in depth in chapter 13, is a major cause of maternal mortality [319, 332, 333].

Major obstetric hemorrhage is defined as blood loss of more than 1,500 ml of blood, or blood loss with signs of shock [345 - 347]. Atonic uterus is the main cause of PPH and is attributed to the "*4 T*" rule: Tone, Trauma, Remnant placental tissue, and Thrombin [348 - 354]. Due to the severity of the patient's underlying condition, continuous monitoring of vital signs and transfusion of blood products is recommended in cases where hemoglobin levels are < 8 g/dL or in patients with coagulation disorders, to ensure hemodynamic stability.

Additional interventions should be used to control the cause of bleeding, including oxytocin 10 U/h, ergometrine 0.5 mg by intravenous or intramuscular injections, and misoprostol rectally (maximum dose 800 mg) combined with uterine massage. The above treatments are considered the optimal modalities for the management of a patient with an atonic uterus and hemorrhage, who is at risk of hypovolemic shock and collapse [355, 356]. If these approaches fail, removal of the uterine artery and hysterectomy by cesarean section are the last resort used to prevent maternal death from severe hemorrhage [357 - 361].

Amniotic fluid embolism (*AFE*) or anaphylactic syndrome of pregnancy is a rare but serious condition associated with significantly high mortality rates of approximately 80%. The pathogenic pathway involves an anaphylactoid inflammatory response to fetal antigens, which occurs due to disruption of the maternal-fetal barrier during delivery and results in increased pulmonary and/or systemic vascular resistance, decreased left ventricular function and coagulopathy. The patient presents with clinical signs of respiratory failure, cardiogenic shock with severe hypoxia, hemodynamic collapse, and coagulopathy [362 - 364]. There is no standard approach to the diagnosis of the disease, and in most cases the diagnosis is based on clinical signs and symptoms [365, 366]. Treatment of AFE is mainly supportive, and includes cardiopulmonary resuscitation, administration of fluids and blood products to correct intravenous coagulopathy, anticoagulant agents, and oxygen support or mechanical ventilation in the case of respiratory failure [362, 367].

To determine the optimal course of management of a woman with obstetric complications and to help decide which group of patients should be admitted to any type of CCU, it is crucial to develop a prognostic and predictive model.

Given their usefulness in non-obstetric patients, established scoring systems such as the Acute Physiological and Chronic Health Evaluation (*APACHE II*), the Sequential Organ Functional Assessment (*SOFA*), the Simplified Acute Physiology Score II (*SAPS II*) and the Mortality Prediction Model (*MPM*) have also been proposed for the assessment of critically ill obstetric populations [368, 369].

The mortality rates predicted by APACHE II, SAPS II and MPM II scores of obstetric patients admitted to intensive care were comparable to those of age-matched non-obstetric patients [370].

The Sepsis in Obstetric Specific score (*SOS*) is a validated pregnancy-specific score to identify the risk of CCU admission for sepsis, with a cut-off score of 6 that has a negative predictive value of 98.6% [371, 372]. A score below 6 excludes the need for intensive care admission [372, 373]. But no differences have been found using the SOS to predict the outcome of septic obstetric patients compared to the performance of the sepsis score in non-obstetric populations [371].

Therefore, although the exact roles of the scoring systems in predicting mortality are still under investigation, and despite their widespread use as a complementary tool, none of the scoring systems has proven to be useful.

This is because physiological changes that occur during pregnancy, including increased heart rate, changes in white blood cell count, and decreased creatinine levels, may result in higher calculated rates in the APACHE scoring system and thus an overestimation of the probability of mortality [331, 368, 369]. In addition to this, the significant improvements that patients show after delivery in most of the parameters assessed are another critical factor that may complicate the estimation of the risk of death and outcome after delivery [368].

The Obstetric Early Warning Score (*OEWS*) has been reported as the most accurate score for estimating the outcome of an obstetric patient in a CCU [374, 375]. The variables taken into account in the calculation of the new clinical OEWS consist of classic early warning signs, such as systolic and diastolic blood pressure, heart and respiratory rate, Fraction of inspired Oxygen (*FiO2*) required to maintain SpO_2 >96 and body temperature in °C, as well as the consciousness level with the mode of delivery (either cesarean or vaginal).

Available evidence shows that this score is able to predict survival in critically ill obstetric patients, which is also confirmed by the American College of Obstetrics and Gynecology and the Royal College of Obstetrics and Gynecology. This suggests that the OEWS is the best available scoring system for this particular patient population [10, 324]. Despite the benefits of OEWS in the obstetric population, its impact on mortality reduction is still inconclusive and further studies are needed [376, 377].

Despite the importance of the above-mentioned scores in predicting the outcome of patients admitted to CCU, their role in patient management remains complementary, and final decisions must combine the wishes of patients and relatives as well as physicians' judgement on the individual case [368, 378, 379].

CONCLUSION

The management of patients with preeclampsia should be multidisciplinary and should be carried out in centres with the necessary technical and human resources to deal with the complications of preeclampsia.

The anaesthetic approach is aimed at providing practices that maintain the mother-infant binomial. Adequate pre-anaesthetic assessment and an early anaesthetic approach are necessary to prevent complications.

Obstetric analgesia techniques can provide an improvement in the hemodynamic pattern, including improvement in blood pressure. There are no significant short-term differences between the anaesthetic techniques available so far.

When general anaesthesia is used, difficult airway management and the risk of aspiration of the pregnant woman must be considered. Analgesic management in the post-partum period must take into account the multi-organ disturbances that can occur in the context of hypertensive disorder, especially in those patients with severe preeclampsia and HELLP syndrome.

CONSENT FOR PUBLICATION

Not applicable.

CONFLICT OF INTEREST

The authors declare no conflict of interest, financial or otherwise.

ACKNOWLEDGEMENT

Declared none.

REFERENCES

[1]   Wallis AB, Saftlas AF, Hsia J, Atrash HK. Secular trends in the rates of preeclampsia, eclampsia, and gestational hypertension, United States, 1987-2004. Am J Hypertens 2008; 21(5): 521-6.
[http://dx.doi.org/10.1038/ajh.2008.20] [PMID: 18437143]

[2]   Knight M. Preeclampsia: increasing incidence but improved outcome? Am J Hypertens 2008; 21(5): 491.
[http://dx.doi.org/10.1038/ajh.2008.33] [PMID: 18437137]

[3]   Duley L. Maternal mortality associated with hypertensive disorders of pregnancy in Africa, Asia, Latin America and the Caribbean. BJOG 1992; 99(7): 547-53.
[http://dx.doi.org/10.1111/j.1471-0528.1992.tb13818.x] [PMID: 1525093]

[4]   Ronsmans C, Campbell O. Quantifying the fall in mortality associated with interventions related to hypertensive diseases of pregnancy. BMC Public Health 2011; 11 (Suppl. 3): S8.
[http://dx.doi.org/10.1186/1471-2458-11-S3-S8] [PMID: 21501459]

[5]   Abalos E, Cuesta C, Carroli G, *et al.* Pre-eclampsia, eclampsia and adverse maternal and perinatal outcomes: a secondary analysis of the World Health Organization Multicountry Survey on Maternal and Newborn Health. BJOG 2014; 121 (Suppl. 1): 14-24.
[http://dx.doi.org/10.1111/1471-0528.12629] [PMID: 24641531]

[6]   Callaghan WM, MacKay AP, Berg CJ. Identification of severe maternal morbidity during delivery hospitalizations, United States, 1991-2003. Am J Obstet Gynecol 2008; 199(2): 133.e1-8.
[http://dx.doi.org/10.1016/j.ajog.2007.12.020] [PMID: 18279820]

[7]   Martin JN Jr, Thigpen BD, Moore RC, Rose CH, Cushman J, May W. Stroke and severe preeclampsia and eclampsia: a paradigm shift focusing on systolic blood pressure. Obstet Gynecol 2005; 105(2): 246-54.
[http://dx.doi.org/10.1097/01.AOG.0000151116.84113.56] [PMID: 15684147]

[8]   Cunningham FG. Severe preeclampsia and eclampsia: systolic hypertension is also important. Obstet Gynecol 2005; 105(2): 237-8.
[http://dx.doi.org/10.1097/01.AOG.0000153144.05885.fa] [PMID: 15684145]

[9]   Demir SC, Evruke C, Ozgunen FT, Urunsak IF, Candan E, Kadayifci O. Factors that influence morbidity and mortality in severe preeclampsia, eclampsia and hemolysis, elevated liver enzymes, and low platelet count syndrome. Saudi Med J 2006; 27(7): 1015-8.
[PMID: 16830022]

[10]   Cantwell R, Clutton-Brock T, Cooper G, *et al.* Saving Mothers' Lives: Reviewing maternal deaths to make motherhood safer: 2006-2008. BJOG 2011; 118 (Suppl. 1): 1-203.
[http://dx.doi.org/10.1111/j.1471-0528.2010.02847.x] [PMID: 21356004]

[11]   Berg CJ, Harper MA, Atkinson SM, *et al.* Preventability of pregnancy-related deaths: results of a state-wide review. Obstet Gynecol 2005; 106(6): 1228-34.
[http://dx.doi.org/10.1097/01.AOG.0000187894.71913.e8] [PMID: 16319245]

[12]   Geller SE, Cox SM, Kilpatrick SJ. A descriptive model of preventability in maternal morbidity and mortality. J Perinatol 2006; 26(2): 79-84.
[http://dx.doi.org/10.1038/sj.jp.7211432] [PMID: 16407964]

[13]   Geller SE, Cox SM, Callaghan WM, Berg CJ. Morbidity and mortality in pregnancy. Womens Health Issues 2006; 16(4): 176-88.
[http://dx.doi.org/10.1016/j.whi.2006.06.003] [PMID: 16920522]

[14]   Clark SL, Belfort MA, Dildy GA, Herbst MA, Meyers JA, Hankins GD. Maternal death in the 21st century: causes, prevention, and relationship to cesarean delivery. Am J Obstet Gynecol. julio de 2008; 199(1): 36.e1-5.

[15]   Kuklina EV, Ayala C, Callaghan WM. Hypertensive disorders and severe obstetric morbidity in the United States. Obstet Gynecol 2009; 113(6): 1299-306.
[http://dx.doi.org/10.1097/AOG.0b013e3181a45b25] [PMID: 19461426]

[16]   Ji L, Brkić J, Liu M, Fu G, Peng C, Wang YL. Placental trophoblast cell differentiation: Physiological regulation and pathological relevance to preeclampsia. Mol Aspects Med 2013; 34(5): 981-1023.
[http://dx.doi.org/10.1016/j.mam.2012.12.008] [PMID: 23276825]

[17]   Red-Horse K, Zhou Y, Genbacev O, *et al.* Trophoblast differentiation during embryo implantation and formation of the maternal-fetal interface. J Clin Invest 2004; 114(6): 744-54.
[http://dx.doi.org/10.1172/JCI200422991] [PMID: 15372095]

[18]   Acar N, Ustunel I, Demir R. Uterine natural killer (uNK) cells and their missions during pregnancy: A review. Acta Histochem 2011; 113(2): 82-91.
[http://dx.doi.org/10.1016/j.acthis.2009.12.001] [PMID: 20047753]

[19]   Bachmayer N, Rafik Hamad R, Liszka L, Bremme K, Sverremark-Ekström E. Aberrant uterine natural killer (NK)-cell expression and altered placental and serum levels of the NK-cell promoting cytokine interleukin-12 in pre-eclampsia. Am J Reprod Immunol Microbiol 2006; 56(5-6): 292-301.
[http://dx.doi.org/10.1111/j.1600-0897.2006.00429.x] [PMID: 17076673]

[20]   Wallace AE, Host AJ, Whitley GS, Cartwright JE. Decidual natural killer cell interactions with trophoblasts are impaired in pregnancies at increased risk of preeclampsia. Am J Pathol 2013; 183(6): 1853-61.
[http://dx.doi.org/10.1016/j.ajpath.2013.08.023] [PMID: 24103555]

[21]   Perez-Sepulveda A, Torres MJ, Khoury M, Illanes SE. Innate immune system and preeclampsia. Front Immunol 2014; 5: 244.
[http://dx.doi.org/10.3389/fimmu.2014.00244] [PMID: 24904591]

[22]   Vargas-Rojas MI, Solleiro-Villavicencio H, Soto-Vega E. Th1, Th2, Th17 and Treg levels in umbilical cord blood in preeclampsia. J Matern Fetal Neonatal Med 2016; 29(10): 1642-5.
[http://dx.doi.org/10.3109/14767058.2015.1057811] [PMID: 26135758]

[23]   Saito S, Nakashima A, Shima T, Ito M. Th1/Th2/Th17 and regulatory T-cell paradigm in pregnancy. Am J Reprod Immunol 2010; 63(6): 601-10.
[http://dx.doi.org/10.1111/j.1600-0897.2010.00852.x] [PMID: 20455873]

[24]   Sammar M, Siwetz M, Meiri H, Sharabi-Nov A, Altevogt P, Huppertz B. Reduced Placental CD24 in Preterm Preeclampsia Is an Indicator for a Failure of Immune Tolerance. Int J Mol Sci 2021; 22(15): 8045.
[http://dx.doi.org/10.3390/ijms22158045] [PMID: 34360811]

[25]   Reslan OM, Khalil RA. Molecular and vascular targets in the pathogenesis and management of the hypertension associated with preeclampsia. Cardiovasc Hematol Agents Med Chem 2010; 8(4): 204-26.
[http://dx.doi.org/10.2174/187152510792481234] [PMID: 20923405]

[26]   Qu H, Khalil RA. Vascular mechanisms and molecular targets in hypertensive pregnancy and preeclampsia. Am J Physiol Heart Circ Physiol 2020; 319(3): H661-81.
[http://dx.doi.org/10.1152/ajpheart.00202.2020] [PMID: 32762557]

[27]   Cox B. Bioinformatic approach to the genetics of preeclampsia. Obstet Gynecol 2014; 124(3): 633.
[http://dx.doi.org/10.1097/AOG.0000000000000436] [PMID: 25162267]

[28]   van Dijk M, Oudejans CBM. STOX1: Key player in trophoblast dysfunction underlying early onset preeclampsia with growth retardation. J Pregnancy 2011; 2011: 1-7.
[http://dx.doi.org/10.1155/2011/521826] [PMID: 21490791]

[29]   Wang X, Wu H, Qiu X. Methylenetetrahydrofolate reductase (MTHFR) gene C677T polymorphism and risk of preeclampsia: an updated meta-analysis based on 51 studies. Arch Med Res 2013; 44(3): 159-68.
[http://dx.doi.org/10.1016/j.arcmed.2013.01.011] [PMID: 23395424]

[30]   Xia X, Chang W, Cao Y. Meta-analysis of the methylenetetrahydrofolate reductase C677T polymorphism and susceptibility to pre-eclampsia. Hypertens Res 2012; 35(12): 1129-34.
[http://dx.doi.org/10.1038/hr.2012.117] [PMID: 22914556]

[31]   Sibai BM. Diagnosis, prevention, and management of eclampsia. Obstet Gynecol 2005; 105(2): 402-10.
[http://dx.doi.org/10.1097/01.AOG.0000152351.13671.99] [PMID: 15684172]

[32]   Wallace K, Harris S, Addison A, Bean C. HELLP Syndrome: Pathophysiology and Current Therapies. Curr Pharm Biotechnol 2018; 19(10): 816-26.
[http://dx.doi.org/10.2174/1389201019666180712115215] [PMID: 29998801]

[33]   del-Rio-Vellosillo M, Garcia-Medina JJ. Anesthetic considerations in HELLP syndrome. Acta Anaesthesiol Scand 2016; 60(2): 144-57.

[http://dx.doi.org/10.1111/aas.12639] [PMID: 26446688]

[34]   Padden MO. HELLP syndrome: recognition and perinatal management. Am Fam Physician 1999; 60(3): 829-836, 839.
[PMID: 10498110]

[35]   Barton JR, Sibai BM. Diagnosis and management of hemolysis, elevated liver enzymes, and low platelets syndrome. Clin Perinatol 2004; 31(4): 807-833, vii.
[http://dx.doi.org/10.1016/j.clp.2004.06.008] [PMID: 15519429]

[36]   Douglas KA, Redman CWG. Eclampsia in the United Kingdom. BMJ 1994; 309(6966): 1395-400.
[http://dx.doi.org/10.1136/bmj.309.6966.1395] [PMID: 7819845]

[37]   Hypertension in pregnancy. report of the american college of obstetricians and gynecologists' task force on hypertension in pregnancy. Obstet Gynecol 2013; 122(5): 1122-31.
[PMID: 24150027]

[38]   Pauli JM, Repke JT. Pitfalls With the New American College of Obstetricians and Gynecologists Task Force on Hypertension in Pregnancy. Clin Obstet Gynecol 2017; 60(1): 141-52.
[http://dx.doi.org/10.1097/GRF.0000000000000247] [PMID: 27977436]

[39]   Menzies J, Magee LA, MacNab YC, *et al.* Current CHS and NHBPEP criteria for severe preeclampsia do not uniformly predict adverse maternal or perinatal outcomes. Hypertens Pregnancy 2007; 26(4): 447-62.
[http://dx.doi.org/10.1080/10641950701521742] [PMID: 18066963]

[40]   Weiler J, Tong S, Palmer KR. Is fetal growth restriction associated with a more severe maternal phenotype in the setting of early onset pre-eclampsia? A retrospective study. PLoS One 2011; 6(10): e26937.
[http://dx.doi.org/10.1371/journal.pone.0026937] [PMID: 22046419]

[41]   Gruslin A, Lemyre B. Pre-eclampsia: Fetal assessment and neonatal outcomes. Best Pract Res Clin Obstet Gynaecol 2011; 25(4): 491-507.
[http://dx.doi.org/10.1016/j.bpobgyn.2011.02.004] [PMID: 21474384]

[42]   Lisonkova S, Sabr Y, Mayer C, Young C, Skoll A, Joseph KS. Maternal morbidity associated with early-onset and late-onset preeclampsia. Obstet Gynecol 2014; 124(4): 771-81.
[http://dx.doi.org/10.1097/AOG.0000000000000472] [PMID: 25198279]

[43]   Engineer N, Kumar S. Perinatal variables and neonatal outcomes in severely growth restricted preterm fetuses. Acta Obstet Gynecol Scand 2010; 89(9): 1174-81.
[http://dx.doi.org/10.3109/00016349.2010.501370] [PMID: 20804344]

[44]   Venkatesh KK, Strauss RA, Westreich DJ, Thorp JM, Stamilio DM, Grantz KL. Adverse maternal and neonatal outcomes among women with preeclampsia with severe features <34 weeks gestation with *versus* without comorbidity. Pregnancy Hypertens 2020; 20: 75-82.
[http://dx.doi.org/10.1016/j.preghy.2020.03.006] [PMID: 32193149]

[45]   Sibai BM. Preeclampsia as a cause of preterm and late preterm (near-term) births. Semin Perinatol 2006; 30(1): 16-9.
[http://dx.doi.org/10.1053/j.semperi.2006.01.008] [PMID: 16549208]

[46]   English FA, Kenny LC, McCarthy FP. Risk factors and effective management of preeclampsia. Integr Blood Press Control 2015; 8: 7-12.
[PMID: 25767405]

[47]   Chaemsaithong P, Sahota DS, Poon LC. First trimester preeclampsia screening and prediction. Am J Obstet Gynecol. 16 de julio de 2020; S0002-9378(20): 30741-9.

[48]   Mission JF, Marshall NE, Caughey AB. Obesity in Pregnancy. Obstet Gynecol Surv 2013; 68(5): 389-99.
[http://dx.doi.org/10.1097/OGX.0b013e31828738ce] [PMID: 23624964]

[49] Mission JF, Marshall NE, Caughey AB. Pregnancy risks associated with obesity. Obstet Gynecol Clin North Am 2015; 42(2): 335-53.
[http://dx.doi.org/10.1016/j.ogc.2015.01.008] [PMID: 26002170]

[50] Overcash RT, Lacoursiere DY. The clinical approach to obesity in pregnancy. Clin Obstet Gynecol 2014; 57(3): 485-500.
[http://dx.doi.org/10.1097/GRF.0000000000000042] [PMID: 25022997]

[51] O'Brien TE, Ray JG, Chan WS. Maternal body mass index and the risk of preeclampsia: a systematic overview. Epidemiology 2003; 14(3): 368-74.
[http://dx.doi.org/10.1097/01.EDE.0000059921.71494.D1] [PMID: 12859040]

[52] Kriebs JM. Obesity as a complication of pregnancy and labor. J Perinat Neonatal Nurs 2009; 23(1): 15-22.
[http://dx.doi.org/10.1097/JPN.0b013e318197bf1b] [PMID: 19209055]

[53] Bujold E, Roberge S, Lacasse Y, et al. Prevention of preeclampsia and intrauterine growth restriction with aspirin started in early pregnancy: a meta-analysis. Obstet Gynecol 2010; 116(2): 402-14.
[http://dx.doi.org/10.1097/AOG.0b013e3181e9322a] [PMID: 20664402]

[54] Roberge S, Nicolaides K, Demers S, Hyett J, Chaillet N, Bujold E. The role of aspirin dose on the prevention of preeclampsia and fetal growth restriction: systematic review and meta-analysis. Am J Obstet Gynecol 2017; 216(2): 110-120.e6.
[http://dx.doi.org/10.1016/j.ajog.2016.09.076] [PMID: 27640943]

[55] Bergeron T, Roberge S, Carpentier C, Sibai B, McCaw-Binns A, Bujold E. Prevention of Preeclampsia with Aspirin in Multiple Gestations: A Systematic Review and Meta-analysis. Am J Perinatol 2016; 33(6): 605-10.
[http://dx.doi.org/10.1055/s-0035-1570381] [PMID: 26731178]

[56] Roberge S, Bujold E, Nicolaides KH. Aspirin for the prevention of preterm and term preeclampsia: systematic review and metaanalysis. Am J Obstet Gynecol 2018; 218(3): 287-293.e1.
[http://dx.doi.org/10.1016/j.ajog.2017.11.561] [PMID: 29138036]

[57] Roberge S, Sibai B, McCaw-Binns A, Bujold E. low-dose aspirin in early gestation for prevention of preeclampsia and small-for-gestational-age neonates: meta-analysis of large randomized trials. Am J Perinatol 2016; 33(8): 781-5.
[http://dx.doi.org/10.1055/s-0036-1572495] [PMID: 26906184]

[58] Wu P, Jordan KP, Chew-Graham CA, et al. Temporal Trends in Pregnancy-Associated Stroke and Its Outcomes Among Women With Hypertensive Disorders of Pregnancy. J Am Heart Assoc 2020; 9(15): e016182.
[http://dx.doi.org/10.1161/JAHA.120.016182] [PMID: 32750300]

[59] Judy AE, McCain CL, Lawton ES, Morton CH, Main EK, Druzin ML. Systolic Hypertension, Preeclampsia-Related Mortality, and Stroke in California. Obstet Gynecol 2019; 133(6): 1151-9.
[http://dx.doi.org/10.1097/AOG.0000000000003290] [PMID: 31135728]

[60] Main EK, McCain CL, Morton CH, Holtby S, Lawton ES. Pregnancy-Related Mortality in California. Obstet Gynecol 2015; 125(4): 938-47.
[http://dx.doi.org/10.1097/AOG.0000000000000746] [PMID: 25751214]

[61] Yoneyama K, Sekiguchi A, Matsushima T, et al. Pregnancy-associated Deaths: 31-year Experience. J Nippon Med Sch 2016; 83(1): 6-14.
[http://dx.doi.org/10.1272/jnms.83.6] [PMID: 26960583]

[62] Leffert LR, Clancy CR, Bateman BT, Bryant AS, Kuklina EV. Hypertensive disorders and pregnancy-related stroke: frequency, trends, risk factors, and outcomes. Obstet Gynecol 2015; 125(1): 124-31.
[http://dx.doi.org/10.1097/AOG.0000000000000590] [PMID: 25560114]

[63] Camargo EC, Singhal AB. Stroke in Pregnancy. Obstet Gynecol Clin North Am 2021; 48(1): 75-96.
[http://dx.doi.org/10.1016/j.ogc.2020.11.004] [PMID: 33573791]

[64]   Moatti Z, Gupta M, Yadava R, Thamban S. A review of stroke and pregnancy: incidence, management and prevention. Eur J Obstet Gynecol Reprod Biol 2014; 181: 20-7.
[http://dx.doi.org/10.1016/j.ejogrb.2014.07.024] [PMID: 25124706]

[65]   van Veen TR, Panerai RB, Haeri S, *et al.* Cerebral autoregulation in different hypertensive disorders of pregnancy. Am J Obstet Gynecol 2015; 212(4): 513.e1-7.
[http://dx.doi.org/10.1016/j.ajog.2014.11.003] [PMID: 25446701]

[66]   Elgendy IY, Bukhari S, Barakat AF, Pepine CJ, Lindley KJ, Miller EC. Maternal Stroke. Circulation 2021; 143(7): 727-38.
[http://dx.doi.org/10.1161/CIRCULATIONAHA.120.051460] [PMID: 33587666]

[67]   https://www.cmqcc.org/resources-tool-kits/toolkits/preeclampsia-toolkit

[68]   Bernstein PS, Martin JN Jr, Barton JR, *et al.* Consensus Bundle on Severe Hypertension During Pregnancy and the Postpartum Period. J Midwifery Womens Health 2017; 62(4): 493-501.
[http://dx.doi.org/10.1111/jmwh.12647] [PMID: 28697534]

[69]   Clark SL, Hankins GDV. Preventing maternal death: 10 clinical diamonds. Obstet Gynecol 2012; 119(2, Part 1): 360-4.
[http://dx.doi.org/10.1097/AOG.0b013e3182411907] [PMID: 22270288]

[70]   Bernstein PS, Martin JN Jr, Barton JR, *et al.* National Partnership for Maternal Safety. Anesth Analg 2017; 125(2): 540-7.
[http://dx.doi.org/10.1213/ANE.0000000000002304] [PMID: 28696959]

[71]   McCoy S, Baldwin K. Pharmacotherapeutic options for the treatment of preeclampsia. Am J Health Syst Pharm 2009; 66(4): 337-44.
[http://dx.doi.org/10.2146/ajhp080104] [PMID: 19202042]

[72]   Magee LA. Oral nifedipine or intravenous labetalol for severe hypertension? BJOG 2016; 123(1): 48.
[http://dx.doi.org/10.1111/1471-0528.13494] [PMID: 26119227]

[73]   Abalos E, Duley L, Steyn DW, Gialdini C. Antihypertensive drug therapy for mild to moderate hypertension during pregnancy. Cochrane Libr 2018; 2018(10): CD002252.
[http://dx.doi.org/10.1002/14651858.CD002252.pub4] [PMID: 30277556]

[74]   Duley L, Meher S, Jones L. Drugs for treatment of very high blood pressure during pregnancy. Cochrane Libr 2013; (7): CD001449.
[http://dx.doi.org/10.1002/14651858.CD001449.pub3] [PMID: 23900968]

[75]   Shekhar S, Gupta N, Kirubakaran R, Pareek P. Oral nifedipine *versus* intravenous labetalol for severe hypertension during pregnancy: a systematic review and meta-analysis. BJOG 2016; 123(1): 40-7.
[http://dx.doi.org/10.1111/1471-0528.13463] [PMID: 26113232]

[76]   Wasim T, Agha S, Saeed K, Riaz A. Oral Nifidepine *versus* IV labetalol in severe preeclampsia: A randomized control trial. Pak J Med Sci 2020; 36(6): 1147-52.
[http://dx.doi.org/10.12669/pjms.36.6.2591] [PMID: 32968371]

[77]   ACOG committee opinion no. 767 summary: emergent therapy for acute-onset, severe hypertension during pregnancy and the post-partum period. Obstet Gynecol 2019; 133(2): 409-12.
[PMID: 30681541]

[78]   Wani-Parekh P, Blanco-Garcia C, Mendez M, Mukherjee D. Guide of Hypertensive Crisis Pharmacotherapy. Cardiovasc Hematol Disord Drug Targets 2017; 17(1): 52-7.
[PMID: 28000548]

[79]   Curran MP, Robinson DM, Keating GM. Intravenous Nicardipine. Drugs 2006; 66(13): 1755-82.
[http://dx.doi.org/10.2165/00003495-200666130-00010] [PMID: 16978041]

[80]   Too GT, Hill JB. Hypertensive crisis during pregnancy and postpartum period. Semin Perinatol 2013; 37(4): 280-7.
[http://dx.doi.org/10.1053/j.semperi.2013.04.007] [PMID: 23916027]

[81]   Sass N, Itamoto CH, Silva MP, Torloni MR, Atallah ÁN. Does sodium nitroprusside kill babies? A systematic review. Sao Paulo Med J 2007; 125(2): 108-11.
[http://dx.doi.org/10.1590/S1516-31802007000200008] [PMID: 17625709]

[82]   ACOG. Patient safety bundle: hypertension 2015. https://ilpqc.org/wp-content/docs/htn/ACOGDIISlideSet/ACOGDII_HTN SlideSetNov2015Updated.pdf

[83]   Fong A, Chau CT, Pan D, Ogunyemi DA. Clinical morbidities, trends, and demographics of eclampsia: a population-based study. Am J Obstet Gynecol 2013; 209(3): 229.e1-7.
[http://dx.doi.org/10.1016/j.ajog.2013.05.050] [PMID: 23727516]

[84]   Liu S, Joseph KS, Liston RM, *et al.* Incidence, risk factors, and associated complications of eclampsia. Obstet Gynecol 2011; 118(5): 987-94.
[http://dx.doi.org/10.1097/AOG.0b013e31823311c1] [PMID: 22015865]

[85]   Fishel Bartal M, Sibai BM. Eclampsia in the 21st century. Am J Obstet Gynecol. 24 de septiembre de 2020; S0002-9378(20): 31128-5.

[86]   Butwick AJ, Druzin ML, Shaw GM, Guo N. Evaluation of US State–Level Variation in Hypertensive Disorders of Pregnancy. JAMA Netw Open 2020; 3(10): e2018741.
[http://dx.doi.org/10.1001/jamanetworkopen.2020.18741] [PMID: 33001203]

[87]   ACOG Practice Bulletin No. 203: Chronic Hypertension in Pregnancy. Obstet Gynecol 2019; 133(1): e26-50.
[http://dx.doi.org/10.1097/AOG.0000000000003020] [PMID: 30575676]

[88]   Sutton ALM, Harper LM, Tita ATN. Hypertensive Disorders in Pregnancy. Obstet Gynecol Clin North Am 2018; 45(2): 333-47.
[http://dx.doi.org/10.1016/j.ogc.2018.01.012] [PMID: 29747734]

[89]   Zeeman GG, Fleckenstein JL, Twickler DM, Cunningham FG. Cerebral infarction in eclampsia. Am J Obstet Gynecol 2004; 190(3): 714-20.
[http://dx.doi.org/10.1016/j.ajog.2003.09.015] [PMID: 15042004]

[90]   y W, M M, y T, *et al.* Eclamptic encephalopathy: MRI, including diffusion-weighted images. Neuroradiology 2002; 44(12): 981-5.
[http://dx.doi.org/10.1007/s00234-002-0867-y] [PMID: 12483442]

[91]   Takeuchi M, Matsuzaki K, Harada M, Nishitani H, Matsuda T. Cerebral hyperperfusion in a patient with eclampsia with perfusion-weighted magnetic resonance imaging. Radiat Med 2005; 23(5): 376-9.
[PMID: 16342911]

[92]   Loureiro R, Leite CC, Kahhale S, *et al.* Diffusion imaging may predict reversible brain lesions in eclampsia and severe preeclampsia: initial experience. Am J Obstet Gynecol 2003; 189(5): 1350-5.
[http://dx.doi.org/10.1067/S0002-9378(03)00651-3] [PMID: 14634567]

[93]   Negro A, Delaruelle Z, Ivanova TA, *et al.* Headache and pregnancy: a systematic review. J Headache Pain 2017; 18(1): 106.
[http://dx.doi.org/10.1186/s10194-017-0816-0] [PMID: 29052046]

[94]   Phipps EA, Thadhani R, Benzing T, Karumanchi SA. Pre-eclampsia: pathogenesis, novel diagnostics and therapies. Nat Rev Nephrol 2019; 15(5): 275-89.
[http://dx.doi.org/10.1038/s41581-019-0119-6] [PMID: 30792480]

[95]   Mol BWJ, Roberts CT, Thangaratinam S, Magee LA, de Groot CJM, Hofmeyr GJ. Pre-eclampsia. Lancet 2016; 387(10022): 999-1011.
[http://dx.doi.org/10.1016/S0140-6736(15)00070-7] [PMID: 26342729]

[96]   Duley L, Henderson-Smart DJ, Walker GJ, Chou D. Magnesium sulphate *versus* diazepam for eclampsia. Cochrane Database Syst Rev 2010; (12): CD000127.
[PMID: 21154341]

[97]   Duley L, Gülmezoglu AM, Henderson-Smart DJ, Chou D. Magnesium sulphate and other

anticonvulsants for women with pre-eclampsia. Cochrane Libr 2010; (11): CD000025.
[http://dx.doi.org/10.1002/14651858.CD000025.pub2] [PMID: 21069663]

[98] Noor S, Halimi M, Faiz NR, Gull F, Akbar N. Magnesium sulphate in the prophylaxis and treatment of eclampsia. J Ayub Med Coll Abbottabad 2004; 16(2): 50-4.
[PMID: 15455618]

[99] Sibai BM. Magnesium sulfate prophylaxis in preeclampsia: lessons learned from recent trials. Am J Obstet Gynecol 2004; 190(6): 1520-6.
[http://dx.doi.org/10.1016/j.ajog.2003.12.057] [PMID: 15284724]

[100] Duley L, Gülmezoglu AM, Chou D. Magnesium sulphate *versus* lytic cocktail for eclampsia. Cochrane Libr 2010; (9): CD002960.
[http://dx.doi.org/10.1002/14651858.CD002960.pub2] [PMID: 20824833]

[101] Duley L, Henderson-Smart DJ, Chou D. Magnesium sulphate *versus* phenytoin for eclampsia. Cochrane Database Syst Rev 2010; (10): CD000128.
[PMID: 20927719]

[102] Taber EB, Tan L, Chao CR, Beall MH, Ross MG. Pharmacokinetics of ionized *versus* total magnesium in subjects with preterm labor and preeclampsia. Am J Obstet Gynecol 2002; 186(5): 1017-21.
[http://dx.doi.org/10.1067/mob.2002.122421] [PMID: 12015530]

[103] Scardo JA, Hogg BB, Newman RB. Favorable hemodynamic effects of magnesium sulfate in preeclampsia. Am J Obstet Gynecol 1995; 173(4): 1249-53.
[http://dx.doi.org/10.1016/0002-9378(95)91364-5] [PMID: 7485331]

[104] Yoshida M, Matsuda Y, Akizawa Y, Ono E, Ohta H. Serum ionized magnesium during magnesium sulfate administration for preterm labor and preeclampsia. Eur J Obstet Gynecol Reprod Biol 2006; 128(1-2): 125-8.
[http://dx.doi.org/10.1016/j.ejogrb.2005.10.036] [PMID: 16337073]

[105] Pergialiotis V, Bellos I, Constantinou T, *et al.* Magnesium sulfate and risk of postpartum uterine atony and hemorrhage: A meta-analysis. Eur J Obstet Gynecol Reprod Biol 2021; 256: 158-64.
[http://dx.doi.org/10.1016/j.ejogrb.2020.11.005] [PMID: 33246200]

[106] Ende HB, Lozada MJ, Chestnut DH, *et al.* risk factors for atonic postpartum hemorrhage. obstet gynecol 2021; 137(2): 305-23.
[http://dx.doi.org/10.1097/AOG.0000000000004228] [PMID: 33417319]

[107] Pippen JL, Adesomo AA, Gonzalez-Brown VM, Schneider PD, Rood KM. Interrupted *versus* continuous magnesium sulfate and blood loss at cesarean delivery. J Matern Fetal Neonatal Med 2020; 1-7.
[http://dx.doi.org/10.1080/14767058.2020.1841162] [PMID: 33179549]

[108] Miller EMS, Sakowicz A, Leger E, Lange E, Yee LM. association between receipt of intrapartum magnesium sulfate and postpartum hemorrhage. ajp rep 2021; 11(1): e21-5.
[http://dx.doi.org/10.1055/s-0040-1721671] [PMID: 33542857]

[109] McDonnell NJ, Muchatuta NA, Paech MJ. Acute magnesium toxicity in an obstetric patient undergoing general anaesthesia for caesarean delivery. Int J Obstet Anesth 2010; 19(2): 226-31.
[http://dx.doi.org/10.1016/j.ijoa.2009.09.009] [PMID: 20219345]

[110] Cavell GF, Bryant C, Jheeta S. Iatrogenic magnesium toxicity following intravenous infusion of magnesium sulfate: risks and strategies for prevention. BMJ Case Rep 2015; 2015: bcr2015209499.
[http://dx.doi.org/10.1136/bcr-2015-209499] [PMID: 26231187]

[111] Bain ES, Middleton PF, Crowther CA. Maternal adverse effects of different antenatal magnesium sulphate regimens for improving maternal and infant outcomes: a systematic review. BMC Pregnancy Childbirth 2013; 13(1): 195.
[http://dx.doi.org/10.1186/1471-2393-13-195] [PMID: 24139447]

[112] Kim LH, Cheng YW, Delaney S, Jelin AC, Caughey AB. Is preeclampsia associated with an increased risk of cesarean delivery if labor is induced? J Matern Fetal Neonatal Med 2010; 23(5): 383-8.
[http://dx.doi.org/10.3109/14767050903168432] [PMID: 19951010]

[113] Pretscher J, Weiss C, Dammer U, *et al.* Influence of Preeclampsia on Induction of Labor at Term: A Cohort Study. In Vivo 2020; 34(3): 1195-200.
[http://dx.doi.org/10.21873/invivo.11892] [PMID: 32354909]

[114] Roland C, Warshak CR, DeFranco EA. Success of labor induction for pre-eclampsia at preterm and term gestational ages. J Perinatol 2017; 37(6): 636-40.
[http://dx.doi.org/10.1038/jp.2017.31] [PMID: 28358381]

[115] Suzuki S. The benefit of labor induction for preeclampsia beyond 37 weeks' gestation. J Matern Fetal Neonatal Med 2010; 23(9): 1072.
[http://dx.doi.org/10.3109/14767050903449928] [PMID: 20803815]

[116] Xenakis E, Piper J, Field N, Conway D, Langer O. Preeclampsia: Is induction of labor more successful? Obstet Gynecol 1997; 89(4): 600-3.
[http://dx.doi.org/10.1016/S0029-7844(97)00043-4] [PMID: 9083320]

[117] Levine LD, Elovitz MA, Limaye M, Sammel MD, Srinivas SK. Induction, labor length and mode of delivery: the impact on preeclampsia-related adverse maternal outcomes. J Perinatol 2016; 36(9): 713-7.
[http://dx.doi.org/10.1038/jp.2016.84] [PMID: 27195978]

[118] Bowers K, Kawakita T. maternal and neonatal outcomes of induction of labor compared with planned cesarean delivery in women with preeclampsia at 34 weeks' gestation or longer. am J perinatol 2018; 35(1): 095-102.
[http://dx.doi.org/10.1055/s-0037-1606185] [PMID: 28838008]

[119] Amorim MMR, Souza ASR, Katz L. Planned caesarean section *versus* planned vaginal birth for severe pre-eclampsia. Cochrane Libr 2017; 2017(10): CD009430.
[http://dx.doi.org/10.1002/14651858.CD009430.pub2] [PMID: 29058762]

[120] Dennis AT. Management of pre-eclampsia: issues for anaesthetists. Anaesthesia 2012; 67(9): 1009-20.
[http://dx.doi.org/10.1111/j.1365-2044.2012.07195.x] [PMID: 22731893]

[121] Lambert G, Brichant JF, Hartstein G, Bonhomme V, Dewandre PY. Preeclampsia: an update. Acta Anaesthesiol Belg 2014; 65(4): 137-49.
[PMID: 25622379]

[122] Rey E, LeLorier J, Burgess E, Lange IR, Leduc L. Report of the Canadian Hypertension Society Consensus Conference: 3. Pharmacologic treatment of hypertensive disorders in pregnancy. CMAJ 1997; 157(9): 1245-54.
[PMID: 9361646]

[123] Coppage K, Sibai B. Treatment of hypertensive complications in pregnancy. Curr Pharm Des 2005; 11(6): 749-57.
[http://dx.doi.org/10.2174/1381612053381864] [PMID: 15777230]

[124] Dymara-Konopka W, Laskowska M, Oleszczuk J. Preeclampsia - Current Management and Future Approach. Curr Pharm Biotechnol 2018; 19(10): 786-96.
[http://dx.doi.org/10.2174/1389201019666180925120109] [PMID: 30255751]

[125] Witcher PM. Preeclampsia: Acute Complications and Management Priorities. AACN Adv Crit Care 2018; 29(3): 316-26.
[http://dx.doi.org/10.4037/aacnacc2018710] [PMID: 30185498]

[126] Hofmeyr R, Matjila M, Dyer R. Preeclampsia in 2017: Obstetric and Anaesthesia Management. Baillieres Best Pract Res Clin Anaesthesiol 2017; 31(1): 125-38.
[http://dx.doi.org/10.1016/j.bpa.2016.12.002] [PMID: 28625300]

[127] Dusse LM, Alpoim PN, Silva JT, Rios DRA, Brandão AH, Cabral ACV. Revisiting HELLP syndrome 2015.
[http://dx.doi.org/10.1016/j.cca.2015.10.024]

[128] Haram K, Svendsen E, Abildgaard U. The HELLP syndrome: Clinical issues and management. A Review. BMC Pregnancy Childbirth 2009; 9(1): 8.
[http://dx.doi.org/10.1186/1471-2393-9-8] [PMID: 19245695]

[129] National Collabourating Centre for Women's and Children's Health (UK). 2010. http://www.ncbi.nlm.nih.gov/books /NBK62652/

[130] Marik PE. Hypertensive disorders of pregnancy. Postgrad Med 2009; 121(2): 69-76.
[http://dx.doi.org/10.3810/pgm.2009.03.1978] [PMID: 19332964]

[131] Deak TM, Moskovitz JB. Hypertension and Pregnancy. Emerg Med Clin North Am 2012; 30(4): 903-17.
[http://dx.doi.org/10.1016/j.emc.2012.08.006] [PMID: 23137402]

[132] Izci B, Riha RL, Martin SE, *et al.* The upper airway in pregnancy and pre-eclampsia. Am J Respir Crit Care Med 2003; 167(2): 137-40.
[http://dx.doi.org/10.1164/rccm.200206-590OC] [PMID: 12411285]

[133] Russell R. Preeclampsia and the anaesthesiologist: current management. Curr Opin Anaesthesiol 2020; 33(3): 305-10.
[http://dx.doi.org/10.1097/ACO.0000000000000835] [PMID: 32049882]

[134] Gogarten W. Preeclampsia and anaesthesia. Curr Opin Anaesthesiol 2009; 22(3): 347-51.
[http://dx.doi.org/10.1097/ACO.0b013e32832a1d05] [PMID: 19318931]

[135] Frerk C, Mitchell VS, McNarry AF, *et al.* Difficult Airway Society 2015 guidelines for management of unanticipated difficult intubation in adults † †This Article is accompanied by Editorials aev298 and aev404. Br J Anaesth 2015; 115(6): 827-48.
[http://dx.doi.org/10.1093/bja/aev371] [PMID: 26556848]

[136] Estcourt LJ, Malouf R, Hopewell S, Doree C, Van Veen J. Use of platelet transfusions prior to lumbar punctures or epidural anaesthesia for the prevention of complications in people with thrombocytopenia. Cochrane Libr 2018; 2018(4): CD011980.
[http://dx.doi.org/10.1002/14651858.CD011980.pub3] [PMID: 29709077]

[137] Thilaganathan B, Kalafat E. Cardiovascular System in Preeclampsia and Beyond. Hypertension 2019; 73(3): 522-31.
[http://dx.doi.org/10.1161/HYPERTENSIONAHA.118.11191] [PMID: 30712425]

[138] Rana S, Lemoine E, Granger JP, Karumanchi SA. Preeclampsia. Circ Res 2019; 124(7): 1094-112.
[http://dx.doi.org/10.1161/CIRCRESAHA.118.313276] [PMID: 30920918]

[139] Paauw ND, Lely AT. Cardiovascular Sequels During and After Preeclampsia. Adv Exp Med Biol 2018; 1065: 455-70.
[http://dx.doi.org/10.1007/978-3-319-77932-4_28] [PMID: 30051401]

[140] Ning S, Kerbel B, Callum J, Lin Y. Safety of lumbar punctures in patients with thrombocytopenia. Vox Sang 2016; 110(4): 393-400.
[http://dx.doi.org/10.1111/vox.12381] [PMID: 26831046]

[141] Osmanağaoğlu MA, Topçuoğlu K, Özeren M, Bozkaya H. Coagulation inhibitors in preeclamptic pregnant women. Arch Gynecol Obstet 2005; 271(3): 227-30.
[http://dx.doi.org/10.1007/s00404-003-0596-4] [PMID: 14735372]

[142] Valera MC, Parant O, Vayssiere C, Arnal JF, Payrastre B. Physiologic and pathologic changes of platelets in pregnancy. Platelets 2010; 21(8): 587-95.
[http://dx.doi.org/10.3109/09537104.2010.509828] [PMID: 20873962]

[143] Leduc L, Wheeler JM, Kirshon B, Mitchell P, Cotton DB. Coagulation profile in severe preeclampsia.

Obstet Gynecol 1992; 79(1): 14-8.
[PMID: 1727573]

[144]   Scardo J, Kiser R, Dillon A, Brost B, Newman R. Hemodynamic comparison of mild and severe preeclampsia: concept of stroke systemic vascular resistance index. J Matern Fetal Neonatal Med 1996; 5(5): 268-72.
[http://dx.doi.org/10.3109/14767059609025433] [PMID: 8930798]

[145]   Nuttall G, Burckhardt J, Hadley A, *et al*. Surgical and Patient Risk Factors for Severe Arterial Line Complications in Adults. Anesthesiology 2016; 124(3): 590-7.
[http://dx.doi.org/10.1097/ALN.0000000000000967] [PMID: 26640979]

[146]   Li YH, Novikova N. Pulmonary artery flow catheters for directing management in pre-eclampsia. Cochrane Libr 2012; (6): CD008882.
[http://dx.doi.org/10.1002/14651858.CD008882.pub2] [PMID: 22696380]

[147]   Bolte AC, Dekker GA, van Eyck J, van Schijndel RS, van Geijn HP. Lack of agreement between central venous pressure and pulmonary capillary wedge pressure in preeclampsia. Hypertens Pregnancy 2000; 19(3): 261-71.
[http://dx.doi.org/10.1081/PRG-100101987] [PMID: 11118399]

[148]   Dennis AT. Transthoracic echocardiography in obstetric anaesthesia and obstetric critical illness. Int J Obstet Anesth 2011; 20(2): 160-8.
[http://dx.doi.org/10.1016/j.ijoa.2010.11.007] [PMID: 21315578]

[149]   Plaat F, Wray S. Role of the anaesthetist in obstetric critical care. Best Pract Res Clin Obstet Gynaecol 2008; 22(5): 917-35.
[http://dx.doi.org/10.1016/j.bpobgyn.2008.06.006] [PMID: 18723402]

[150]   Bateman RM, Sharpe MD, Jagger JE, *et al*. 36th International Symposium on Intensive Care and Emergency Medicine. Crit Care 2016; 20(S2) (Suppl. 2): 94.
[http://dx.doi.org/10.1186/s13054-016-1208-6] [PMID: 27885969]

[151]   Regitz-Zagrosek V, Roos-Hesselink JW, Bauersachs J, *et al*. 2018 ESC Guidelines for the management of cardiovascular diseases during pregnancy. Kardiol Pol 2019; 77(3): 245-326.
[http://dx.doi.org/10.5603/KP.2019.0049] [PMID: 30912108]

[152]   Griffiths SE, Waight G, Dennis AT. Focused transthoracic echocardiography in obstetrics. BJA Educ 2018; 18(9): 271-6.
[http://dx.doi.org/10.1016/j.bjae.2018.06.001] [PMID: 33456844]

[153]   Ferrazzani S, De Carolis S, Pomini F, Testa AC, Mastromarino C, Caruso A. The duration of hypertension in the puerperium of preeclamptic women: Relationship with renal impairment and week of delivery. Am J Obstet Gynecol 1994; 171(2): 506-12.
[http://dx.doi.org/10.1016/0002-9378(94)90290-9] [PMID: 8059832]

[154]   Raheem IA, Saaid R, Omar SZ, Tan PC. Oral nifedipine *versus* intravenous labetalol for acute blood pressure control in hypertensive emergencies of pregnancy: a randomised trial. BJOG 2012; 119(1): 78-85.
[http://dx.doi.org/10.1111/j.1471-0528.2011.03151.x] [PMID: 21985500]

[155]   Amaral LM, Wallace K, Owens M, LaMarca B. Pathophysiology and Current Clinical Management of Preeclampsia. Curr Hypertens Rep 2017; 19(8): 61.
[http://dx.doi.org/10.1007/s11906-017-0757-7] [PMID: 28689331]

[156]   Kattah AG, Garovic VD. The management of hypertension in pregnancy. Adv Chronic Kidney Dis 2013; 20(3): 229-39.
[http://dx.doi.org/10.1053/j.ackd.2013.01.014] [PMID: 23928387]

[157]   Ascarelli MH, Johnson V, McCreary H, Cushman J, May WL, Martin JN Jr. Postpartum preeclampsia management with furosemide: a randomized clinical trial. Obstet Gynecol 2005; 105(1): 29-33.
[http://dx.doi.org/10.1097/01.AOG.0000148270.53433.66] [PMID: 15625138]

[158] Sibai BM, Mercer BM, Schiff E, Friedman SA. Aggressive *versus* expectant management of severe preeclampsia at 28 to 32 weeks' gestation: A randomized controlled trial. Am J Obstet Gynecol 1994; 171(3): 818-22.
[http://dx.doi.org/10.1016/0002-9378(94)90104-X] [PMID: 8092235]

[159] Ahn HK, Nava-Ocampo AA, Han JY, *et al.* Exposure to amlodipine in the first trimester of pregnancy and during breastfeeding. Hypertens Pregnancy 2007; 26(2): 179-87.
[http://dx.doi.org/10.1080/10641950701204554] [PMID: 17469008]

[160] Kernaghan D, Duncan AC, McKay GA. Hypertension in pregnancy: a review of therapeutic options. Obstet Med 2012; 5(2): 44-9.
[http://dx.doi.org/10.1258/om.2011.110061] [PMID: 27579135]

[161] Firoz T, Magee LA, MacDonell K, *et al.* Oral antihypertensive therapy for severe hypertension in pregnancy and postpartum: a systematic review. BJOG 2014; 121(10): 1210-8.
[http://dx.doi.org/10.1111/1471-0528.12737] [PMID: 24832366]

[162] Clark SM, Dunn HE, Hankins GDV. A review of oral labetalol and nifedipine in mild to moderate hypertension in pregnancy. Semin Perinatol 2015; 39(7): 548-55.
[http://dx.doi.org/10.1053/j.semperi.2015.08.011] [PMID: 26344738]

[163] Sridharan K, Sequeira RP. Drugs for treating severe hypertension in pregnancy: a network meta-analysis and trial sequential analysis of randomized clinical trials. Br J Clin Pharmacol 2018; 84(9): 1906-16.
[http://dx.doi.org/10.1111/bcp.13649] [PMID: 29974489]

[164] Naden RP, Redman CWG. Antihypertensive drugs in pregnancy. Clin Perinatol 1985; 12(3): 521-38.
[http://dx.doi.org/10.1016/S0095-5108(18)30853-4] [PMID: 2865023]

[165] Rosenthal T, Oparil S. The effect of antihypertensive drugs on the fetus. J Hum Hypertens 2002; 16(5): 293-8.
[http://dx.doi.org/10.1038/sj.jhh.1001400] [PMID: 12082488]

[166] Vest AR, Cho LS. Hypertension in Pregnancy. Cardiol Clin 2012; 30(3): 407-23.
[http://dx.doi.org/10.1016/j.ccl.2012.04.005] [PMID: 22813366]

[167] Ghanem FA, Movahed A. Use of antihypertensive drugs during pregnancy and lactation. Cardiovasc Ther 2008; 26(1): 38-49.
[PMID: 18466419]

[168] Beardmore KS, Morris JM, Gallery EDM. Excretion of antihypertensive medication into human breast milk: a systematic review. Hypertens Pregnancy 2002; 21(1): 85-95.
[http://dx.doi.org/10.1081/PRG-120002912] [PMID: 12044345]

[169] James PR, Nelson-Piercy C. Management of hypertension before, during, and after pregnancy. Heart 2004; 90(12): 1499-504.
[http://dx.doi.org/10.1136/hrt.2004.035444] [PMID: 15547046]

[170] McDonald S, Fernando R, Ashpole K, Columb M. Maternal cardiac output changes after crystalloid or colloid coload following spinal anesthesia for elective cesarean delivery: a randomized controlled trial. Anesth Analg 2011; 113(4): 803-10.
[http://dx.doi.org/10.1213/ANE.0b013e31822c0f08] [PMID: 21890886]

[171] Anthony J, Schoeman LK. Fluid management in pre-eclampsia. Obstet Med 2013; 6(3): 100-4.
[http://dx.doi.org/10.1177/1753495X13486896] [PMID: 27708700]

[172] Engelhardt T, MacLennan FM. Fluid management in pre-eclampsia. Int J Obstet Anesth 1999; 8(4): 253-9.
[http://dx.doi.org/10.1016/S0959-289X(99)80106-X] [PMID: 15321120]

[173] Pretorius T, van Rensburg G, Dyer RA, Biccard BM. The influence of fluid management on outcomes in preeclampsia: a systematic review and meta-analysis. Int J Obstet Anesth 2018; 34: 85-95.

[http://dx.doi.org/10.1016/j.ijoa.2017.12.004] [PMID: 29398426]

[174] Ripollés Melchor J, Espinosa Á, Martínez Hurtado E, *et al.* Colloids *versus* crystalloids in the prevention of hypotension induced by spinal anesthesia in elective cesarean section. A systematic review and meta-analysis. Minerva Anestesiol 2015; 81(9): 1019-30.
[PMID: 25501602]

[175] Loubert C. Fluid and vasopressor management for Cesarean delivery under spinal anesthesia: Continuing Professional Development. Can J Anaesth 2012; 59(6): 604-19.
[http://dx.doi.org/10.1007/s12630-012-9705-9] [PMID: 22528166]

[176] Duley L, Williams J, Henderson-Smart DJ. Plasma volume expansion for treatment of women with pre-eclampsia. Cochrane Database Syst Rev 2000; (2): CD001805.
[PMID: 10796272]

[177] Ganzevoort W, Rep A, Bonsel GJ, *et al.* A randomised controlled trial comparing two temporising management strategies, one with and one without plasma volume expansion, for severe and early onset pre-eclampsia. BJOG 2005; 112(10): 1358-68.
[http://dx.doi.org/10.1111/j.1471-0528.2005.00687.x] [PMID: 16167938]

[178] Williams D. Pre-eclampsia and long-term maternal health. Obstet Med 2012; 5(3): 98-104.
[http://dx.doi.org/10.1258/om.2012.120013] [PMID: 27582864]

[179] Dhariwal NK, Lynde GC. update in the management of patients with preeclampsia. anesthesiol clin 2017; 35(1): 95-106.
[http://dx.doi.org/10.1016/j.anclin.2016.09.009] [PMID: 28131123]

[180] Sobhy S, Dharmarajah K, Arroyo-Manzano D, *et al.* Type of obstetric anesthesia administered and complications in women with preeclampsia in low- and middle-income countries: A systematic review. Hypertens Pregnancy 2017; 36(4): 326-36.
[http://dx.doi.org/10.1080/10641955.2017.1389951] [PMID: 29125378]

[181] Jones L, Othman M, Dowswell T, *et al.* Pain management for women in labour: an overview of systematic reviews. Cochrane Database Syst Rev 2012; (3): CD009234.
[PMID: 22419342]

[182] Henke VG, Bateman BT, Leffert LR. Focused review: spinal anesthesia in severe preeclampsia. Anesth Analg 2013; 117(3): 686-93.
[http://dx.doi.org/10.1213/ANE.0b013e31829eeef5] [PMID: 23868886]

[183] Beilin Y, Katz DJ. Analgesia use among 984 women with preeclampsia: A retrospective observational single-center study. J Clin Anesth 2020; 62: 109741.
[http://dx.doi.org/10.1016/j.jclinane.2020.109741] [PMID: 32062527]

[184] Anim-Somuah M, Smyth RMD, Cyna AM, Cuthbert A. Epidural *versus* non-epidural or no analgesia for pain management in labour. Cochrane Libr 2018; 2018(5): CD000331.
[http://dx.doi.org/10.1002/14651858.CD000331.pub4] [PMID: 29781504]

[185] Hofmeyr GJ, Cyna AM, Middleton P. Prophylactic intravenous preloading for regional analgesia in labour. Cochrane Libr 2004; (4): CD000175.
[http://dx.doi.org/10.1002/14651858.CD000175.pub2] [PMID: 15494990]

[186] Patel P, Desai P, Gajjar F. Labor epidural analgesia in pre-eclampsia: A prospective study. J Obstet Gynaecol Res 2005; 31(4): 291-5.
[http://dx.doi.org/10.1111/j.1447-0756.2005.00290.x] [PMID: 16018774]

[187] Head BB, Owen J, Vincent RD Jr, Shih G, Chestnut DH, Hauth JC. A randomized trial of intrapartum analgesia in women with severe preeclampsia. Obstet Gynecol 2002; 99(3): 452-7.
[PMID: 11864673]

[188] Halpern SH, Muir H, Breen TW, *et al.* A multicenter randomized controlled trial comparing patient-controlled epidural with intravenous analgesia for pain relief in labor. Anesth Analg 2004; 99(5): 1532-8.

[http://dx.doi.org/10.1213/01.ANE.0000136850.08972.07] [PMID: 15502060]

[189] El-Kerdawy H, Farouk A. Labor analgesia in preeclampsia: remifentanil patient controlled intravenous analgesia *versus* epidural analgesia. Middle East J Anaesthesiol 2010; 20(4): 539-45.
[PMID: 20394251]

[190] van Wijk MJ, Boer K, van der Meulen ET, Bleker OP, Spaan JAE, VanBavel E. Resistance artery smooth muscle function in pregnancy and preeclampsia. Am J Obstet Gynecol 2002; 186(1): 148-54.
[http://dx.doi.org/10.1067/mob.2002.119184] [PMID: 11810101]

[191] Clark VA, Sharwood-Smith GH, Stewart AVG. Ephedrine requirements are reduced during spinal anaesthesia for caesarean section in preeclampsia. Int J Obstet Anesth 2005; 14(1): 9-13.
[http://dx.doi.org/10.1016/j.ijoa.2004.08.002] [PMID: 15627532]

[192] Wimalasundera RC, Thom SAM, Regan L, Hughes AD. Effects of vasoactive agents on intracellular calcium and force in myometrial and subcutaneous resistance arteries isolated from preeclamptic, pregnant, and nonpregnant woman. Am J Obstet Gynecol 2005; 192(2): 625-32.
[http://dx.doi.org/10.1016/j.ajog.2004.07.040] [PMID: 15696013]

[193] Chooi C, Cox JJ, Lumb RS, *et al.* Techniques for preventing hypotension during spinal anaesthesia for caesarean section. Cochrane Database Syst Rev 2020; 7: CD002251.
[PMID: 32619039]

[194] Wallace D, Leveno KJ, Cunningham FG, Giesecke AH, Shearer VE, Sidawi JE. Randomized comparison of general and regional anesthesia for cesarean delivery in pregnancies complicated by severe preeclampsia. Obstet Gynecol 1995; 86(2): 193-9.
[http://dx.doi.org/10.1016/0029-7844(95)00139-I] [PMID: 7617349]

[195] Visalyaputra S, Rodanant O, Somboonviboon W, Tantivitayatan K, Thienthong S, Saengchote W. Spinal *versus* epidural anesthesia for cesarean delivery in severe preeclampsia: a prospective randomized, multicenter study. Anesth Analg 2005; 101(3): 862-8.
[http://dx.doi.org/10.1213/01.ANE.0000160535.95678.34] [PMID: 16116005]

[196] Balki M, Wong CA. Refractory uterine atony: still a problem after all these years. Int J Obstet Anesth 2021; 48: 103207.
[http://dx.doi.org/10.1016/j.ijoa.2021.103207] [PMID: 34391025]

[197] Preeclampsia, HELLP and eclampsia [Internet]. Clinical Pain Advisor. 2019 [citado 1 de septiembre de 2021]. Disponible en: https://www.clinicalpainadvisor.com/home/decision-support--n-medicine/anesthesiology/preeclampsia-hellp-and-eclampsia

[198] Turner J. Diagnosis and management of pre-eclampsia: an update. Int J Womens Health 2010; 2: 327-37.
[http://dx.doi.org/10.2147/IJWH.S8550] [PMID: 21151680]

[199] Rath W. Prevention of postpartum haemorrhage with the oxytocin analogue carbetocin. Eur J Obstet Gynecol Reprod Biol 2009; 147(1): 15-20.
[http://dx.doi.org/10.1016/j.ejogrb.2009.06.018] [PMID: 19616358]

[200] Reyes OA, Gonzalez GM. Carbetocin *versus* oxytocin for prevention of postpartum hemorrhage in patients with severe preeclampsia: a double-blind randomized controlled trial. J Obstet Gynaecol Can 2011; 33(11): 1099-104.
[http://dx.doi.org/10.1016/S1701-2163(16)35077-0] [PMID: 22082783]

[201] Nucci B, Aya AGM, Aubry E, Ripart J. Carbetocin for prevention of postcesarean hemorrhage in women with severe preeclampsia: a before-after cohort comparison with oxytocin. J Clin Anesth 2016; 35: 321-5.
[http://dx.doi.org/10.1016/j.jclinane.2016.08.017] [PMID: 27871550]

[202] Pisani I, Tiralongo GM, Gagliardi G, *et al.* The maternal cardiovascular effect of carbetocin compared to oxytocin in women undergoing caesarean section. Pregnancy Hypertens 2012; 2(2): 139-42.
[http://dx.doi.org/10.1016/j.preghy.2012.01.002] [PMID: 26105099]

[203]   https://www.medicines.org.uk/emc/product/172/smpc

[204]   AEMPS. https://cima.aemps.es/cima/pdfs/es/ft/79228/79228_ft.pdf

[205]   https://www.tga.gov.au/sites/default/files/auspar-carbetocin-180823-pi.docx

[206]   Salati JA, Leathersich SJ, Williams MJ, Cuthbert A, Tolosa JE. Prophylactic oxytocin for the third stage of labour to prevent postpartum haemorrhage. Cochrane Libr 2019; 2019(4): CD001808.
        [http://dx.doi.org/10.1002/14651858.CD001808.pub3] [PMID: 31032882]

[207]   Nahar S, Rasul CH, Sayed A, Azim AKMA. Utility of misoprostol for labor induction in severe pre-eclampsia and eclampsia. J Obstet Gynaecol Res 2004; 30(5): 349-53.
        [http://dx.doi.org/10.1111/j.1447-0756.2004.00207.x] [PMID: 15327446]

[208]   Liabsuetrakul T, Choobun T, Peeyananjarassri K, Islam QM. Prophylactic use of ergot alkaloids in the third stage of labour. Cochrane Libr 2018; 2018(6): CD005456.
        [http://dx.doi.org/10.1002/14651858.CD005456.pub3] [PMID: 29879293]

[209]   Smakosz A, Kurzyna W, Rudko M, Dąsal M. The Usage of Ergot (*Claviceps purpurea* (fr.) Tul.) in Obstetrics and Gynecology: A Historical Perspective. Toxins (Basel) 2021; 13(7): 492.
        [http://dx.doi.org/10.3390/toxins13070492] [PMID: 34357964]

[210]   Cheng C, Liao AHW, Chen CY, Lin YC, Kang YN. A systematic review with network meta-analysis on mono strategy of anaesthesia for preeclampsia in caesarean section. Sci Rep 2021; 11(1): 5630.
        [http://dx.doi.org/10.1038/s41598-021-85179-5] [PMID: 33707559]

[211]   Hood DD, Curry R. Spinal *versus* epidural anesthesia for cesarean section in severely preeclamptic patients: a retrospective survey. Anesthesiology 1999; 90(5): 1276-82.
        [http://dx.doi.org/10.1097/00000542-199905000-00009] [PMID: 10319773]

[212]   Sumikura H, Niwa H, Sato M, Nakamoto T, Asai T, Hagihira S. Rethinking general anesthesia for cesarean section. J Anesth 2016; 30(2): 268-73.
        [http://dx.doi.org/10.1007/s00540-015-2099-4] [PMID: 26585767]

[213]   Littleford J. Effects on the fetus and newborn of maternal analgesia and anesthesia: a review. Can J Anaesth 2004; 51(6): 586-609.
        [http://dx.doi.org/10.1007/BF03018403] [PMID: 15197123]

[214]   Hess PE. What's New in Obstetric Anesthesia. Anesth Analg 2017; 124(3): 863-71.
        [http://dx.doi.org/10.1213/ANE.0000000000001681] [PMID: 28212182]

[215]   Wilińska M, Walas W, Kamińska E, Malec Milewska M, Sękowska A, Stankiewicz J, et al. Do drugs used in obstetric anesthesia interfere with early breastfeeding? Characteristics of the pharmacodynamic and pharmacokinetic properties of certain drugs. Part 2. J Mother Child. 29 de enero de 2021; 23(4): 233-44.

[216]   Mitchell J, Jones W, Winkley E, Kinsella SM. Guideline on anaesthesia and sedation in breastfeeding women 2020. Anaesthesia 2020; 75(11): 1482-93.
        [http://dx.doi.org/10.1111/anae.15179] [PMID: 32737881]

[217]   Bloor M, Paech M. Nonsteroidal anti-inflammatory drugs during pregnancy and the initiation of lactation. Anesth Analg 2013; 116(5): 1063-75.
        [http://dx.doi.org/10.1213/ANE.0b013e31828a4b54] [PMID: 23558845]

[218]   Yoshimura M. Dexmedetomidine in breast milk. Anaesthesia 2021; 76(2): 289.
        [http://dx.doi.org/10.1111/anae.15280] [PMID: 33095443]

[219]   Arzola C, Perlas A, Siddiqui NT, Carvalho JCA. Bedside Gastric Ultrasonography in Term Pregnant Women Before Elective Cesarean Delivery. Anesth Analg 2015; 121(3): 752-8.
        [http://dx.doi.org/10.1213/ANE.0000000000000818] [PMID: 26097988]

[220]   Hakak S, McCaul CL, Crowley L. Ultrasonographic evaluation of gastric contents in term pregnant women fasted for six hours. Int J Obstet Anesth 2018; 34: 15-20.

[http://dx.doi.org/10.1016/j.ijoa.2018.01.004] [PMID: 29519668]

[221] Rouget C, Chassard D, Bonnard C, Pop M, Desgranges FP, Bouvet L. Changes in qualitative and quantitative ultrasound assessment of the gastric antrum before and after elective caesarean section in term pregnant women: a prospective cohort study. Anaesthesia 2016; 71(11): 1284-90.
[http://dx.doi.org/10.1111/anae.13605] [PMID: 27561371]

[222] Van de Putte P, Perlas A. Gastric sonography in the severely obese surgical patient: a feasibility study. Anesth Analg 2014; 119(5): 1105-10.
[http://dx.doi.org/10.1213/ANE.0000000000000373] [PMID: 25054584]

[223] Wong CA, McCarthy RJ, Fitzgerald PC, Raikoff K, Avram MJ. Gastric emptying of water in obese pregnant women at term. Anesth Analg 2007; 105(3): 751-5.
[http://dx.doi.org/10.1213/01.ane.0000278136.98611.d6] [PMID: 17717235]

[224] Wong CA, Loffredi M, Ganchiff JN, Zhao J, Wang Z, Avram MJ. Gastric emptying of water in term pregnancy. Anesthesiology 2002; 96(6): 1395-400.
[http://dx.doi.org/10.1097/00000542-200206000-00019] [PMID: 12170052]

[225] Emergent Therapy for Acute-Onset, Severe Hypertension During Pregnancy and the Postpartum Period. Obstet Gynecol 2017; 129(4): e90-5.
[http://dx.doi.org/10.1097/AOG.0000000000002019] [PMID: 28333820]

[226] Shields LE, Wiesner S, Klein C, Pelletreau B, Hedriana HL. Early standardized treatment of critical blood pressure elevations is associated with a reduction in eclampsia and severe maternal morbidity. Am J Obstet Gynecol 2017; 216(4): 415.e1-5.
[http://dx.doi.org/10.1016/j.ajog.2017.01.008] [PMID: 28153655]

[227] Alexander JM, McIntire DD, Leveno KJ, Cunningham FG. Selective magnesium sulfate prophylaxis for the prevention of eclampsia in women with gestational hypertension. Obstet Gynecol 2006; 108(4): 826-32.
[http://dx.doi.org/10.1097/01.AOG.0000235721.88349.80] [PMID: 17012442]

[228] Czarnetzki C, Lysakowski C, Elia N, Tramèr MR. Time course of rocuronium-induced neuromuscular block after pre-treatment with magnesium sulphate: a randomised study. Acta Anaesthesiol Scand 2010; 54(3): 299-306.
[http://dx.doi.org/10.1111/j.1399-6576.2009.02160.x] [PMID: 19919585]

[229] Czarnetzki C, Tassonyi E, Lysakowski C, Elia N, Tramèr MR. Efficacy of sugammadex for the reversal of moderate and deep rocuronium-induced neuromuscular block in patients pretreated with intravenous magnesium: a randomized controlled trial. Anesthesiology 2014; 121(1): 59-67.
[http://dx.doi.org/10.1097/ALN.0000000000000204] [PMID: 24608361]

[230] Pinard AM, Donati F, Martineau R, Denault AY, Taillefer J, Carrier M. Magnesium potentiates neuromuscular blockade with cisatracurium during cardiac surgery. Can J Anaesth 2003; 50(2): 172-8.
[http://dx.doi.org/10.1007/BF03017852] [PMID: 12560310]

[231] Williamson RM, Mallaiah S, Barclay P. Rocuronium and sugammadex for rapid sequence induction of obstetric general anaesthesia. Acta Anaesthesiol Scand 2011; 55(6): 694-9.
[http://dx.doi.org/10.1111/j.1399-6576.2011.02431.x] [PMID: 21480829]

[232] Richardson MG, Raymond BL. sugammadex administration in pregnant women and in women of reproductive potential. anesth analg 2020; 130(6): 1628-37.
[http://dx.doi.org/10.1213/ANE.0000000000004305] [PMID: 31283616]

[233] Kessell G, Trapp JN. Rocuronium and sugammadex for rapid sequence induction of obstetric general anaesthesia. Acta Anaesthesiol Scand 2012; 56(3): 394.
[http://dx.doi.org/10.1111/j.1399-6576.2011.02530.x] [PMID: 22221068]

[234] Odor PM, Bampoe S, Moonesinghe SR, *et al.* General anaesthetic and airway management practice for obstetric surgery in England: a prospective, multicentre observational study. Anaesthesia 2021; 76(4): 460-71.

[http://dx.doi.org/10.1111/anae.15250] [PMID: 32959372]

[235]   Donati F, Bevan DR. Succinylcholine in Obstetrics. Anesth Analg 1983; 62(11): 1051-2.
[http://dx.doi.org/10.1213/00000539-198311000-00029] [PMID: 6625214]

[236]   Smith JM, Lowe RF, Fullerton J, Currie SM, Harris L, Felker-Kantor E. An integrative review of the side effects related to the use of magnesium sulfate for pre-eclampsia and eclampsia management. BMC Pregnancy Childbirth 2013; 13(1): 34.
[http://dx.doi.org/10.1186/1471-2393-13-34] [PMID: 23383864]

[237]   Lu JF, Nightingale CH. Magnesium sulfate in eclampsia and pre-eclampsia: pharmacokinetic principles. Clin Pharmacokinet 2000; 38(4): 305-14.
[http://dx.doi.org/10.2165/00003088-200038040-00002] [PMID: 10803454]

[238]   Duffy JMN, Hirsch M, Pealing L, *et al.* Inadequate safety reporting in pre-eclampsia trials: a systematic evaluation. BJOG 2018; 125(7): 795-803.
[http://dx.doi.org/10.1111/1471-0528.14969] [PMID: 29030992]

[239]   Brown CM, Garovic VD. Drug treatment of hypertension in pregnancy. Drugs 2014; 74(3): 283-96.
[http://dx.doi.org/10.1007/s40265-014-0187-7] [PMID: 24554373]

[240]   Easterling TR. Pharmacological management of hypertension in pregnancy. Semin Perinatol 2014; 38(8): 487-95.
[http://dx.doi.org/10.1053/j.semperi.2014.08.016] [PMID: 25311173]

[241]   Leavitt K, Običan S, Yankowitz J. treatment and prevention of hypertensive disorders during pregnancy. clin perinatol 2019; 46(2): 173-85.
[http://dx.doi.org/10.1016/j.clp.2019.02.002] [PMID: 31010554]

[242]   Chourdakis E, Oikonomou N, Fouzas S, Hahalis G, Karatza AA. preeclampsia emerging as a risk factor of cardiovascular disease in women. high blood press cardiovasc prev 2021; 28(2): 103-14.
[http://dx.doi.org/10.1007/s40292-020-00425-7] [PMID: 33660234]

[243]   Shi Q, Leng W, Yao Q, Mi C, Xing A. Oral nifedipine *versus* intravenous labetalol for the treatment of severe hypertension in pregnancy. Int J Cardiol 2015; 178: 162-4.
[http://dx.doi.org/10.1016/j.ijcard.2014.10.111] [PMID: 25464243]

[244]   Sanghavi M, Rutherford JD. Cardiovascular physiology of pregnancy. Circulation 2014; 130(12): 1003-8.
[http://dx.doi.org/10.1161/CIRCULATIONAHA.114.009029] [PMID: 25223771]

[245]   Ouzounian JG, Elkayam U. Physiologic changes during normal pregnancy and delivery. Cardiol Clin 2012; 30(3): 317-29.
[http://dx.doi.org/10.1016/j.ccl.2012.05.004] [PMID: 22813360]

[246]   Kumari A, Kumar K, Kumar Sinha A. The pattern of valvular heart diseases in india during pregnancy and its outcomes. cureus 2021; 13(7): e16394.
[http://dx.doi.org/10.7759/cureus.16394] [PMID: 34408947]

[247]   Liu S, Elkayam U, Naqvi TZ. Echocardiography in Pregnancy: Part 1. Curr Cardiol Rep 2016; 18(9): 92.
[http://dx.doi.org/10.1007/s11886-016-0760-7] [PMID: 27491768]

[248]   Echocardiography in Pregnancy. https://pubmed.ncbi.nlm.nih.gov/27457084/

[249]   Moors S, van Oostrum NHM, Rabotti C, *et al.* Speckle Tracking Echocardiography in Hypertensive Pregnancy Disorders: A Systematic Review. Obstet Gynecol Surv 2020; 75(8): 497-509.
[http://dx.doi.org/10.1097/OGX.0000000000000811] [PMID: 32856716]

[250]   Keser N. Echocardiography in pregnant women. Anadolu Kardiyol Derg 2006; 6(2): 169-73.
[PMID: 16766283]

[251]   Campos O, Andrade JL, Bocanegra J, *et al.* Physiologic multivalvular regurgitation during pregnancy: a longitudinal Doppler echocardiographic study. Int J Cardiol 1993; 40(3): 265-72.

[http://dx.doi.org/10.1016/0167-5273(93)90010-E] [PMID: 8225661]

[252] Melchiorre K, Sharma R, Thilaganathan B. Cardiovascular implications in preeclampsia: an overview. Circulation 2014; 130(8): 703-14.
[http://dx.doi.org/10.1161/CIRCULATIONAHA.113.003664] [PMID: 25135127]

[253] Melchiorre K, Sutherland GR, Liberati M, Thilaganathan B. Preeclampsia is associated with persistent postpartum cardiovascular impairment. Hypertension 2011; 58(4): 709-15.
[http://dx.doi.org/10.1161/HYPERTENSIONAHA.111.176537] [PMID: 21844489]

[254] Shahul S, Rhee J, Hacker MR, *et al.* Subclinical left ventricular dysfunction in preeclamptic women with preserved left ventricular ejection fraction: a 2D speckle-tracking imaging study. Circ Cardiovasc Imaging 2012; 5(6): 734-9.
[http://dx.doi.org/10.1161/CIRCIMAGING.112.973818] [PMID: 22891044]

[255] Tasar O, Kocabay G, Karagoz A, *et al.* Evaluation of Left Atrial Functions by 2-dimensional Speckle-Tracking Echocardiography During Healthy Pregnancy. J Ultrasound Med 2019; 38(11): 2981-8.
[http://dx.doi.org/10.1002/jum.15004] [PMID: 30927311]

[256] Shivananjiah C, Nayak A, Swarup A. Echo changes in hypertensive disorder of pregnancy. J Cardiovasc Echogr 2016; 26(3): 94-6.
[http://dx.doi.org/10.4103/2211-4122.187961] [PMID: 28465970]

[257] Ying W, Catov JM, Ouyang P. Hypertensive Disorders of Pregnancy and Future Maternal Cardiovascular Risk. J Am Heart Assoc 2018; 7(17): e009382.
[http://dx.doi.org/10.1161/JAHA.118.009382] [PMID: 30371154]

[258] Orabona R, Vizzardi E, Sciatti E, *et al.* Maternal cardiac function after HELLP syndrome: an echocardiography study. Ultrasound Obstet Gynecol 2017; 50(4): 507-13.
[http://dx.doi.org/10.1002/uog.17358] [PMID: 28971558]

[259] Ambrozic J, Brzan Simenc G, Prokselj K, Tul N, Cvijic M, Lucovnik M. Lung and cardiac ultrasound for hemodynamic monitoring of patients with severe pre-eclampsia. Ultrasound Obstet Gynecol 2017; 49(1): 104-9.
[http://dx.doi.org/10.1002/uog.17331] [PMID: 27736042]

[260] Ambrožič J, Lučovnik M, Prokšelj K, Toplišek J, Cvijić M. Dynamic changes in cardiac function before and early postdelivery in women with severe preeclampsia. J Hypertens 2020; 38(7): 1367-74.
[http://dx.doi.org/10.1097/HJH.0000000000002406] [PMID: 32195819]

[261] Weiniger CF, Sharoni L. The use of ultrasound in obstetric anesthesia. Curr Opin Anaesthesiol 2017; 30(3): 306-12.
[http://dx.doi.org/10.1097/ACO.0000000000000450] [PMID: 28291128]

[262] Lee A. Ultrasound in obstetric anesthesia. Semin Perinatol 2014; 38(6): 349-58.
[http://dx.doi.org/10.1053/j.semperi.2014.07.006] [PMID: 25155870]

[263] Lee A, Loughrey JPR. The role of ultrasonography in obstetric anesthesia. Baillieres Best Pract Res Clin Anaesthesiol 2017; 31(1): 81-90.
[http://dx.doi.org/10.1016/j.bpa.2016.12.001] [PMID: 28625308]

[264] Ecimovic P, Loughrey JPR. Ultrasound in obstetric anaesthesia: a review of current applications. Int J Obstet Anesth 2010; 19(3): 320-6.
[http://dx.doi.org/10.1016/j.ijoa.2010.03.006] [PMID: 20605438]

[265] Ghossein-Doha C, van Neer J, Wissink B, *et al.* Pre-eclampsia: an important risk factor for asymptomatic heart failure. Ultrasound Obstet Gynecol 2017; 49(1): 143-9.
[http://dx.doi.org/10.1002/uog.17343] [PMID: 27804179]

[266] Zieleskiewicz L, Contargyris C, Brun C, *et al.* Lung ultrasound predicts interstitial syndrome and hemodynamic profile in parturients with severe preeclampsia. Anesthesiology 2014; 120(4): 906-14.
[http://dx.doi.org/10.1097/ALN.0000000000000102] [PMID: 24694847]

[267] Valensise H, Lo Presti D, Gagliardi G, *et al.* Persistent Maternal Cardiac Dysfunction After Preeclampsia Identifies Patients at Risk for Recurrent Preeclampsia. Hypertension 2016; 67(4): 748-53.
[http://dx.doi.org/10.1161/HYPERTENSIONAHA.115.06674] [PMID: 26902488]

[268] Lichtenstein DA, Mezière GA, Lagoueyte JF, Biderman P, Goldstein I, Gepner A. A-Lines and B-Lines. Chest 2009; 136(4): 1014-20.
[http://dx.doi.org/10.1378/chest.09-0001] [PMID: 19809049]

[269] Lichtenstein DA. BLUE-protocol and FALLS-protocol: two applications of lung ultrasound in the critically ill. Chest 2015; 147(6): 1659-70.
[http://dx.doi.org/10.1378/chest.14-1313] [PMID: 26033127]

[270] Picano E, Pellikka PA. Ultrasound of extravascular lung water: a new standard for pulmonary congestion. Eur Heart J 2016; 37(27): 2097-104.
[http://dx.doi.org/10.1093/eurheartj/ehw164] [PMID: 27174289]

[271] Lichtenstein D. Lung ultrasound in the critically ill. Curr Opin Crit Care 2014; 20(3): 315-22.
[http://dx.doi.org/10.1097/MCC.0000000000000096] [PMID: 24758984]

[272] Brown MC, Best KE, Pearce MS, Waugh J, Robson SC, Bell R. Cardiovascular disease risk in women with pre-eclampsia: systematic review and meta-analysis. Eur J Epidemiol 2013; 28(1): 1-19.
[http://dx.doi.org/10.1007/s10654-013-9762-6] [PMID: 23397514]

[273] Brouwers L, van der Meiden-van Roest AJ, Savelkoul C, *et al.* Recurrence of pre-eclampsia and the risk of future hypertension and cardiovascular disease: a systematic review and meta-analysis. BJOG 2018; 125(13): 1642-54.
[http://dx.doi.org/10.1111/1471-0528.15394] [PMID: 29978553]

[274] Turbeville HR, Sasser JM. Preeclampsia beyond pregnancy: long-term consequences for mother and child. Am J Physiol Renal Physiol 2020; 318(6): F1315-26.
[http://dx.doi.org/10.1152/ajprenal.00071.2020] [PMID: 32249616]

[275] Vatten LJ, Skjaerven R. Is pre-eclampsia more than one disease? BJOG 2004; 111(4): 298-302.
[http://dx.doi.org/10.1111/j.1471-0528.2004.00071.x] [PMID: 15008762]

[276] Too G, Wen T, Boehme AK, *et al.* Timing and Risk Factors of Postpartum Stroke. Obstet Gynecol 2018; 131(1): 70-8.
[http://dx.doi.org/10.1097/AOG.0000000000002372] [PMID: 29215510]

[277] Al-Safi Z, Imudia AN, Filetti LC, Hobson DT, Bahado-Singh RO, Awonuga AO. Delayed postpartum preeclampsia and eclampsia: demographics, clinical course, and complications. Obstet Gynecol 2011; 118(5): 1102-7.
[http://dx.doi.org/10.1097/AOG.0b013e318231934c] [PMID: 21979459]

[278] Lindley KJ, Conner SN, Cahill AG, Novak E, Mann DL. impact of preeclampsia on clinical and functional outcomes in women with peripartum cardiomyopathy. circ heart fail 2017; 10(6): e003797.
[http://dx.doi.org/10.1161/CIRCHEARTFAILURE.116.003797] [PMID: 28572214]

[279] McDermott M, Miller EC, Rundek T, Hurn PD, Bushnell CD. Preeclampsia. Stroke 2018; 49(3): 524-30.
[http://dx.doi.org/10.1161/STROKEAHA.117.018416] [PMID: 29438078]

[280] Silverberg O, Park AL, Cohen E, Fell DB, Ray JG. Premature Cardiac Disease and Death in Women Whose Infant Was Preterm and Small for Gestational Age. JAMA Cardiol 2018; 3(3): 247-51.
[http://dx.doi.org/10.1001/jamacardio.2017.5206] [PMID: 29387888]

[281] Lykke JA, Langhoff-Roos J, Sibai BM, Funai EF, Triche EW, Paidas MJ. Hypertensive pregnancy disorders and subsequent cardiovascular morbidity and type 2 diabetes mellitus in the mother. Hypertension 2009; 53(6): 944-51.
[http://dx.doi.org/10.1161/HYPERTENSIONAHA.109.130765] [PMID: 19433776]

[282] Simmons D. Diabetes and obesity in pregnancy. Best Pract Res Clin Obstet Gynaecol 2011; 25(1): 25-36.
[http://dx.doi.org/10.1016/j.bpobgyn.2010.10.006] [PMID: 21247811]

[283] Grandi SM, Vallée-Pouliot K, Reynier P, *et al.* Hypertensive Disorders in Pregnancy and the Risk of Subsequent Cardiovascular Disease. Paediatr Perinat Epidemiol 2017; 31(5): 412-21.
[http://dx.doi.org/10.1111/ppe.12388] [PMID: 28816365]

[284] Grandi SM, Reynier P, Platt RW, Basso O, Filion KB. The timing of onset of hypertensive disorders in pregnancy and the risk of incident hypertension and cardiovascular disease. Int J Cardiol 2018; 270: 273-5.
[http://dx.doi.org/10.1016/j.ijcard.2018.06.059] [PMID: 29950283]

[285] Haug EB, Horn J, Markovitz AR, *et al.* Association of Conventional Cardiovascular Risk Factors With Cardiovascular Disease After Hypertensive Disorders of Pregnancy. JAMA Cardiol 2019; 4(7): 628-35.
[http://dx.doi.org/10.1001/jamacardio.2019.1746] [PMID: 31188397]

[286] Bellamy L, Casas JP, Hingorani AD, Williams DJ. Pre-eclampsia and risk of cardiovascular disease and cancer in later life: systematic review and meta-analysis. BMJ 2007; 335(7627): 974.
[http://dx.doi.org/10.1136/bmj.39335.385301.BE] [PMID: 17975258]

[287] Behrens I, Basit S, Melbye M, *et al.* Risk of post-pregnancy hypertension in women with a history of hypertensive disorders of pregnancy: nationwide cohort study. BMJ 2017; 358: j3078.
[http://dx.doi.org/10.1136/bmj.j3078] [PMID: 28701333]

[288] Barrett HL, Callaway LK. Hypertensive disorders of pregnancy. BMJ 2017; 358: j3245.
[http://dx.doi.org/10.1136/bmj.j3245] [PMID: 28705906]

[289] Groenhof TKJ, van Rijn BB, Franx A, Roeters van Lennep JE, Bots ML, Lely AT. Preventing cardiovascular disease after hypertensive disorders of pregnancy: Searching for the how and when. Eur J Prev Cardiol 2017; 24(16): 1735-45.
[http://dx.doi.org/10.1177/2047487317730472] [PMID: 28895439]

[290] Groenhof TKJ, Zoet GA, Franx A, *et al.* trajectory of cardiovascular risk factors after hypertensive disorders of pregnancy. hypertension 2019; 73(1): 171-8.
[http://dx.doi.org/10.1161/HYPERTENSIONAHA.118.11726] [PMID: 30571544]

[291] Nerenberg KA, Park AL, Vigod SN, *et al.* Long-term Risk of a Seizure Disorder After Eclampsia. Obstet Gynecol 2017; 130(6): 1327-33.
[http://dx.doi.org/10.1097/AOG.0000000000002364] [PMID: 29112665]

[292] Alsnes IV, Vatten LJ, Fraser A, *et al.* Hypertension in Pregnancy and Offspring Cardiovascular Risk in Young Adulthood. Hypertension 2017; 69(4): 591-8.
[http://dx.doi.org/10.1161/HYPERTENSIONAHA.116.08414] [PMID: 28223467]

[293] Magnussen EB, Vatten LJ, Smith GD, Romundstad PR. Hypertensive disorders in pregnancy and subsequently measured cardiovascular risk factors. Obstet Gynecol 2009; 114(5): 961-70.
[http://dx.doi.org/10.1097/AOG.0b013e3181bb0dfc] [PMID: 20168095]

[294] Podymow T, August P. Postpartum course of gestational hypertension and preeclampsia. Hypertens Pregnancy 2010; 29(3): 294-300.
[http://dx.doi.org/10.3109/10641950902777747] [PMID: 20670153]

[295] Mikami Y, Takagi K, Itaya Y, *et al.* Post-partum recovery course in patients with gestational hypertension and pre-eclampsia. J Obstet Gynaecol Res 2014; 40(4): 919-25.
[http://dx.doi.org/10.1111/jog.12280] [PMID: 24428339]

[296] Macdonald-Wallis C, Lawlor DA, Fraser A, May M, Nelson SM, Tilling K. Blood pressure change in normotensive, gestational hypertensive, preeclamptic, and essential hypertensive pregnancies. Hypertension 2012; 59(6): 1241-8.
[http://dx.doi.org/10.1161/HYPERTENSIONAHA.111.187039] [PMID: 22526257]

[297] Mgawadere F, Kana T, van den Broek N. Measuring maternal mortality: a systematic review of methods used to obtain estimates of the maternal mortality ratio (MMR) in low- and middle-income countries. Br Med Bull 2017; 121(1): 121-34.
[http://dx.doi.org/10.1093/bmb/ldw056] [PMID: 28104630]

[298] Browne JL, Vissers KM, Antwi E, *et al.* Perinatal outcomes after hypertensive disorders in pregnancy in a low resource setting. Trop Med Int Health 2015; 20(12): 1778-86.
[http://dx.doi.org/10.1111/tmi.12606] [PMID: 26426071]

[299] Chen L, Feng P, Shaver L, Wang Z. Maternal mortality ratio in China from 1990 to 2019: trends, causes and correlations. BMC Public Health 2021; 21(1): 1536.
[http://dx.doi.org/10.1186/s12889-021-11557-3] [PMID: 34380436]

[300] Bauserman M, Thorsten VR, Nolen TL, *et al.* Maternal mortality in six low and lower-middle income countries from 2010 to 2018: risk factors and trends. Reprod Health 2020; 17(S3) (Suppl. 3): 173.
[http://dx.doi.org/10.1186/s12978-020-00990-z] [PMID: 33334343]

[301] Sobhy S, Zamora J, Dharmarajah K, *et al.* Anaesthesia-related maternal mortality in low-income and middle-income countries: a systematic review and meta-analysis. Lancet Glob Health 2016; 4(5): e320-7.
[http://dx.doi.org/10.1016/S2214-109X(16)30003-1] [PMID: 27102195]

[302] Say L, Chou D, Gemmill A, *et al.* Global causes of maternal death: a WHO systematic analysis. Lancet Glob Health 2014; 2(6): e323-33.
[http://dx.doi.org/10.1016/S2214-109X(14)70227-X] [PMID: 25103301]

[303] Khan KS, Wojdyla D, Say L, Gülmezoglu AM, Van Look PFA. WHO analysis of causes of maternal death: a systematic review. Lancet 2006; 367(9516): 1066-74.
[http://dx.doi.org/10.1016/S0140-6736(06)68397-9] [PMID: 16581405]

[304] Troiano NH, Witcher PM. Maternal Mortality and Morbidity in the United States. J Perinat Neonatal Nurs 2018; 32(3): 222-31.
[http://dx.doi.org/10.1097/JPN.0000000000000349] [PMID: 30036304]

[305] Chang J, Elam-Evans LD, Berg CJ, *et al.* Pregnancy-related mortality surveillance--United States, 1991--1999. MMWR Surveill Summ 2003; 52(2): 1-8.
[PMID: 12825542]

[306] Zieleskiewicz L, Chantry A, Duclos G, *et al.* Intensive care and pregnancy: Epidemiology and general principles of management of obstetrics ICU patients during pregnancy. Anaesth Crit Care Pain Med 2016; 35 (Suppl. 1): S51-7.
[http://dx.doi.org/10.1016/j.accpm.2016.06.005] [PMID: 27386763]

[307] Hogan MC, Foreman KJ, Naghavi M, *et al.* Maternal mortality for 181 countries, 1980–2008: a systematic analysis of progress towards Millennium Development Goal 5. Lancet 2010; 375(9726): 1609-23.
[http://dx.doi.org/10.1016/S0140-6736(10)60518-1] [PMID: 20382417]

[308] Neal S, Mahendra S, Bose K, *et al.* The causes of maternal mortality in adolescents in low and middle income countries: a systematic review of the literature. BMC Pregnancy Childbirth 2016; 16(1): 352.
[http://dx.doi.org/10.1186/s12884-016-1120-8] [PMID: 27836005]

[309] Souza JP, Cecatti JG, Haddad SM, *et al.* The WHO maternal near-miss approach and the maternal severity index model (MSI): tools for assessing the management of severe maternal morbidity. PLoS One 2012; 7(8): e44129.
[http://dx.doi.org/10.1371/journal.pone.0044129] [PMID: 22952897]

[310] Cecatti JG, Costa ML, Haddad SM, *et al.* Network for Surveillance of Severe Maternal Morbidity: a powerful national collaboration generating data on maternal health outcomes and care. BJOG 2016; 123(6): 946-53.
[http://dx.doi.org/10.1111/1471-0528.13614] [PMID: 26412586]

[311] Lima HMP, Carvalho FHC, Feitosa FEL, Nunes GC. Factors associated with maternal mortality among patients meeting criteria of severe maternal morbidity and near miss. Int J Gynaecol Obstet 2017; 136(3): 337-43.
[http://dx.doi.org/10.1002/ijgo.12077] [PMID: 28099693]

[312] Gaffney A. Critical care in pregnancy—Is it different? Semin Perinatol 2014; 38(6): 329-40.
[http://dx.doi.org/10.1053/j.semperi.2014.07.002] [PMID: 25176639]

[313] Koukoubanis K, Prodromidou A, Stamatakis E, Valsamidis D, Thomakos N. Role of Critical Care Units in the management of obstetric patients (Review). Biomed Rep 2021; 15(1): 58.
[http://dx.doi.org/10.3892/br.2021.1434] [PMID: 34007451]

[314] Honiden S, Abdel-Razeq SS, Siegel MD. The management of the critically ill obstetric patient. J Intensive Care Med 2013; 28(2): 93-106.
[http://dx.doi.org/10.1177/0885066611411408] [PMID: 21841145]

[315] Shapiro JM. Critical care of the obstetric patient. J Intensive Care Med 2006; 21(5): 278-86.
[http://dx.doi.org/10.1177/0885066606290390] [PMID: 16946443]

[316] Munnur U, Bandi V, Guntupalli KK. Management principles of the critically ill obstetric patient. Clin Chest Med 2011; 32(1): 53-60.
[http://dx.doi.org/10.1016/j.ccm.2010.10.003] [PMID: 21277449]

[317] Minville V, Vidal F, Loutrel O, Castel A, Jacques L, Vayssière C, *et al.* Identifying predictive factors for admitting patients with severe preeclampsia to intensive care unit. J Matern Fetal Neonatal Med 2020; 1-7.
[PMID: 32900240]

[318] Thakur M, Gonik B, Gill N, Awonuga AO, Rocha FG, Gonzalez JM. Intensive Care Admissions in Pregnancy: Analysis of a Level of Support Scoring System. Matern Child Health J 2016; 20(1): 106-13.
[http://dx.doi.org/10.1007/s10995-015-1808-9] [PMID: 26318180]

[319] Maged AM, Elsherief A, Hassan H, *et al.* Maternal, fetal, and neonatal outcomes among different types of hypertensive disorders associating pregnancy needing intensive care management. J Matern Fetal Neonatal Med 2020; 33(2): 314-21.
[http://dx.doi.org/10.1080/14767058.2018.1491030] [PMID: 29914278]

[320] Bokslag A, van Weissenbruch M, Mol BW, de Groot CJM. Preeclampsia; short and long-term consequences for mother and neonate. Early Hum Dev 2016; 102: 47-50.
[http://dx.doi.org/10.1016/j.earlhumdev.2016.09.007] [PMID: 27659865]

[321] Crozier T. General Care of the Pregnant Patient in the Intensive Care Unit. Semin Respir Crit Care Med 2017; 38(2): 208-17.
[http://dx.doi.org/10.1055/s-0037-1600905] [PMID: 28561252]

[322] Kazma JM, van den Anker J, Allegaert K, Dallmann A, Ahmadzia HK. Anatomical and physiological alterations of pregnancy. J Pharmacokinet Pharmacodyn 2020; 47(4): 271-85.
[http://dx.doi.org/10.1007/s10928-020-09677-1] [PMID: 32026239]

[323] Baird SM, Martin S. Framework for Critical Care in Obstetrics. J Perinat Neonatal Nurs 2018; 32(3): 232-40.
[http://dx.doi.org/10.1097/JPN.0000000000000348] [PMID: 30036305]

[324] ACOG Practice Bulletin No. 211: Critical Care in Pregnancy. Obstet Gynecol 2019; 133(5): e303-19.
[http://dx.doi.org/10.1097/AOG.0000000000003241] [PMID: 31022122]

[325] Farr A, Lenz-Gebhart A, Einig S, *et al.* Outcomes and trends of peripartum maternal admission to the intensive care unit. Wien Klin Wochenschr 2017; 129(17-18): 605-11.
[http://dx.doi.org/10.1007/s00508-016-1161-z] [PMID: 28101669]

[326] Einav S, Leone M. Epidemiology of obstetric critical illness. Int J Obstet Anesth 2019; 40: 128-39.

[http://dx.doi.org/10.1016/j.ijoa.2019.05.010] [PMID: 31257034]

[327] Pollock W, Rose L, Dennis CL. Pregnant and postpartum admissions to the intensive care unit: a systematic review. Intensive Care Med 2010; 36(9): 1465-74.
[http://dx.doi.org/10.1007/s00134-010-1951-0] [PMID: 20631987]

[328] Edwards Z, Lucas DN, Gauntlett R. Is training in obstetric critical care adequate? An international comparison. Int J Obstet Anesth 2019; 37: 96-105.
[http://dx.doi.org/10.1016/j.ijoa.2018.08.011] [PMID: 30482716]

[329] Pollock WE. Caring for pregnant and postnatal women in intensive care: What do we know? Aust Crit Care 2006; 19(2): 54-65, 57-65.
[http://dx.doi.org/10.1016/S1036-7314(06)80010-X] [PMID: 16764153]

[330] Bhorat I. Pre-eclampsia and the foetus: a cardiovascular perspective. Cardiovasc J Afr 2018; 29(6): 387-93.
[http://dx.doi.org/10.5830/CVJA-2017-039] [PMID: 31199427]

[331] Vasquez DN, Estenssoro E, Canales HS, *et al.* Clinical characteristics and outcomes of obstetric patients requiring ICU admission. Chest 2007; 131(3): 718-24.
[http://dx.doi.org/10.1378/chest.06-2388] [PMID: 17356085]

[332] Guntupalli KK, Karnad DR, Bandi V, Hall N, Belfort M. Critical Illness in Pregnancy. Chest 2015; 148(5): 1333-45.
[http://dx.doi.org/10.1378/chest.14-2365] [PMID: 26020727]

[333] Guntupalli KK, Hall N, Karnad DR, Bandi V, Belfort M. Critical illness in pregnancy: part I: an approach to a pregnant patient in the ICU and common obstetric disorders. Chest 2015; 148(4): 1093-104.
[http://dx.doi.org/10.1378/chest.14-1998] [PMID: 26020613]

[334] Jayaratnam S, Jacob-Rodgers S, Costa C. Characteristics and preventability of obstetric intensive care unit admissions in Far North Queensland. Aust N Z J Obstet Gynaecol 2020; 60(6): 871-6.
[http://dx.doi.org/10.1111/ajo.13198] [PMID: 32557552]

[335] Aoyama K, Pinto R, Ray JG, *et al.* Variability in intensive care unit admission among pregnant and postpartum women in Canada: a nationwide population-based observational study. Crit Care 2019; 23(1): 381.
[http://dx.doi.org/10.1186/s13054-019-2660-x] [PMID: 31775866]

[336] Zhao Z, Han S, Yao G, *et al.* Pregnancy-Related ICU Admissions From 2008 to 2016 in China. Crit Care Med 2018; 46(10): e1002-9.
[http://dx.doi.org/10.1097/CCM.0000000000003355] [PMID: 30059363]

[337] Chawla S, Jose T, Paul M. Critical Care in Obstetrics: Where are We. J Obstet Gynaecol India 2018; 68(3): 155-63.
[http://dx.doi.org/10.1007/s13224-018-1109-5] [PMID: 29895993]

[338] Lam MC, Dierking E. Intensive Care Unit issues in eclampsia and HELLP syndrome. Int J Crit Illn Inj Sci 2017; 7(3): 136-41.
[http://dx.doi.org/10.4103/IJCIIS.IJCIIS_33_17] [PMID: 28971026]

[339] Williams J, Mozurkewich E, Chilimigras J, Van De Ven C. Critical care in obstetrics: pregnancy-specific conditions. Best Pract Res Clin Obstet Gynaecol 2008; 22(5): 825-46.
[http://dx.doi.org/10.1016/j.bpobgyn.2008.06.003] [PMID: 18775679]

[340] Brown CE, Cunningham FG, Pritchard JA. Convulsions in hypertensive, proteinuric primiparas more than 24 hours after delivery. Eclampsia or some other cause? J Reprod Med 1987; 32(7): 499-503.
[PMID: 3625613]

[341] Lakshmi R, Upreti D, Agrawal A, Raina A. Late postpartum eclampsia at five weeks post-delivery. Singapore Med J 2007; 48(10): 946-7.
[PMID: 17909682]

[342]   Chhabra S, Tyagi S, Bhavani M, Gosawi M. Late postpartum eclampsia. J Obstet Gynaecol 2012; 32(3): 264-6.
[http://dx.doi.org/10.3109/01443615.2011.639467] [PMID: 22369401]

[343]   Al-Shoha M, Klair JS, Girotra M, Garcia-Saenz-de-Sicilia M. magnesium toxicity-induced ileus in a postpartum patient treated for preeclampsia with magnesium sulphate. ACG case rep J 2015; 2(1): 227-9.
[http://dx.doi.org/10.14309/crj.2015.67] [PMID: 26203447]

[344]   Leetheeragul J, Boriboonhirunsarn D, Reesukumal K, Srisaimanee N, Horrasith S, Wataganara T. A retrospective review of on-admission factors on attainment of therapeutic serum concentrations of magnesium sulfate in women treated for a diagnosis of preeclampsia. J Matern Fetal Neonatal Med 2020; 33(2): 258-66.
[http://dx.doi.org/10.1080/14767058.2018.1489531] [PMID: 29898629]

[345]   Agarwal S, Laycock HC. The debate ROTEMs on – the utility of point-of-care testing and fibrinogen concentrate in postpartum haemorrhage. Anaesthesia 2020; 75(9): 1247-51.
[http://dx.doi.org/10.1111/anae.15193] [PMID: 32662889]

[346]   Mallaiah S, Barclay P, Harrod I, Chevannes C, Bhalla A. Introduction of an algorithm for ROTEM-guided fibrinogen concentrate administration in major obstetric haemorrhage. Anaesthesia 2015; 70(2): 166-75.
[http://dx.doi.org/10.1111/anae.12859] [PMID: 25289791]

[347]   Leal-Noval SR, Fernández Pacheco J, Casado Méndez M, Cuenca-Apolo D, Múñoz-Gómez M. Current perspective on fibrinogen concentrate in critical bleeding. Expert Rev Clin Pharmacol 2020; 13(7): 761-78.
[http://dx.doi.org/10.1080/17512433.2020.1776608] [PMID: 32479129]

[348]   Gilmandyar D, Thornburg LL. Surgical management of postpartum hemorrhage. Semin Perinatol 2019; 43(1): 27-34.
[http://dx.doi.org/10.1053/j.semperi.2018.11.006] [PMID: 30578144]

[349]   Dohbit JS, Foumane P, Nkwabong E, *et al.* Uterus preserving surgery *versus* hysterectomy in the treatment of refractory postpartum haemorrhage in two tertiary maternity units in Cameroon: a cohort analysis of perioperative outcomes. BMC Pregnancy Childbirth 2017; 17(1): 158.
[http://dx.doi.org/10.1186/s12884-017-1346-0] [PMID: 28558661]

[350]   Mohan B, Wander G, Bansal R, *et al.* Intra-operative uterine artery embolization with caesarean delivery in an adjoining operating theatre and catheter lab (OT/CL) complex *vs.* conventional management in patients with abnormally invasive placenta: a retrospective case control study. J Obstet Gynaecol 2020; 40(3): 324-9.
[http://dx.doi.org/10.1080/01443615.2019.1621817] [PMID: 31340698]

[351]   Condous GS, Arulkumaran S. Medical and conservative surgical management of postpartum hemorrhage. J Obstet Gynaecol Can 2003; 25(11): 931-6.
[http://dx.doi.org/10.1016/S1701-2163(16)30241-9] [PMID: 14608443]

[352]   Said Ali A, Faraag E, Mohammed M, *et al.* The safety and effectiveness of Bakri balloon in the management of postpartum hemorrhage: a systematic review. J Matern Fetal Neonatal Med 2021; 34(2): 300-7.
[http://dx.doi.org/10.1080/14767058.2019.1605349] [PMID: 30957590]

[353]   Wright C, Abuhamad A, Chauhan S. Bakri balloon in the management of postpartum hemorrhage: a review. Am J Perinatol 2014; 31(11): 957-64.
[http://dx.doi.org/10.1055/s-0034-1372422] [PMID: 24705972]

[354]   Suarez S, Conde-Agudelo A, Borovac-Pinheiro A, *et al.* Uterine balloon tamponade for the treatment of postpartum hemorrhage: a systematic review and meta-analysis. Am J Obstet Gynecol 2020; 222(4): 293.e1-293.e52.
[http://dx.doi.org/10.1016/j.ajog.2019.11.1287] [PMID: 31917139]

[355] Sorensen BL, Rasch V, Massawe S, Nyakina J, Elsass P, Nielsen BB. Advanced Life Support in Obstetrics (ALSO) and post-partum hemorrhage: a prospective intervention study in Tanzania. Acta Obstet Gynecol Scand 2011; 90(6): 609-14.
[http://dx.doi.org/10.1111/j.1600-0412.2011.01115.x] [PMID: 21388368]

[356] McGready R, Rijken MJ, Turner C, *et al.* A mixed methods evaluation of Advanced Life Support in Obstetrics (ALSO) and Basic Life Support in Obstetrics (BLSO) in a resource-limited setting on the Thailand-Myanmar border. Wellcome Open Res 2021; 6: 94.
[http://dx.doi.org/10.12688/wellcomeopenres.16599.1] [PMID: 34195384]

[357] Dinc G, Oğuz Ş. The efficacy of pelvic arterial embolisation for the treatment in massive vaginal haemorrhage in obstetric and gynaecological emergencies: a single-centre experience. J Obstet Gynaecol 2019; 39(6): 774-81.
[http://dx.doi.org/10.1080/01443615.2019.1586858] [PMID: 31023116]

[358] Spreu A, Abgottspon F, Baumann MU, Kettenbach J, Surbek D. Efficacy of pelvic artery embolisation for severe postpartum hemorrhage. Arch Gynecol Obstet 2017; 296(6): 1117-24.
[http://dx.doi.org/10.1007/s00404-017-4554-y] [PMID: 28993867]

[359] Ruiz Labarta FJ, Pintado Recarte MP, Alvarez Luque A, *et al.* Outcomes of pelvic arterial embolization in the management of postpartum haemorrhage: a case series study and systematic review. Eur J Obstet Gynecol Reprod Biol 2016; 206: 12-21.
[http://dx.doi.org/10.1016/j.ejogrb.2016.07.510] [PMID: 27612214]

[360] Zhang XQ, Chen XT, Zhang YT, Mai CX. The Emergent Pelvic Artery Embolization in the Management of Postpartum Hemorrhage: A Systematic Review and Meta-analysis. Obstet Gynecol Surv 2021; 76(4): 234-44.
[http://dx.doi.org/10.1097/OGX.0000000000000887] [PMID: 33908615]

[361] Vegas G, Illescas T, Muñoz M, Pérez-Piñar A. Selective pelvic arterial embolization in the management of obstetric hemorrhage. Eur J Obstet Gynecol Reprod Biol 2006; 127(1): 68-72.
[http://dx.doi.org/10.1016/j.ejogrb.2005.09.008] [PMID: 16229935]

[362] Clark SL. Amniotic fluid embolism. Obstet Gynecol 2014; 123(2): 337-48.
[http://dx.doi.org/10.1097/AOG.0000000000000107] [PMID: 24402585]

[363] Shamshirsaz AA, Clark SL. Amniotic Fluid Embolism. Obstet Gynecol Clin North Am 2016; 43(4): 779-90.
[http://dx.doi.org/10.1016/j.ogc.2016.07.001] [PMID: 27816160]

[364] Nawaz N, Raheem Buksh A. Amniotic Fluid Embolism. J Coll Physicians Surg Pak 2018; 28(6): S107-9.
[http://dx.doi.org/10.29271/jcpsp.2018.06.S107] [PMID: 29866238]

[365] Sultan P, Seligman K, Carvalho B. Amniotic fluid embolism. Curr Opin Anaesthesiol 2016; 29(3): 288-96.
[http://dx.doi.org/10.1097/ACO.0000000000000328] [PMID: 27153475]

[366] Clark SL, Romero R, Dildy GA, *et al.* Proposed diagnostic criteria for the case definition of amniotic fluid embolism in research studies. Am J Obstet Gynecol 2016; 215(4): 408-12.
[http://dx.doi.org/10.1016/j.ajog.2016.06.037] [PMID: 27372270]

[367] McBride AM. Clinical Presentation and Treatment of Amniotic Fluid Embolism. AACN Adv Crit Care 2018; 29(3): 336-42.
[http://dx.doi.org/10.4037/aacnacc2018419] [PMID: 30185500]

[368] Dean Gopalan P, Muckart DJJ. The critically ill obstetric patient: what's the score? Int J Obstet Anesth 2004; 13(3): 144-5.
[http://dx.doi.org/10.1016/j.ijoa.2004.04.005] [PMID: 15321391]

[369] Pryn A, Young S. APACHE II: for one or for all? Int J Obstet Anesth 2005; 14(1): 81-2.
[http://dx.doi.org/10.1016/j.ijoa.2004.10.002] [PMID: 15627553]

[370] El-Solh AA, Grant BJB. A comparison of severity of illness scoring systems for critically ill obstetric patients. Chest 1996; 110(5): 1299-304.
[http://dx.doi.org/10.1378/chest.110.5.1299] [PMID: 8915238]

[371] Aarvold ABR, Ryan HM, Magee LA, von Dadelszen P, Fjell C, Walley KR. Multiple Organ Dysfunction Score Is Superior to the Obstetric-Specific Sepsis in Obstetrics Score in Predicting Mortality in Septic Obstetric Patients. Crit Care Med 2017; 45(1): e49-57.
[http://dx.doi.org/10.1097/CCM.0000000000002018] [PMID: 27618276]

[372] Albright CM, Has P, Rouse DJ, Hughes BL. internal validation of the sepsis in obstetrics score to identify risk of morbidity from sepsis in pregnancy. obstet gynecol 2017; 130(4): 747-55.
[http://dx.doi.org/10.1097/AOG.0000000000002260] [PMID: 28885400]

[373] Albright CM, Ali TN, Lopes V, Rouse DJ, Anderson BL. The Sepsis in Obstetrics Score: a model to identify risk of morbidity from sepsis in pregnancy. Am J Obstet Gynecol 2014; 211(1): 39.e1-8.
[http://dx.doi.org/10.1016/j.ajog.2014.03.010] [PMID: 24613756]

[374] Carle C, Alexander P, Columb M, Johal J. Design and internal validation of an obstetric early warning score: secondary analysis of the Intensive Care National Audit and Research Centre Case Mix Programme database. Anaesthesia 2013; 68(4): 354-67.
[http://dx.doi.org/10.1111/anae.12180] [PMID: 23488833]

[375] Smith GB, Prytherch DR. Obstetric early warning scores: much more work required. Anaesthesia 2013; 68(7): 778-9.
[http://dx.doi.org/10.1111/anae.12320] [PMID: 24044394]

[376] Shields LE, Wiesner S, Klein C, Pelletreau B, Hedriana HL. Use of Maternal Early Warning Trigger tool reduces maternal morbidity. Am J Obstet Gynecol 2016; 214(4): 527.e1-6.
[http://dx.doi.org/10.1016/j.ajog.2016.01.154] [PMID: 26924745]

[377] Blumenthal EA, Hooshvar N, Tancioco V, Newman R, Senderoff D, McNulty J. implementation and evaluation of an electronic maternal early warning trigger tool to reduce maternal morbidity. am J perinatol 2021; 38(9): 869-79.
[http://dx.doi.org/10.1055/s-0040-1721715] [PMID: 33368094]

[378] Zuckerwise LC, Lipkind HS. Maternal early warning systems—Towards reducing preventable maternal mortality and severe maternal morbidity through improved clinical surveillance and responsiveness. Semin Perinatol 2017; 41(3): 161-5.
[http://dx.doi.org/10.1053/j.semperi.2017.03.005] [PMID: 28416176]

[379] Senanayake H, Dias T, Jayawardena A. Maternal mortality and morbidity: Epidemiology of intensive care admissions in pregnancy. Best Pract Res Clin Obstet Gynaecol 2013; 27(6): 811-20.
[http://dx.doi.org/10.1016/j.bpobgyn.2013.07.002] [PMID: 23992951]

CHAPTER 15

Air and Amniotic Fluid Embolism

Clara Isabel Fernandez Sánchez[1,*], **Adriana Carolina Orozco Vinasco**[1], **Monica San Juan Alvarez**[1] and **Marta Chacón Castillo**[1]

[1] *Department of Anaesthesiology, Hospital Universitario Severo Ochoa, Leganés. Madrid, Spain*

Abstract: Amniotic fluid embolism (*AFE*) is an uncommon pathology, whose incidence ranges from 2 to 8 per 100,000 births, depending on the country. This syndrome has four cardinal symptoms: circulatory collapse, respiratory distress, cyanosis and coma. If the patient survives cardiorespiratory failure, disseminated intravascular coagulopathy occurs, leading to incoercible bleeding and eventually death. Clinical diagnosis is based on Clark's four criteria: sudden cardiorespiratory arrest, established disseminated intravascular coagulation prior to bleeding, and all of these occurring peripartum in the absence of fever. The two main differential diagnosis syndromes are pulmonary thromboembolism and myocardial infarction. Treatment consists of cardiopulmonary support of the patient. Despite aggressive measures, such as the placement of ventricular assist devices and external oxygenation membranes, the prognosis continues to be poor. The main death cause is incoercible bleeding caused by disseminated intravascular coagulopathy.

Keywords: Amniotic Fluid Embolism, Cardiopulmonary Arrest, Coma, Cyanosis, Death, Disseminated Intravascular Coagulopathy, Embolism, Extracorporeal Membrane Oxygenation, Myocardial Infarction, Postpartum Hemorrhage, Pulmonary Embolism, Respiratory Distress Syndrome, Ventricular Assist Devices.

INTRODUCTION

Amniotic fluid embolism (*AFE*) is a disease that has a fatal prognosis, for both the mother and the fetus, because sadly it is an untreatable disease. Fortunately, its occurrence is very rare [1].

JR Meyer first published amniotic fluid embolism as a case report in the Brazilian Medical Journal in 1926. It is not found in the literature again until 1941, when Steiner and Luschbaugh described it as a sudden peripartum shock syndrome with acute pulmonary edema in eight parturients. After an autopsy, they were found to

---

* **Corresponding author Clara Isabel Fernandez Sánchez:** Department of Anaesthesiology, Hospital Universitario Severo Ochoa, Leganés, Madrid, Spain; Email: clarisa1988@hotmail.com

Eugenio Daniel Martinez-Hurtado, Monica Sanjuan-Alvarez & Marta Chacon-Castillo (Eds.)
All rights reserved-© 2022 Bentham Science Publishers

have fetal squamous cells in the pulmonary vascular tree. All eight women had died unexpectedly and suddenly during labor [2, 3].

Nowadays, although the morbimortality of many pregnancy conditions, such as preeclampsia, has been reduced, amniotic fluid embolism syndrome continues to be devastating. This is the result of an unknown pathogenesis. Its diagnosis is only confirmed with an autopsy having no specific treatment; its prognosis is calamitous.

INCIDENCE AND MORTALITY

Amniotic fluid embolism is a usually devastating obstetric syndrome with an incidence that is difficult to estimate due to its high mortality and the impossibility of diagnosis until autopsy.

Its incidence ranges from 2 to 8 cases per 100 000 habitats in different countries. It is one of the main causes of death directly related to labor, accounting for 5 to 15% of death cases worldwide. In Australia, it is the first cause of death and the second in the United Kingdom [4] (Table **1**).

Table 1. Amniotic fluid embolism incidence. Modified according to Rath *et al* [4].

Country	Period	Incidence (n/100.000 Birth)	Case-related Mortality	Perinatal Mortality
Australia	2001 to 2007	3.3	35%	32%
USA	1999 to 2003	7.7	21.6%	No data
UK	1991 to 2002	6	13%	No data
The Netherlands	2005 to 2009	2	20%	13.5%

Recurrence rate is unknown due to the rarity of the syndrome and its high mortality rate. According to the literature, in the few survival cases that have had a new pregnancy, it has been normal. A history of amniotic fluid embolism seems to not predispose to a new episode of this type of embolism, so no relationship with recurrence has been found.

AMNIOTIC FLUID CHARACTERISTICS

The volume of amniotic fluid increases from an average of 50 ml at 12 weeks to 1000 ml at 38 weeks, after which it begins to decrease.

At the beginning of pregnancy, amniotic fluid is a kind of dialysate of maternal serum, so the electrolytes have the same concentration found in maternal blood. As pregnancy progresses, amniotic fluid is diluted with fetal urine and it becomes more hypotonic. Other components such as urea, creatinine and uric acid are twice as high as in maternal blood, there is no fibrinogen or bilirubin, but prostaglandins can be found [1]. Fetal materials such as skin flakes, lanugo hair and intestinal mucin can be found in amniotic fluid.

The volume of fluid needed to pass into maternal circulation to produce symptom is unknown.

RISK FACTORS

Knowing the risk factors of the disease would be very beneficial in order to be alert and prevent this syndrome with such high mortality (Table **2**).

Table 2. Amniotic fluid embolism risk factors. Modified from Fitzpatrick [5].

- Advanced maternal age
- Multiple pregnancy
- Polyhydramnios
- Placenta previa
- Placental abruption
- Labor induction
- For postnatal syndrome: cesarean section and instrumental delivery

Unfortunately, owing to such a high mortality rate, it is difficult to find associated risk factors; therefore, articles from multicenter studies should be analyzed [5].

PATHOGENESIS

Amniotic fluid enters the bloodstream through a tear in the membranes that opens the decidual vessels in an abnormal manner. This can occur in different situations such as cesarean section, ruptured uterus or placenta accreta. Some cases are devoid of any detectable underlying mechanism.

Three processes occur as a result:

1. *Pulmonary artery obstruction*: this acute obstruction produces dilatation of the right ventricle and atrium, leading to a displacement of the septum and thus hindering blood outflow from the left ventricle. This results in systolic dysfunction and finally hypotension.

2. Ventilation-perfusion mismatch produces severe anoxia, which explains cyanosis, tachypnea, altered mental function and seizures. Blood replacement by the amniotic fluid is also involved in anoxia [1].

Hypoxemia and hypotension lead to a sudden cardiovascular collapse.

3. Amniotic fluid activates platelet factor III, stimulates platelet aggregation and activates coagulation factor Xa, leading to pathological activation of the coagulation and fibrinolytic pathways and thus causing severe coagulopathy. Disseminated Intravascular Coagulation (*DIC*) occurs in 80% of patients and can result in fatal bleeding [6].

4. Studies show that the presence of amniotic fluid in the blood leads to accelerated clot formation. Nevertheless, there is no evidence of fibrinolysis activation, so it is considered that coagulopathy occurs by consumption [7].

5. *Anaphylactoid reaction*: as there are similar clinical features, some authors have tried to compare amniotic fluid embolism with anaphylactic shock. They suggest that the fetal elements present in the maternal blood generate an anaphylactic reaction, but no study has been able to demonstrate mast cell degranulation or histamine release in this population.

However, some studies suggest that there may be a complement-mediated immune response elicited by a foreign body, as several studies have shown decreased c3 and c4 in patients with amniotic fluid embolism syndrome. Therefore, it would be reasonable to question whether anaphylaxis plays a role in the pathogenesis of amniotic fluid embolism.

CLINICAL MANIFESTATIONS

AE is a very rare syndrome and there are four cardinal symptoms that should always be present: ***respiratory distress, cyanosis, circulatory collapse*** and ***coma*** [1].

Onset is usually very nonspecific, starting with vague symptoms such as vomiting or malaise, which delay suspicion. Sometimes seizures can be present before cardiorespiratory failure, which could lead to an erroneous eclampsia diagnosis.

The onset of a severe form usually begins with respiratory failure and cyanosis, along with hypotension that does not correspond to the actual bleeding. Finally, cardiorespiratory collapse occurs. This is, unfortunately, always present in the syndrome. If the patient survives the cardiorespiratory failure, DIC may develop, resulting in incoercible bleeding.

Other symptoms are:

- Acute pulmonary edema, related to the vigorous resuscitation performed.
- Renal failure due to sustained hypotension.

The outcome is fatal. Up to 50% of women are not able to survive the first two hours. The few long-term survivors have permanent neurological sequelae due to sustained hypoxia and low cardiac output.

DIAGNOSIS

A definitive diagnosis is made upon finding fetal remains in the maternal right circulation, unfortunately this usually happens at autopsy. These fetal remains are composed of epithelial debris of fetal skin; lanugo hairs, fat from the caseous vernix, mucin from the fetal intestine and bile containing meconium. In fatal cases, this fetal material may be found in the maternal brain, kidneys or coronary arteries [1].

Since definitive diagnosis is made at autopsy, a consensus on core clinical characteristics must be met, in order to make the diagnosis while the patient is still alive. To achieve this aim, the symptoms of mothers who died from AFE were retrospectively collected and defined at a consensus symposium by the Maternal-Fetal Medicine Committee of the Society for Maternal-Fetal Medicine and the Amniotic Fluid Embolism Foundation described by Clark *et al* in 2016 as [8]:

1. *Sudden onset of cardiorespiratory arrest* or hypotension along with respiratory compromise (desaturation below 90%, dyspnea, and cyanosis).
2. *Disseminated intravascular coagulation* not explained by blood loss or dilutional coagulopathy. Coagulopathy is critical to differentiate amniotic fluid embolism from other conditions that may present with clinical cardiorespiratory failure, such as myocardial infarction or anaphylaxis.
   Physiological hypercoagulability, occurring in all pregnancies, must be taken into account at diagnosis.
3. Clinical manifestations must appear during labor or within 30 minutes after placental delivery. The diagnosis may be delayed in women who are undergoing cesarean section under general anesthesia, because they are already under hemodynamic and respiratory support.
4. Absence of fever. It is the only sign that differentiates sepsis and septic shock since all other features may be present.

Diagnostic tests

Diagnostic tests employees are [9]:

- Chest X-ray may be normal despite a catastrophic clinical situation. Sometimes, findings compatible with acute pulmonary edema may be seen. It is unspecific and of little help to establish a diagnosis.

- *Laboratory tests:*
  - *Blood gases*: drop in pH, drop in pO_2, increase in CO_2.
  - Coagulation must be assessed to detect early coagulopathy: elongated PT, shortened aPTT, thrombocytopenia. Decreased fibrinogen.
  - Decreased hemoglobin occurs because of bleeding and levels should be periodically monitored.
- *ECG* will show tachycardia with ST-segment and T-segment changes, as well as signs of right heart overload.
- *Transthoracic or transesophageal echocardiography* will show right ventricular dilatation, wall motion abnormalities, overload and tricuspid valve regurgitation. Septum flattening produces left ventricular obstruction and systolic dysfunction.

In the last year, efforts have been made in order to identify serum markers that help in the diagnosis of this disease. This is, however, very difficult, because comparison is usually made with healthy obstetric patients and not with critically ill obstetric patients of other causes.

DIFFERENTIAL DIAGNOSIS

Differential diagnosis of this syndrome includes any pathology that produces respiratory failure and excessive bleeding during labor or in the immediate aftermath.

Among them we can find [9] (Table **3**):

1. **Pulmonary thromboembolism**: it usually presents with chest pain and without coagulopathy. Heart disease is accompanied by alterations in ST-T due to right ventricular overload.
2. **Septic shock**: it is accompanied by an inflammatory response (*SIRS*) and evidence of infection without a cardiovascular collapse as sudden as that of amniotic fluid embolism.
3. **Myocardial infarction**: ECG will show ST alterations with an elevation of myocardial enzymes and altered myocardial wall contractility.
4. **Mendelson's syndrome**: it is usually accompanied by bronchospasm, which in amniotic fluid embolism syndrome does not usually occur.
5. **Eclampsia**: the presence of seizures can lead to an erroneous diagnosis of eclampsia, but this disease produces elevated blood pressure, proteinuria and edema.
6. **Anaphylaxis**: it usually begins with rash and urticaria.
7. **Total spinal anesthesia**: presents with hypotension, bradycardia and high blocked sensory level.

PREVENTION

Preventive measures are very difficult to implement because of the rarity of this syndrome. Mortality is very high in a short period of time, which impedes the identification of associated factors.

The only precaution that can be taken is avoidance of unnecessary trauma, such as rupture of membranes, placental incisions during cesarean section and excessive uterine activity [1].

Table 3. Differential diagnoses by clinical symptoms. Modified from Rath *et al* [4].

Symptoms	Amniotic Fluid Embolism	Pulmonary Embolism	Myocardial Infarction
Manifestations	During labor/birth	2 to 15 times more common during labor than pregnancy	21% peripartum 34% postpartum
Cardiac arrest	++	+ / ++	+
Chest pain	-	++ / +++	+++
Heart arrhythmia	+ / ++	++ / +++	+++
Dyspnea	+++	+ / +++	+ / ++
Hypotension	+++	+ / ++	+ / ++
Neurological symptoms	++	Secondary	Secondary
Coagulopathy	++	-	-
Acute fetal distress	+ / ++	Secondary	Secondary

TREATMENT

It is important to know that there is no specific treatment for amniotic fluid embolism. The only thing that can be done is to provide supportive care measures, such as cardiopulmonary assistance. That is why it has such a high mortality rate.

Thanks to advances in recent years, the possibility of more aggressive measures for cardiopulmonary support is feasible. By virtue of ventricular assist device placement and extracorporeal membrane oxygenation, survival has been achieved in some cases; although the long-term prognosis, due to the severity of the condition, continues to be ominous.

DIC continues to be the main cause of death in these patients, as there is currently no treatment that can stop the chain of events.

Patient Monitoring and Management [4]

A pulmonary artery catheter can be used to assess pulmonary arterial pressure and cardiac output, among other useful parameters, such as vascular resistances and oxygen delivery and consumption.

Cannulation of a peripheral artery allows a continuous arterial pressure measurement and readily available arterial samples for analysis. Central venous access is indicated to determine venous pressures and for vasoactive drug administration. A large bore peripheral access allows the rapid infusion of a substantial amount of fluids. Urinary catheterization is useful for diuresis control.

For its management, the most important things are:

1. Perform *early extraction of the fetus* if it has not been performed, as this increases the survival of mother and fetus.
2. Perform *rapid and effective cardiopulmonary resuscitation*: fluid administration should be done cautiously, because an excessive amount of fluids can exacerbate coagulopathy and anemia on a dilutional basis. Therefore, vasoactive drugs should be used promptly.

Nitric oxide or sildenafil can be used to decrease pulmonary vascular resistance.

In case of cardiogenic shock refractory to VAD, a ventricular assist device remains an option.

1. Perform *effective mechanical ventilation* to keep the patient well oxygenated.

If refractory cardiogenic shock with the impossibility to oxygenate the patient supervenes, extracorporeal membrane oxygenation is the last line and most aggressive treatment [10].

Disseminated Intravascular Coagulopathy Treatment

As mentioned before, fluid administration must be done carefully. Fresh frozen plasma, coagulation factor concentrates and complexes, fibrinogen (trying to maintain values above 200 mg/dL) and tranexamic acid should be all started early in order to enhance coagulation and diminish fibrinolysis.

Correct monitoring of coagulopathy involves the evaluation of coagulation status in a dynamic way. Viscoelastic tests are very useful for this, as they are performed bedside on whole blood.

Some studies suggest that Rivaroxaban, as a factor Xa antagonist, is able to reverse coagulopathy and stop consumption [11]. Incoercible obstetric bleeding can be treated with uterine artery embolization, although the most definitive treatment is obstetric hysterectomy. At the onset of bleeding, administration of packed red blood cells and platelet concentrates will be required. The situation of low cardiac output and maintained anoxia will lead to multiorgan failure. The resulting renal failure may require renal replacement therapy.

CONCLUSION

Fortunately, Amniotic fluid embolism is a rare pathology, but has a high morbimortality for both, mother and fetus.

Under physiological conditions, we can find fetal material in the amniotic fluid such as: skin flakes, lanugo hair and intestinal mucin.

Due to its high mortality, it is very difficult to identify associated risk factors. The most important ones seem to be: advanced maternal age, multiple pregnancy, polyhydramnios, placenta previa, and placental abruption.

Due to an abnormal rupture of the uterine vessels, the amniotic fluid enters the maternal circulation producing obstruction of the pulmonary artery and an alteration in ventilation-perfusion leading to cardiopulmonary arrest.

The four cardinal symptoms are cardiorespiratory arrest, respiratory distress, cyanosis and coma; followed by disseminated intravascular coagulopathy unrelated to previous bleeding. A definitive diagnosis is made when fetal cells are found in the pulmonary circulation of the mother.

In order to make an early diagnosis, Clark's criteria are used: sudden cardiorespiratory arrest, disseminated intravascular coagulopathy prior to bleeding, absence of fever, and all of these occurring peripartum.

The main differential diagnoses are pulmonary thromboembolism and myocardial infarction. The only possible treatment is cardiopulmonary support for the patient. In spite of the progress and aggressive measures, the prognosis of the disease continues to be unfavorable for both the mother and the fetus.

CONSENT FOR PUBLICATION

Not applicable.

CONFLICT OF INTEREST

The authors declare no conflict of interest, financial or otherwise.

ACKNOWLEDGEMENT

Declared none.

REFERENCES

[1]   Morgan M. Amniotic fluid embolism. Anaesthesia 1979; 34(1): 20-32.
        [http://dx.doi.org/10.1111/j.1365-2044.1979.tb04862.x] [PMID: 371460]

[2]   Meyer JR. Embolia pulmonar amnio caseosa. Bras Med 1926; 2: 301-2.

[3]   Steiner P, Lushbaugh CC. Maternal pulmonary embolism by amniotic fluid as a cause of obstetric
        shock and unexpected death in obstetrics. J Am Med Assoc 1941; 117(15): 1245-54.
        [http://dx.doi.org/10.1001/jama.1941.02820410023008]

[4]   Rath WH, Hoferr S, Sinicina I. Amniotic fluid embolism: an interdisciplinary challenge:
        epidemiology, diagnosis and treatment. Dtsch Arztebl Int 2014; 111(8): 126-32.
        [PMID: 24622759]

[5]   Fitzpatrick KE, van den Akker T, Bloemenkamp KWM, *et al.* Risk factors, management, and
        outcomes of amniotic fluid embolism: A multicountry, population-based cohort and nested case-
        control study. PLoS Med 2019; 16(11): e1002962.
        [http://dx.doi.org/10.1371/journal.pmed.1002962] [PMID: 31714909]

[6]   Sharma SK, Philip J, Wiley J. Thromboelastographic changes in healthy parturients and postpartum
        women. Anesth Analg 1997; 85(1): 94-8.
        [PMID: 9212129]

[7]   Harnett MJ P, Hepner DL, Datta S, *et al.* Effect of amniotic fluid on coagulation and platelet function
        in pregnancy: an evaluation using tromboelastography 2005; 60: 1068-72.

[8]   Clark SL, Romero R, Dildy GA, *et al.* Proposed diagnostic criteria for the case definition of amniotic
        fluid embolism in research studies. Am J Obstet Gynecol 2016; 215(4): 408-12.
        [http://dx.doi.org/10.1016/j.ajog.2016.06.037] [PMID: 27372270]

[9]   Kiranpreet K, Mamta B, *et al.* Amniotic fluid embolism. 2016; 32: 153-9.

[10]   Eiras M, Taboada M, *et al.* venoarterial extracorporeal membrane oxygenation and ventricular
        assistance with impella CP in an amniotic fluid embolism. rev esp cardiol 2019; 72(8): 677-93.
        [PMID: 30173948]

[11]   Xiao-Yan X, Ming-Long T, *et al.* Successful treatment of amniotic fluid embolism complicated by
        disseminated intravascular coagulation with rivaroxaban. Case Rep Med 2020; 99: 1-4.

CHAPTER 16

Postoperative Management of Postnatal Complications

Ligia María Pérez Cubías[1,*], Yobanys Rodríguez Téllez[1], Carolina Forero Cortés[1] and Clara Hernández Cera[1]

[1] *Department of Maternal and Child Anesthesiology, Hospital Sant Joan de Déu, Esplugues, Barcelona, Spain*

Abstract: The postpartum period is the time after delivery when physiological changes by the pregnancy return to the previous state. Primary postpartum haemorrhage takes place during the first 24 hours, and secondary postpartum haemorrhage occurs between 24 hours and 6 weeks after delivery.

Many disorders can occur in the immediate postpartum period, there is a considerable source of morbidity and mortality in women of reproductive age, which can be mild to severe and life-threatening.

Protocols aimed at the multidisciplinary management of postpartum haemorrhage, and together with the use of coadjuvant hemostatic agents, the activation of massive transfusion protocols in a responsible manner, and surgical management have improved the prognosis of these patients.

Keywords: Amniotic Fluid Embolism, Postpartum Complications, Postanesthetic Complications, Postpartum Haemorrhage, Postpartum Thromboembolism, Preeclampsia.

INTRODUCTION

Primary postpartum haemorrhage takes place during the first 24 hours, and secondary postpartum haemorrhage occurs between 24 hours and 6 weeks after delivery [1, 2].

It is one of the main causes of maternal morbidity and mortality worldwide and represents an approximate incidence of 4-6% of pregnancies [3]. It can be classified as mild (500-1000 ml), moderate (1001-2000 ml) and severe (greater than 2000 ml) [4]. Early identification and its etiology are essential for its imme-

* **Corresponding author Ligia María Pérez Cubías:** Department of Maternal and Child Anesthesiology, Hospital Sant Joan de Déu, Esplugues, Barcelona, Spain; E-mail: ligiamaria.perez@hsjdbcn.es

Eugenio Daniel Martinez-Hurtado, Monica Sanjuan-Alvarez & Marta Chacon-Castillo (Eds.)
All rights reserved-© 2022 Bentham Science Publishers

diate management and treatment. Maternal predisposing factors include, obesity (body mass index greater than 35 kg/m^2), advanced maternal age (more than 35 years), hypertensive states or diabetes mellitus [5].

The implementation of protocols aimed at the multidisciplinary management of postpartum haemorrhage has improved the prognosis of these patients. In addition to specific treatment according to the cause, the use of coadjuvant haemostatic agents, the activation of massive transfusion protocols in a responsible manner, and surgical management should be considered if necessary. An overview of obstetric management of postpartum haemorrhage is presented in Fig. (**1**).

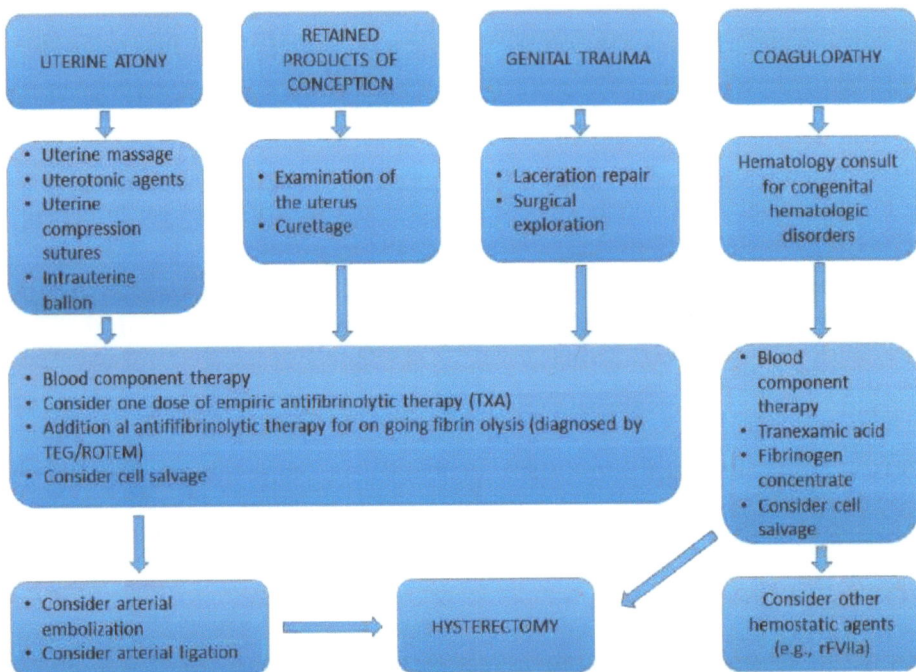

Fig (1). Obstetric management of postpartum hemorrhage.

Uterine Atony

It is the most common cause of postpartum haemorrhage (over 70% of cases). Risk factors are uterine overdistension, precipitous or prolonged labour or administration of oxytocin augmentation dosage, magnesium sulphate or halogenated anesthetic agents.

Uterotonic Treatment

The choice of the therapeutic agent to be used should be based on the comorbidities of the patient and the clinical judgment of the practitioners involved in the case [6].

Oxytocin

Oxytocin is almost universally accepted as the more effective uterotonic agent in the management and prevention of uterine atony after vaginal and operative delivery. Adverse effects include hemodynamic instability (hypotension, tachycardia, myocardial ischemia, and arrhythmias), nausea, vomiting, headache, and flushing. They are generally related to the dose and rate of administration. Routes for administration are intravenous (immediate onset of action) or intramuscular (onset between 3-7 minutes, 10 units after delivery of the placenta).

An optimal regimen may be the application of the *"Rule of Threes"* algorithm [7, 8]:

• Initial dose of 3 units given over 5 seconds after delivery of the fetus, uterine tone is assessed every 3 minutes. 3 units of oxytocin is given if inadequate tone is observed after each 3-minute interval. If a third bolus of oxytocin is ineffective, it is often appropriate to administer a second-line uterotonic agent).
• A continuous intravenous infusion is required to maintain the uterus in a contracted state and it takes approximately 20 to 30 minutes to reach a steady-state in plasma. The usual dose is 20 IU in 500 mL of crystalloid solution, with the dosage rate adjusted according to response.

Carbetocin

Carbetocin is administrated in a single dose either intravenously or intramuscularly (Table 1) [9, 10]. Side effects include, headaches, tremor, hypotension, flushing, nausea, abdominal pain, pruritus and a feeling of warmth.

Table 1. Carbetocin usage criteria.

MATERNAL	FETAL OR PLACENTAL
- More than 4 deliveries or 2 caesarean sections in the past - Uterine surgery in the past or clinical suspicion of large uterine fibroids - Postpartum haemorrhage or uterine atony in the past - BMI > 35 kg/m^2 - Haematocrit < 35%, fibrinogen < 4 g/L or Platelet count < 100000/m^3	- Polyhydramnios - Suspected fetal macrosomia - Multiple pregnancy - Placenta previa/accreta

Methylergonovine and Carboprost

Both are second-line treatment.

Methylergonovine 0.2 mg is administered intramuscularly at a frequency of 2 to 4 hours as needed. It is associated with severe vasoconstriction that may lead to hypertension, headaches or seizures ; contraindicated for hypertensive patients or with risk factors for coronary artery disease (smoking, obesity, diabetes, and high cholesterol). Intravenous injection is not recommended due to the potential for hypertensive or cerebrovascular events. If necessary, as a lifesaving measure, it should be given slowly over a period of more than 60 seconds with close blood pressure monitoring.

Carboprost administration is performed intramuscularly. The recommended dose is 250 mg and may be repeated every 15 to 30 minutes (total dose should not exceed 2 mg or 8 dosages). The main side effect is severe bronchospasm, contraindicated in patients with asthma.

Misoprostol

Misoprostol can be administered orally, sublingually, buccally, vaginally or rectally. Less effective. Adverse effects include nausea, vomiting and diarrhoea.

Non-Pharmacological Management

Manual uterine massage, together with oxytocin are recommended as the first-line treatments for uterine atony [11].

Uterine Compression Sutures

B-Lynch suture placement can be easily achieved at the time of caesarean delivery.

Balloon Tamponade

Rusch catheter, Sengstaken-Blakemore (C.R. Bard, Inc, Covington, GA) tube, and the Bakri catheter (Cook Medical, Inc, Bloomington, IN). It could be used in combination with a brace suture.

Surgical Interventions

The ultimate step to be considered is surgical interventions such as ligation of the uterine or hypogastric arteries or peripartum hysterectomy, in order to preserve fertility in young women as much as possible.

Retained Products of Conception

The most common risk factors are abortions, previous uterine surgery, uterine malformations, preterm or induced labour advanced maternal age, multiparity, infection and preeclampsia [12]. The first-line active management involves oxytocin administration, manual massage of the uterus and controlled traction of the umbilical cord. If the placenta has not been expelled spontaneously up to 30 minutes after delivery despite active management, manual removal of the placenta should be carried out under anaesthesia (by giving an epidural reinforcement dose, or under sedation or general anesthesia if necessary).

Genital Trauma

The most common injuries during childbirth are lacerations and hematomas of the perineum, vagina, and cervix.

Pelvic hematomas can be divided into three types: vaginal, vulvar, and retroperitoneal.

- Vaginal hematoma risk increases in instrumented vaginal deliveries. Risk factors: nulliparity, advanced maternal age, macrosoma (> 4 kg), multiple gestation, preeclampsia, vulvovaginal varicosities, prolonged second stage of labour.
- Vulvar hematoma usually results from injury to branches of the pudendal artery. Large hematomas should be suspected if the patient reports extreme pain or clinical manifestations of hypovolemia secondary to blood loss, should be drained and injured vessels ligated. In most cases, the origin of the bleeding is not identified. Currently, arterial embolization is an increasingly used technique, displacing surgical exploration to very specific cases and as the last therapeutic alternative. Volume resuscitation and transfusion are often required.
- Retroperitoneal hematomas are the least common but the most dangerous. Injury
to the hypogastric artery typically occurs after caesarean section or very rarely after rupture of a low transverse uterine scar during labour. This entity should be suspected if an unexpected decrease in haematocrit or tachycardia and hypotension is observed in the postpartum period with no other obvious symptoms.

PULMONAR EMBOLISM IN POST PARTUM

In the post-partum period, the pulmonary embolism (*PE*) can be a thromboembolism associated to thromboembolic disease or an amniotic fluid embolism.

Pulmonary Thromboembolism

Venous thromboembolism remains one of the main causes of maternal death in developed countries. It includes two related entities: deep venous thrombosis and pulmonary thromboembolism. The risk of the venous thromboembolism is four to five times higher in pregnant women than in non-pregnant at the same age [13, 14].

The pathogenesis is based on the Virchow triad: A hypercoagulable state, vascular damage and venous stasis. Approximately half of the episodes related to pregnancy occur during the six weeks post-partum period. The diagnostic approach will be based on clinical suspicion, screening tests and confirmatory tests (Table **2**) [15, 16].

Table 2. Protocol for diagnosis of suspected venous thromboembolism in pregnant women.

SCREENING TESTS (Recommendation C)	CONFIRMATORY TESTS
- Electrocardiogram (most frequent finding in the electrocardiogram is sinus tachycardia. Other findings are unspecified investment of T wave, depression of ST, right bundle branch block. The electrocardiographic pattern S1Q3T3 it is rare). - Thorax X-ray is abnormal only in 17% of cases. (The real value is to discard other pleuropulmonary pathologies). - In pregnancy D-dimer not shown a thrombotic process, but low values (< 500 ng/ml) suggest about the process does not exist.	- Suspected pulmonary embolism + symptoms and signs of deep venous thrombosis (*DVT*), compression duplex ultrasound should be performed. If confirms the presence of DVT, no further investigation is necessary and treatment for venous thromboembolism should continue. - Without symptoms of DVT a ventilation/perfusion (V/Q) scan or CTPA (with a low radiation dose protocol) should be performed. CTPA is preferable when chest X-ray is abnormal.

Clinical Suspicion

Symptoms and signs can include dyspnoea, tachycardia, tachypnoea, pleuritic pain, fever, anxiety, pleural touch, sweating, cyanosis and sometimes haemoptysis. Most of them can be confused whit normal symptoms in the pregnancy.

Every hospital should have an agreed protocol for the objective diagnosis of suspected venous thromboembolism in pregnant women.

Treatment

The management of pulmonary thromboembolism needs a multidisciplinary approach [17] (Table **3**). Treatment must start using anticoagulant treatment in patient´s with high diagnostic suspicion (unless exist a formal contraindication).

Oral anticoagulants as maintenance treatment will be preferable in the onset in puerperium. New anticoagulants (*DOACs*) are contraindicated in pregnancy and lactation.

Table 3. Venous thromboembolism treatment in pregnant women.

General	- Vital sign monitoring. Intravenous catheter. Baseline blood investigations. Oxygen therapy. Analgesia.
Low-molecular-weight heparin (*LMWH*)	- First choice in deep venous thrombosis and stable pulmonary embolism. Some recommendations: Enoxaparin 1mg/kg/12 hrs or Dalteparin 100U/kg/12 hrs or Tanzaparin 175U/kg/24 hrs. - Routine measurement of peak anti-Xa activity is not recommended except in women at extremes of body weight (< 50 kg or > 90 kg) or with complicated factors (renal impairment, recurrent thrombosis). - It should be clear local guidelines for the dosage of LMWH to use.
Unfractionated Heparin	- High haemorrhagic risk, imminent surgical intervention, unstable PE or massive PE. - Renal impairment. - Intravenous route. Bolus 5000 UI or 80 UI/kg, followed by continuous perfusion 18 UI/kg/hour. Dose adjustment by TTPa every 6 hours to get TTPa ratio values of 1.5 – 2. - Maternity units should develop guidelines for treatment whit intravenous unfractionated heparin.
Other Therapies	- Inferior vein cava filter (contraindicated drug anticoagulation, ineffective conventional anticoagulation, anticoagulation complication, pulmonary vascular territory significantly compromised) - Thrombolytic therapy. Increased risk of bleeding. It is essential to have a high diagnostic certainty.

Duration of anticoagulant treatment shall be:

* A minimum of 6 weeks post-partum with minimal total duration.
* 6 months: Women with transitory risk factors.
* 6 months based on recurrences, added risk factors and etiology.

In addition, it is an important criterion for anticoagulant-related bleeding events and the type of anaesthesia used in delivery or caesarean.

Amniotic Fluid Embolism

Amniotic fluid embolism (*AFE*), also termed as anaphylactoid syndrome of pregnancy, is a rare but catastrophic complication of pregnancy or immediate postpartum [18 - 20]. It has been dealt with in detail in chapter 15.

The events are triggered by entrance into the maternal circulation of amniotic fluid, fetal cells, hair or other debris, resulting in an abnormal activation of proinflammatory mediator systems.

It is considered an unpredictable and unpreventable event with an unknown cause.It may occur during labor, caesarean section, abnormal vaginal delivery, and in the second trimester of pregnancy up to 48 hours postdelivery. It may also occur during abortion, and after abdominal trauma during amnioinfusion.

Diagnosis Approach

The diagnosis is clinical. Typical presentation includes sudden hypoxia, hypotension followed in many cases by coagulopathy in relation to labor and delivery [21].

Nonspecific symptoms: headaches, chest pain, cough, sweating, nausea, vomiting. Dyspnea, tachypnea, hypotension, tachycardia, and cyanosis. Fetal bradycardia

Sudden cardiovascular collapse or cardiac arrest, seizures, encephalopathy, severe respiratory difficulty, hypoxia particularly if events are followed by coagulopathy that cannot be otherwise explained

Arterial Blood Gases (*ABG*). Baseline blood investigations (PT is prolonged). Blood reserve in the anticipation of the requirement for a transfusion. In Chest X-ray, findings are usually nonspecific, and main anomalies are diffuse bilateral areas of increased opacity. A 12-lead electrocardiogram may show findings consistent with right ventricle strain.

Increased serum tryptase, urinary histamine concentration and significantly lower complement concentrations suggest an anaphylactoid process.

Management

The most important factors are early recognition, prompt resuscitation, and delivery of the fetus [21]. Management is primary supportive and resuscitative (*CPR*).

General Management

* Maintaining vital signs.
* Oxigenation and control of the airway.
* Fluid resuscitation. Optimization of preload (isotonic crystalloid and colloids solutions). Avoid excessive fluid resuscitation.
* Echocardiography can guide fluid therapy, early phase commonly characterized by right ventricular failure, second phase characterized by left ventricular failure

and cardiogenic pulmonary edema. An arterial line or pulmonary catheter can also help.
- Correcting coagulopathy (platelets < 20000 or bleeding and platelets 20000-50000, transfuse platelets 1-3 U/10kg/day; Fresh frozen plasma to normalize the PT; Fibrinogen if it is < 100 mg/dl).

Pharmacological Management

- Vasopressors and inotropic support are generally needed. The choice of the vasopressor drug depends on the clinical scenario. The early phase is commonly characterized by right ventricular failure, while the second phase is characterized by left ventricular failure and cardiogenic pulmonary edema.
- Hydrocortisone.
- Uterotonics.
- Aprotinin, other antifibrinolytic drugs.

Is recommended that a multidisciplinary team including anaesthesia, respiratory therapy, critical care, and maternal-fetal medicine should be involved in ongoing care of women with AFE (Best Practice).

PRE-ECLAMPSIA / ECLAMPSIA

Preeclampsia is a multisystem disorder characterized by the appearance of hypertension in a previously normotensive pregnant woman, after 20 weeks of gestation with or without organ dysfunction, probably caused by vascular dysfunction of the placenta [22, 23]. It has been dealt with in detail in chapter 14.

Classification of hypertensive disorders of pregnancy (*HDP*) in pregnant women, according to the American College of Obstetrics and Gynecology (*ACOG*):

- *Chronic hypertension*: defined as systolic blood pressure (*SBP*) 140 mmHg and / or diastolic blood pressure (*DBP*) 90 mmHg that precedes pregnancy or occurs before 20 weeks of gestation (at least in two blood pressure intakes) or that persists 12 weeks after postpartum.
- *Gestational hypertension*: defined as new-onset hypertension (SBP 140 mmHg and/or DBP 90 mmHg) without proteinuria or another sign of Preeclampsia, develops after 20 weeks of gestation. This should be resolved after 12 weeks postpartum.
- *Preeclampsia-Eclampsia*: refers to the increase in blood pressure (*BP*), after 20 weeks of gestation in a previously normotension pregnant woman, (SBP 140 mmHg and / or DBP 90 mmHg), accompanied by proteinuria > 300 mg / day, radio protein / creatinine > 0.3, and / or organic dysfunction.
  □ *Mild Preeclampsia*: Preeclampsia with proteinuria.

□*Severe Preeclampsia*: Preeclampsia with one or more of the following aspects:
▪ Appearance of new brain or visual disorders.
▪ Liver dysfunction (upper quadrant pain or increased serum transaminases ≥ twice normal or both.
▪ Severe elevated BP (SBP ≥ 160 mmHg and/or DBP ≥ 110 mmHg).
▪ Thrombocytopenia (<100,000/mL).
▪ Progressive renal impairment (serum creatinine (*Crs*) > 1.1 mg/dL or twice the concentration of Crs in the absence of other kidney diseases.
▪ Pulmonary edema.
▪ This classification does not include proteinuria > 5g /24 h. and neither restriction on fetal growth; aspects to consider.
□*Eclampsia*: refers to seizure type of great mal in a woman with PEC, in the absence of other causes that justify seizures.
•*Chronic Hypertension with over added Preeclampsia*: Pregnant woman diagnosed with hypertension who after 20 weeks of gestation shows proteinuria and/or organ dysfunction.
Medical management includes the prevention of seizures and hypertension [24]:
•*Magnesium Sulfate* (MgSO$_4$), employs Preeclampsia/Eclampsia prevention and treatment and as a fetal neuroprotectant.

Loading dose of 4 g intravenous (IV) in 20 minutes and maintenance of an IV infusion of 12g/h.

It should be maintained from diagnosis to 24 hours after delivery and during caesarean section.

Monitor renal, cardiovascular, respiratory and neurological function. Due to the possible toxicity of MgSO$_4$ the limits should be maintained between 4-6 mg/dL.

Toxicity is treated with calcium gluconate 1g per 10 minutes.

•*Antihypertensive*:
□ Labetalol 20 mg IV every 30 min, increments between 5-10 mg (maximum 300 mg).
□ Nifedipine 5-10 mg oral.
□ Hydralazine 5 mg EV every 30 min (maximum 45 mg).
•*Corticosteroids*:
□ Intramuscular betamethasone (*IM*), 2 doses.

Anesthetic Management

History and detailed physical examination, insist on the forecast of difficult airway and risk of full stomach. We need to monitor cardiovascular, respiratory, neurological and renal function. If severe cardiorespiratory dysfunction is observed, consider arterial and/or venous line for fluid and inotropic management [25, 26].

Neuraxial anesthesia is the first option if maternal/fetal clinical conditions allow it.

* Epidural anesthesia: avoid anesthetics that contain epinephrine.
* Spinal anesthesia: hyperbaric Bupivacaine 10-12 mg plus opiates. If spinal hypotension bolus of phenylephrine (40-80 mcg) or infusion of 40-80 mcg/min, associating fluid therapy with crystalloids.

If general anesthesia is required:

* Consider rapid sequence induction and arterial line.
* $MgSO_4$ interacts with neuromuscular depolarizers, fasciculations may not occur after succinylcholine is administered. It also interacts with non-depolarizing muscles, they can prolong their effect. Peripheral nerve monitoring is recommended.
* Fluid therapy judiciously to avoid pulmonary edema.
* Uterine atony. Methylergonovine (Methergine). It can cause coronary spasms and myocardial infarction. It should not be used in Preeclampsia.

Very close monitoring, invasive if necessary. Respiratory and airway support. Oxygenation. Anticonvulsant therapy. Antihypertensive blood pressure control therapy. Left side position (in pregnant women). Isotonic Fluids 700 ml/day.

Second line of treatment will be phenytoin, diazepam 5-10 mg or lorazepam 2-4 mg every 2-5 min. Other potent antihypertensive medications, such as sodium nitroprusside or nitroglycerin, can be used but are rarely required.

Pain Management

Multimodal analgesia should be used: neuraxial opioids if possible or IV (prophylaxis of nausea and vomiting), acetaminophen; caution with NSAIDs, verify renal, cardiovascular and hematological function.

Consider abdominal transverse plane block (*TAP*), if the platelet count is normal. HELLP syndrome is a severe form of preeclampsia that includes hemolytic anemia, elevated liver tests, and decreased platelet count.

Early evaluation should be performed to predict cardiopulmonary stability, the risks of aspiration are increased and edema in the airway can cause a difficult airway, associated with increased intracranial pressure during intubation and extubation.

About 10% of women with eclampsia will have an additional seizure after receiving magnesium sulfate. Another 2 g bolus of magnesium may be given in these cases. For the rare patient who continues to have seizure activity while receiving adequate magnesium therapy, seizures may be treated with sodium amobarbital, 250 mg IV over 3-5 minutes. Alternatively, lorazepam or diazepam may be administered (as described above) for status epilepticus. However, these drugs can be associated with prolonged neonatal neurologic depression.

POSTANESTHETIC COMPLICATIONS

Postpartum Headache

It is defined as a complaint of cephalic, neck or shoulder pain occurring during the first 6 weeks after delivery [27]. Postdural-dural puncture headache (*PDPH*) is one of the most common postpartum complications of neuraxial anesthesia [28, 29]. Differential diagnosis of this postanesthetic complication and other types of postpartum headaches must be considered.

PDPH is defined as a headache occurring within 5 days of a lumbar puncture, caused by cerebrospinal fluid (*CSF*) leakage through the dural puncture. The rate of PDPH after dural puncture varies widely across patient populations; young pregnant women with a low body mass index (*BMI*) are at the highest risk.

Conservative management with symptomatic therapy (*e.g.*, oral analgesics, caffeine) may be indicated if the patient does not desire an epidural blood patch (*EBP*) or if the headache is not severe. Rare but serious complications may occur following dural puncture and PDPH, including subdural hematoma, cerebral venous sinus thrombosis, chronic headache, diplopia and hearing loss.

Backache

Localized back pain related to tissue trauma at the site of a neuraxial procedure may be present for several days, but prospective studies have consistently reported no correlation between neuraxial analgesia and long-term backache.

Postpartum Neuropathy

Neurologic complications associated with neuraxial anesthesia are extremely rare. Neurologic injury can be the result of needle or catheter trauma, drug toxicity, spinal epidural hematoma, or infection, and may involve injury to the spinal cord, nerve roots, or neuraxial vasculature.

Postpartum neuropathies usually have obstetric etiologies, and are often due to compression of nerves of the lumbosacral plexus by the descending fetal head, extrinsic neural compression (*i.e.*, by stirrup supports) or from ischemia due to prolonged stretching of nerves (*i.e.*, extreme hip flexion) during the second stage of labor [30].

Severe Infection

Epidural abscess and meningitis are uncommon but potentially catastrophic complications of neuraxial anesthesia procedures. Epidural abscess is more likely to occur after epidural techniques, particularly after prolonged epidural catheterization, whereas meningitis typically occurs after the dura has been punctured, either intentionally as part of a spinal anesthetic or unintentionally as a complication of an epidural procedure [30].

CONCLUSION

All hospitals should have protocols for the objective diagnosis and treatment of severe postpartum complications, as well as established pathways for the timeline management of massive bleeding, respiratory support, sepsis, *etc*.

The management of serious postpartum complications requires a multidisciplinary team. The anticipation and early diagnosis of postpartum complications are key to proper management and better outcomes.

CONSENT FOR PUBLICATION

Not applicable.

CONFLICT OF INTEREST

The authors declare no conflict of interest, financial or otherwise.

ACKNOWLEDGEMENT

Declared none.

REFERENCES

[1]   Postpartum hemorrhage. Practice Bulletin No. 183. American College of Obstetricians and Gynecologists. Obstet Gynecol 2017; 130: e168-86.
        [http://dx.doi.org/10.1097/AOG.0000000000002351]

[2]   Chestnut DH. Chestnut's Obstetric Anesthesia: Principles and Practice. 6th ed., Philadelphia, PA: Elsevier 2020.

[3]   Say L, Chou D, Gemmill A, *et al*. Global causes of maternal death: a WHO systematic analysis. Lancet Glob Health 2014; 2(6): e323-33.

[http://dx.doi.org/10.1016/S2214-109X(14)70227-X] [PMID: 25103301]

[4]   Higgins N, Patel SK, Toledo P. Postpartum hemorrhage revisited. Curr Opin Anaesthesiol 2019; 32(3): 278-84.
[http://dx.doi.org/10.1097/ACO.0000000000000717] [PMID: 31045634]

[5]   Feduniw S, Warzecha D, Szymusik I, Wielgos M. Epidemiology, prevention and management of early postpartum hemorrhage — a systematic review. Ginekol Pol 2020; 91(1): 38-44.
[http://dx.doi.org/10.5603/GP.2020.0009] [PMID: 32039467]

[6]   Vallera C, Choi LO, Cha CM. Uterotonic medications: oxytocin, methylergonovine, carboprost, misoprostol. 2017; 35(2): P207-19.
[http://dx.doi.org/10.1016/j.anclin.2017.01.007]

[7]   Kovacheva VP, Soens MA, Tsen LC. A randomized, double-blinded trial of a "rule of threes" algorithm versus continuous infusion of oxytocin during elective cesarean delivery. Anesthesiology 2015; 123(1): 92-100.
[http://dx.doi.org/10.1097/ALN.0000000000000682] [PMID: 25909969]

[8]   Breathnach F, Geary M. Uterine atony: definition, prevention, nonsurgical management, and uterine tamponade. Semin Perinatol 2009; 33(2): 82-7.
[PMID: 19324236]

[9]   Theunissen FJ, Chinery L, Pujar YV. Current research on carbetocin and implications for prevention of postpartum haemorrhage. Reprod Health 2018; 15(S1) (Suppl. 1): 94.
[http://dx.doi.org/10.1186/s12978-018-0529-0] [PMID: 29945640]

[10] Chen YT, Chen SF, Hsieh TT, Lo LM, Hung TH. A comparison of the efficacy of carbetocin and oxytocin on hemorrhage-related changes in women with cesarean deliveries for different indications. Taiwan J Obstet Gynecol 2018; 57(5): 677-82.
[http://dx.doi.org/10.1016/j.tjog.2018.08.011] [PMID: 30342650]

[11] Urner F, Zimmermann R, Krafft A. Manual removal of the placenta after vaginal delivery: an unsolved problem in Obstetrics J Pregnancy 2014; 2014: 274651.
[http://dx.doi.org/10.1155/2014/274651]

[12] Mousa HA, Blum J, Abou El Senoun G, Shakur H, Alfirevic Z. Treatment for primary postpartum haemorrhage. Cochrane Database Syst Rev 2014; (2): CD003249.
[PMID: 24523225]

[13] Protocolos SEGO. Complicaciones tromboembólicas de la gestación. Progresos de Obstetricia y Ginecología 2008; 51(3): 181-92.
[http://dx.doi.org/10.1016/S0304-5013(08)71074-4]

[14] Protocols medicina maternofetal. Protocolo tromboembolismo venoso en la gestación y el puerperio. Hospital Clinic - Hospital Sant Joan de Déu – Universitat de Barcelona. 2018.
[PMID: 19324236]

[15] RCOG. Thromboembolic disease in pregnancy and the puerperium: acute management 2015.

[16] Rojas-Sánchez AG, Navarro-de la Rosa G, Mijangos-Méndez JC, Campos-Cerda R. Tromboembolia pulmonar en el embarazo y puerperio. Neumol Cir Torax 2014; 73(1): 42-8.
[http://dx.doi.org/10.35366/48972]

[17] Wiegers HMG, Middeldorp S. Contemporary best practice in the management of pulmonary embolism during pregnancy. Ther Adv Respir Dis 2020; 14
[http://dx.doi.org/10.1177/1753466620914222] [PMID: 32425105]

[18] Baldisseri M, Clark S. Amniotic fluid embolism 2020.

[19] Clark SL. Amniotic fluid embolism. Obstet Gynecol 2014; 123(2): 337-48.
[http://dx.doi.org/10.1097/AOG.0000000000000107] [PMID: 24402585]

[20] Kaur K, Bhardwaj M, Kumar P, Singhal S, Singh T, Hooda S. Amniotic fluid embolism. J

Anaesthesiol Clin Pharmacol 2016; 32(2): 153-9.
[http://dx.doi.org/10.4103/0970-9185.173356] [PMID: 27275041]

[21]   Pacheco LD, Saade G, Hankins G, Clark S. Amniotic fluid embolism: diagnosis and management
Society for maternal – fetal medicine Clinical guidelines No 9.

[22]   Hofmeyr R, Matjila M, Dyer R. Preeclampsia in 2017: obstetric and anaesthesia management.
baillieres best pract res clin anaesthesiol 2017; 31(1): 125-38.
[http://dx.doi.org/10.1016/j.bpa.2016.12.002]

[23]   Consults in Obstetric Anesthesiology Suzanne K.W. Mankowits, MD ISBN 978-3-319-2 Hypertensive
diseases Victoria Danhakl, Ruth Landau capt 83 pag 289-293.
[http://dx.doi.org/10.1007/978-3-319-59680-8]

[24]   Sepúlveda-Martínez A, Rencoret G, Silva MC, *et al.* First trimester screening for preterm and term
pre-eclampsia by maternal characteristics and biophysical markers in a low-risk population. J Obstet
Gynaecol Res 2019; 45(1): 104-12.
[http://dx.doi.org/10.1111/jog.13809] [PMID: 30230132]

[25]   Michael G. Ross, MD, MPD; Chief editor: Ronald M Ramus. Obstetrics & Ginecology. Eclampsia.
Medscape. Update: 2019.

[26]   Gestational Hypertension and Preeclampsia. Gestational Hypertension and Preeclampsia. Obstet
Gynecol 2020; 135(6): 1492-5.
[PMID: 32443077]

[27]   Headache Classification Committee of the International Headache Society (HIS). The International
classification of headache disorders 2018. https://ichd-3.org/

[28]   de Almeida SM, Shumaker SD, LeBlanc SK, *et al.* Incidence of post-dural puncture headache in
research volunteers. Headache 2011; 51(10): 1503-10.
[http://dx.doi.org/10.1111/j.1526-4610.2011.01959.x] [PMID: 21797856]

[29]   Choi PT, Galinski SE, Takeuchi L, Lucas S, Tamayo C, Jadad AR. PDPH is a common complication
of neuraxial blockade in parturients: a meta-analysis of obstetrical studies. Can J Anaesth 2003; 50(5):
460-9.
[http://dx.doi.org/10.1007/BF03021057] [PMID: 12734154]

[30]   D'Angelo R, Smiley RM, Riley ET, Segal S. Serious complications related to obstetric anesthesia: the
serious complication repository project of the Society for Obstetric Anesthesia and Perinatology.
Anesthesiology 2014; 120(6): 1505-12.
[http://dx.doi.org/10.1097/ALN.0000000000000253] [PMID: 24845921]

CHAPTER 17

Analgesia after Labor and Cesarean Section: Chronic Pain after Pregnancy

Carmen Gomar Sancho[1,*], **Ana Plaza Moral**[1], **Marina Vendrell Jordà**[1], **Antonio López Hernández**[1] and **Irene León Carsí**[1]

[1] *Hospital Clinic, University of Barcelona and University Vic-Central de Catalonia, Barcelona, Spain*

Abstract: Chronic pain (*CP*) conditions after childbirth include persistent pain after caesarean section (*CPCS*), perineal pain after instrumental vaginal delivery, lower back pain and pelvic girdle pain. Any type of CP before or during pregnancy increases the risk of CP after delivery. Scar pain is the most recognized etiology for CPCS with a neuropathic component, although it is less frequent than in other surgeries. Reported CPCS incidence ranges from 1 to 23%. Pain intensity is moderate and decreases with time in all studies. The severity and duration of peripartum pain are the main risk factors for CP and its control is the most recommended strategy for reducing risk. Fear of fetal and neonatal adverse events means that CP is often undertreated, but after delivery, pharmacological restrictions disappear and many pain drugs are compatible with breastfeeding. Education of obstetric teams about early detection and referral to specialized consultation of women with CP is the key. In this chapter, available information in the recent literature, mainly during the last years, is presented. This chapter focuses on CP conditions after childbirth, as analgesia for labor and childbirth and immediate pain after CS and vaginal delivery are covered in other chapters of this book.

Keywords: Chronic pain, Obstetric patient, Incidence, Postpartum, Risk Factors, Treatment.

INTRODUCTION

Women´s health-related to maternity is recognized as of utmost importance due to the number of childbirths worldwide and the characteristics of the affected population: young women at an active and productive stage of their life both in their families and productive fields of all societies.

After delivery, chronic pain (*CP*) may be due to different types and causes, but

* **Corresponding author Carmen Gomar Sancho:** Hospital Clinic, University of Barcelona and University Vic-Central de Catalonia, Barcelona, Spain; Email: cgomar@umanresa.cat

Eugenio Daniel Martinez-Hurtado, Monica Sanjuan-Alvarez & Marta Chacon-Castillo (Eds.)
All rights reserved-© 2022 Bentham Science Publishers

mainly includes persistent pain after cesarean section (*CPCS*), perineal pain after vaginal delivery, lower back pain, and pelvic girdle pain. The risk to present any of these pain conditions is increased in women with any type of CP before or during pregnancy.

Pain present in the postpartum period can be related to the delivery mode, such as operational assisted vaginal delivery or cesarean section (*CS*). It may have originated during pregnancy such as low back pain, pelvic girdle pain, or headaches, or correspond to a previous history of any type of CP. Rarely, CP conditions present before pregnancy improve after childbirth, except for migraine.

Most research in postpartum CP has been dedicated to persistent or chronic pain after CS (*CPCS*). Little information is available regarding the overall prevalence of pre-existing CP disorders in pregnant women and their course during pregnancy and after delivery, although their negative impact on pregnancy and the postpartum period is recognized [1].

In addition to the scarcity of research on postpartum CP in relation to the high prevalence of childbirths, there is another issue in obstetric pain management: it is widely acknowledged that pain management teams and clinics frequently discharge or decline to manage women during pregnancy, and transition of care is frequently referred to the obstetrical team, which has inadequate training and limited time to manage patients with CP. Therefore, pregnancy and early postpartum period can turn into periods of suboptimal medical care of pre-existing pain due to both the lack of evidence-based treatment guidelines, limited formal training and expertise of the obstetric team, and the patient's acceptance of pain due to her fear of harming her child with any treatment [1].

However, obstetric pain management is considered an indicator of the quality of health organizations. Well-informed obstetrical teams and mothers must come in advance for specialized pain consultation since established post-surgical CP is difficult to treat. Awareness that CPCS is associated with other CP conditions and psychological and emotional problems should be part of the obstetric team's education on CPSC prognosis, as well as that any other CP condition improves with the earliest reference to the pain clinic.

POSTPARTUM CHRONIC PAIN RELATED TO DELIVERY METHOD

The relevance and available pieces of evidence of postpartum CP have been comprehensively exposed in the recent reviews by Lavand'Homme P and Komatsu R et al [2, 3]. The reported incidence of persistent pain after childbirth varies depending on the method of delivery, study population, and, above all, the study design.

Chronic Pain After Cesarean Section

Persistent pain after CS and vaginal delivery is considered a type of postsurgical CP. The terms *"persistent pain"* or *"chronic pain"* are used indistinctly after surgery. It is defined as *"pain that develops or increases in intensity after a surgical procedure and persists beyond the healing process, i.e.,* at least 3 months after the initiating event", and it frequently has a neuropathic component. Some studies have considered two months of pain persistence in the definition. Postsurgical CP develops in one out of ten surgical patients and becomes an intolerable pain condition after one of every 100 operations – an incidence that has not changed over time. It represents more than 22% of pain clinic consultations [4].

The development of any postsurgical CP is due to complex neurophysiologic mechanisms, which are only partly known, and which appear and develop after the surgical wound or other severe tissue trauma. The type of surgery influences the incidence of postsurgical CP. Cesarean section is in the ninth position in frequency in the list of surgeries causing CP [2] behind thoracic, orthopedic, and abdominal surgical procedures.

The detailed description of the neurobiological changes causing the transition from acute to chronic pain after surgery and trauma is beyond the scope of this chapter. We refer the readers to excellent published reviews [4 - 8].

In Fig. (**1**), the locations in the peripheral and central nervous system where the sensitization mechanisms responsible for the transition from acute to chronic pain take place are outlined. Neural sensitization is triggered by nociceptive inputs from the inflammation and nerve lesion at the surgical location. The resulting local molecular changes lead to peripheral neural pain sensitisation in the form of primary hyperalgesia and allodynia.

Peripheral sensitization increases pain transmission, which in turn ensures maladaptive neuroplastic changes in primary sensory neurons of the dorsal root ganglia and at the spinal dorsal horn and/or higher central nervous system structures known as central sensitization.

Central sensitization reflects the interaction of multiple factors, neurotransmitters, activation of neurons and microglia at the spinal dorsal horn, called *"wind up"* that is manifested by neuro-sensitive changes in the wound surroundings. It´s called secondary hyperalgesia and allodynia. Sustained hypersensitivity to pain has developed in the peripheral and central nervous systems [2, 9, 10]. The descending inhibitory modulation of noxious signalling in the spinal pathways is compromised and maladaptive changes in the brain function and structure develop. N-methyl-D-aspartate receptors' activation has a key role in the central sensitization mechanisms.

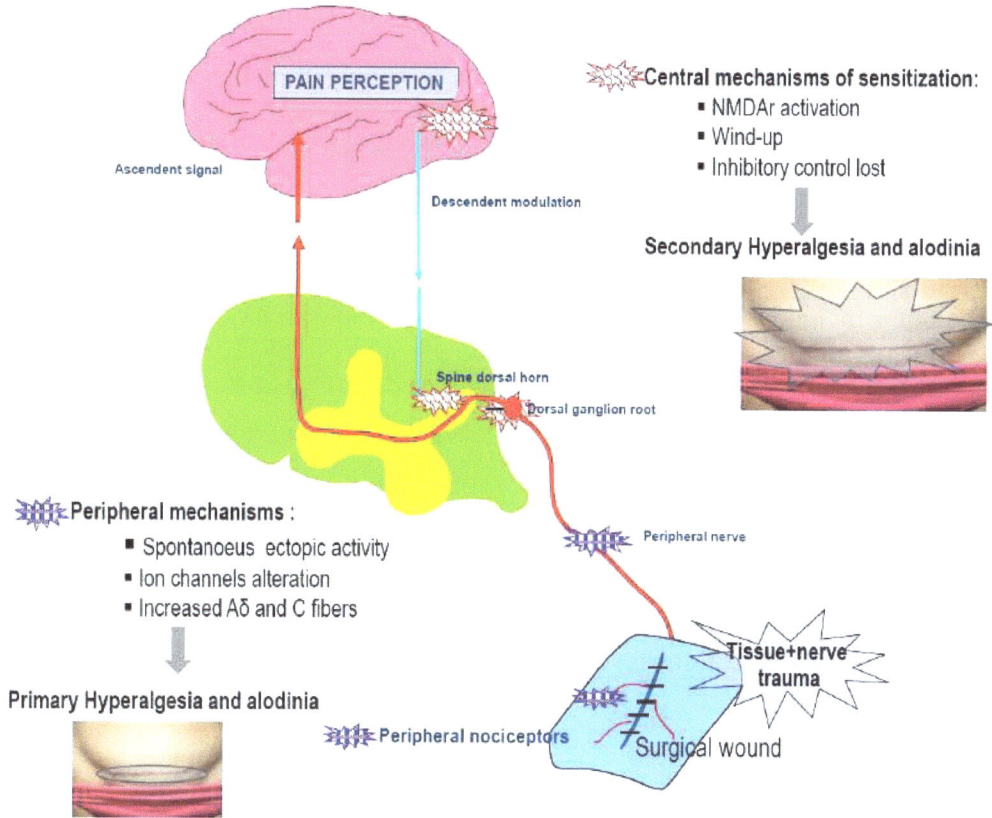

Fig. (1). Schematic representation of the mechanisms of transition of postoperative pain to chronic pain. The hatched marks indicate the locations where neurobiological changes causing neurosensitization are marked, blue for peripheral neurosentization and red for central sensitization. ***Primary hyperalgesia*** and allodynia close to the wound manifest peripheral noxious *via* nerve damage and tissue inflammation. Exaggerated pain transmission arriving at the primary neuron in the dorsal ganglion route and spinal dorsal horn activates N-methyl-D-aspartate receptors among other molecular factors, magnifying the reception area at the spinal dorsal horn. That, together with a poor descendent, causes ***secondary hyperalgesia and allodynia***. The area of ***secondary hyperalgesia and allodynia*** has a direct relationship with the risk of CP.

Scar pain is the most identified etiology for persistent pain after CS. The common horizontal suprapubic scar (Pfannenstiel) can entrap the ilio-inguinal or ilio-hypogastric nerves, initiating diffuse persistent neuropathic pain. The neuropathic component of CPCS is present in 50% of women with CPCS, less than in other types of surgery. Pain intensity is usually mild or moderate; a pain score of more than 3/10 is found in about 2% of cases; and, in all studies, both CPSC incidence and intensity decrease with time [2, 3].

The clinical relevance of CPCS is important since the number of CS procedures has increased dramatically both in developed and developing countries in recent decades. The calculated number of CS performed in 2015 worldwide is calculated at 29 million, an increase of 16 million since the year 2000 [11].

As happens with other types of post-surgical CP, the differences in the design of research studies make it difficult to get evidence on the incidence and risk factors of CPCS [10, 12]. Therefore, the reported incidence of CPCS one year after surgery is highly variable, ranging from less than 1% to 23% [13].

A systematic review published in 2016 found 17 studies specifically aimed at assessing the incidence of CPCS with a follow-up period of more than 2 months. The studies included 4932 records overall, and the incidence of CPCS was highly variable among the studies, ranging between 4% and 41.8%. The reported factors that influence CPCS were inconsistent among studies, except for the presence of a higher intensity of pain on postoperative day 1 [14].

Another meta-analysis published in 2016 found a clinically relevant incidence of CPCS ranging from 15% at 3 months to 11% at 12 months or longer [15]. This incidence has remained largely stable, with a tendency towards a decrease in recent years [16], perhaps due to better control of immediate postoperative pain. It is still generally accepted by pain specialists that women are reluctant to report pain in the context of childbirth, and the reported incidence may be underrated.

CPCS affects the daily activities and quality of life of mothers during a period in which they are overloaded with caring for their babies. Therefore, it is considered a relevant clinical and social problem due to the high and increasing frequency of CS and the vulnerability of the affected population [3]. The World Health Organization has included CPCS in the new International Classification of Diseases (ICD-11) and its prevention is now considered an indicator of the quality of health care [17]. Furthermore, CPCS is often associated with chronic use of analgesics like opioids, and there is currently a growing concern about persistent opioid use after not only major but also minor surgical procedures, including postpartum pain [2, 18].

Chronic Pain After Vaginal Delivery

The persistence of pain after vaginal delivery has been little assessed. Reported incidence increases from 2% to 10% at six months and later, almost exclusively in mothers who have had an instrumentalized vaginal birth and is related to the magnitude of the perineal trauma [19]. Chronic pain related to instrumentalized vaginal delivery has been scarcely investigated and is not included as a high-risk CP procedure.

As it has been speculated that tissue damage and inflammation are potential mechanisms for postpartum vaginal and perineal pain, it is considered predominantly nociceptive pain [3]. The nature of persistent vaginal and perineal pain is less well characterized than after CS, but when it occurs, it is of higher intensity, longer duration, and affects more of the quality of life and mood than CPCS. Women often complain of pain in the perineal area and buttocks, as well as deep abdominal and pelvic pain. Nevertheless, long-lasting dyspareunia, an evoked CP type, that women are reluctant to complain about, is frequent after both spontaneous and assisted vaginal delivery [19]. Vaginal delivery has been associated with a higher incidence of chronic pelvic girdle pain than CS [20].

In a limited sample of Spanish women, an incidence of 12.5% of perineal CP in vaginal deliveries with episiotomy without any other instrumentation was described, confirming older reports. This supports the current trend of not considering episiotomy harmless [21].

Influencing Factors on Postpartum Chronic Pain

Several papers have identified factors associated with a higher incidence of CPCS. Uncontrolled immediate postoperative pain and the time spent in severe pain are the most consistent independent predictors of CPSP, as happens with other post-surgical CP [5, 9, 11, 12].

Recently, the intensity of pain on movement, also known as dynamic pain, on postpartum day 1 has been associated with CPCS incidence at 6 months and with CPCS intensity at 1 year [16]. This information offers an important opportunity for intervention to reduce the risk of CPCS by applying aggressive postoperative analgesia techniques.

Besides the above-described neurobiological process, there are also individual factors that affect the propensity for the persistence of acute pain, but there is still a lot of unknown information. A direct relationship between the degree of tissue trauma and the severity of acute postpartum pain is evident, this being a robust risk factor for CP. Nevertheless, a direct relationship between tissue trauma and CP development after delivery is less clear [2, 3]. It is accepted that individual-related factors such as an exaggerated reaction to tissue trauma and failed neuro-adaptation in different pain dimensions modulate the risk of postpartum CP. On the other hand, CS causes very complex surgical trauma. It occurs in a state of exaggerated hormonal stimulation and changes in the mother's immune system. And opening of the pregnant uterus and the manipulation of the placenta may have unique inflammatory effects of unknown impact.

A previous history of pain affecting the area of the CS incision or in other body parts (*i.e.* neuropathy, fibromyalgia, low back pain, pelvic pain, chronic headaches) triples the risk of CPCS [22], as well as depression before and during pregnancy. On the other hand, it has been reported that women with CPCS have a higher risk of developing other CP pain conditions after delivery [2, 3, 16]. Pre-partum anxiety, smoking, and longer CS surgical time have been related to a greater risk for CPCS in some studies [16]. A second CS does not increase CPCS, but it is a significant risk factor for the development of CPCS after a later-life hysterectomy [23]. To date, there is no evidence that the type of peripartum anaesthesia (general or neuraxial) and analgesia (epidural or intravenous) have an influence on postpartum CP, particularly in the context of CS. However, a recent Cochrane Review including 601 patients found that the use of effective intrawound infiltration and parietal blocks reduce CP after CS [24].

Genetic factors have been considered as potential contributing factors in the setting of acute postoperative pain, including acute postpartum pain. Recently, an association between gene polymorphism (CCL2 gene rs4586, CALCA rs3781719, CX3CL1 rs614230) and CPCS has been described in Chinese Han women [25]. The research on genetic factors influencing pain is of great interest, but its complexity makes transference to the clinical practice a long-term feat.

Hormonal changes during pregnancy are also considered to influence pain. High oestrogen and progesterone concentrations induce dramatic changes in the maternal immune system. Pregnancy-induced analgesia has been shown in animals and suggested in women [26]. An interesting observation has been that CPCS incidence is lower in comparison with that occurring after some general surgical procedures in similar locations in women. Women with previous CP condition can improve during pregnancy and return to previous pain level after delivery.

A very well-designed study in young adult female mice with induced neuropathic and inflammatory CP has demonstrated a switch from a microglia-independent to a microglia-dependent pain hypersensitivity mechanism in early weeks of pregnancy; in late pregnancy, the evidence of CP disappeared [26]. This pregnancy-induced analgesia in mice was dependent on pregnancy hormones (oestrogen and progesterone), opioid receptors, and T cells of the adaptive immune system.

These findings are relevant for understanding CP changes observed during pregnancy, but also add to growing evidence of sex-specific T-cell involvement in CP. It has not been studied if the pregnancy-related analgesia persists after delivery.

Women want and need to recover faster after delivery, and more attention should be paid to the postpartum recovery period in which pain persists and functional recovery is a goal for patients and health providers. Recently, the subacute period of recovery is considered a *"key period"* in the chronification of postoperative pain because of the increased involvement of psycho-social factors that include the psychological burden of pain in some patients [4, 27].

Interventions for Decreasing the Risk of Postpartum Chronic Pain

There is no evidence of direct or effective interventions for reducing CP risk or for treating it, but some recommendations have been made based on decreasing acute postoperative pain burden, a consistent severe postoperative pain risk factor.

More aggressive use of labor epidural analgesia for decreasing both the pain during labor and the need for general anaesthesia in the case of urgent intrapartum CS is recommended, as well as opiates added to intrathecal local anaesthetics, increasing intrathecal local anaesthetic doses when opiates are contraindicated, wound infiltrations, and parietal blocks [3, 4, 24]. Since some of these recommendations go against the current trend towards minimally medicalized delivery, it is important to detect patients at risk of postpartum CP to make decisions.

Aggressive postpartum pain treatment and detection of women with CP history, together with educational measures for helping women to communicate postpartum pain, seem like logical interventions according to current evidence [2]. Pain education of the obstetric team is crucial since they are in charge of postpartum follow-up. They should be trained in acute pain assessment, both upon movement and at rest, control of severe pain, and the importance of subacute pain in the recovery period, an emergent field of interest in preventing CP that requires balancing pain against the need for fast recovery [27].

CHRONIC PAIN AFTER CHILDBIRTH UNRELATED TO DELIVERY METHOD

One recent publication by Komatsu R *et al.* in 2020 has updated the available evidence on post-delivery CP of any type [3]. After delivery, women can present any CP conditions found in the general population, as well as previous CP conditions that could have persisted during pregnancy, or a return to previous characteristics in case these changed during pregnancy. Low back pain, pelvic girdle pain, and migraine appearance are the most characteristic of this period [28].

Low Back Pain

Low back pain (*LBP*) is the most frequent pain condition during pregnancy and postpartum, reaching a prevalence of 50% [29]. It is the most common reason for the referral of pregnant women to pain consultations in Spain [30].

In most women, LBP started during pregnancy disappears during the postpartum period, but it persists in about 10% several years after delivery, even up until old age. When LBP is associated with visceral pelvic pain or pelvic girdle pain, its prognosis is worse [31]. The cause of LBP in pregnancy is considered multifactorial and associated with biomechanical, vascular, and hormonal changes during pregnancy [32]. A considerable number of pregnant women who had previously only occasionally presented with LBP complain about daily pain during pregnancy.

LBP during and after pregnancy share some predisposing factors. The most robust predisposing factors are past LBP before pregnancy, obesity, and excessive weight gain during pregnancy. Other factors with weaker evidence are LBP in previous pregnancies, number of previous pregnancies, earliest LBP onset in pregnancy, back pain during menstruation, a younger age, and lack of physical activity [3, 33].

Neither the delivery method (emergent or planned CS, spontaneous or instrumented vaginal delivery) nor the type of analgesia-anaesthesia technique (epidural anaesthesia/analgesia) seems to influence LBP incidence after delivery. As Komatsu *et al*. points out, sample size of prospective studies is too small to assure that the relevance of some predisposing factors has not been missed [3].

The influence of hormonal changes of pregnancy in patients' conditions favouring LBP is an interesting fact. Finger joint laxity, as a reflection of connective tissue constitutional weakness, is an early predictor of LBP in pregnancy [34], but there is no information on whether this influence persists to some extent in the postpartum period.

Significant disability due to LBP only affects a small proportion during pregnant and postpartum women [33] but when LBP is associated with depression and anxiety, which happens in 15% of the cases, it has a negative impact that increases over time, increasing the probability of labor inductions and CS, preterm birth, and low birth weight [29]. After delivery, maternal depression associated with LBP affects her well-being and perhaps her ability to take care of the newborn. Evidence for depression should be explored in women with LBP before and after delivery.

Pelvic Girdle Pain

Pelvic girdle pain (*PGP*) together with LBP is the most frequent pain condition in the obstetric population. The association of PGP, LBP and leg pain is relatively frequent. Pelvic girdle pain is a multifactorial condition of unknown etiology with a significant negative impact on women's psychological and physical wellbeing, both during and after pregnancy. PGP is a musculoskeletal pain that should not be confused with pelvic pain caused by the pelvic intra-abdominal viscera [2, 35, 36]. PGP may exist before pregnancy, begin during it, or appear postpartum.

Pregnancy related PGP ranges from 23 to 65% and produces severe physical disability in about 10% of women [37]. The Spanish Pain Research Network reported a prevalence of 64.7% of PGP at four weeks after delivery [30]. As with other CP conditions, pregnancy represents a gap in specialized pain management for many women. There is very little information about PGP assessment during pregnancy, and there is not a clear definition of PGP in the context of pregnancy changes [38].

In PGP, pain is located at the posterior iliac crest and the gluteal fold, particularly in the vicinity of the sacroiliac joints and reproducible by specific clinical tests that are also reproducible in pregnant women [39]. The positive elicited clinical responses of PGP during pregnancy predict its long-term persistence after delivery [40].

Most frequently, PGP that first appears during pregnancy improves in the first postpartum weeks, but in pregnant women with a previous history of chronic PGP, this pain will reappear after a few weeks. Recently, Gausel AM *et al.* have conducted a prospective study on 130 women with severe-moderate pregnancy related PGP to investigate the subjective recovery after delivery [41]. Substantial pain relief was found in 83% of women 6 weeks after delivery, in almost half of them, this occurred during the first two weeks. Risk factors for poor recovery were PGP during the year before pregnancy, severe pain during pregnancy, and multiparity. When PGP does not improve after delivery, it has a negative emotional and psychological impact on women, affecting their daily life, sense of identity, and ability to care for their children [42].

Some evidence suggests that vaginal delivery is associated with less postpartum PGP incidence than urgent or planned CS [20]. A recently published review on risk factors for postpartum PGP, including 22 studies, described risk factors that can be easily detectable during pregnancy. Three months after delivery, PGP persistence was associated with pain intensity and disability due to PGP during pregnancy, positive provocation tests and other detectable physical symptoms [40]. In the subgroup of women presenting PGP associated with LBP, only one third recovered after delivery. Psychosocial characteristics influence the risk of long-lasting lumbo-pelvic CP related to pregnancy [28]. PGP which persists even after 12 years postpartum, has been associated with interpersonally distressed and dysfunctional personality traits. In fact, the bio-psycho-social model has become the leading theory for the development and management of chronic pain [31].

Other Pain Conditions

Migraine prevalence in women of reproductive age reaches 18%, but during pregnancy, pre-existing migraines largely improve with a reported incidence of about 5%, 25% of them with a previous history of migraines [43]. Pregnancy and the postpartum period present a high-risk period for secondary headaches due to vascular or neurological severe complications. Headache onset in late pregnancy and postpartum should be carefully investigated to discard any subjacent medical problems.

Chronic headache or LBP CP after postdural puncture headache in intrathecal or epidural techniques has not been the subject of publications in obstetric patients, despite the high frequency of this complication in obstetric population. Therefore, it can be considered that the risk of CP is negligible. Recently, a pilot study with a small sample of obstetric patients treated with an epidural blood patch for postdural puncture headache was found to present a greater risk of chronic LBP [44].

This unspecific etiology of vulvodynia makes it hard to diagnose and treat; with young women in their early reproductive years at greatest risk of developing it [45]. Pre-existing vulvodynia has a variable course during pregnancy, either getting worse, stabilizing, or improving. The latter is more frequent during the third gestational trimester. Elective cesarean section is frequently planned and there is little information about neuraxial anaesthetic techniques for vaginal delivery in these women. In the postpartum period, vulvodynia usually presents with the same pain characteristics as before pregnancy [46].

CHRONIC PAIN TREATMENT AFTER DELIVERY

After delivery, restrictions on the prescription of analgesics taken during pregnancy due to adverse effects on the fetus and childbirth disappear. In the postpartum period, the main concern regarding pharmacological treatment is breastfeeding and the possible adverse effects on the baby. Fortunately, many analgesics and adjuvant drugs used for pain management are quite safe during lactation, and therefore, it is not at all justifiable to leave pain insufficiently treated.

The Relevance of Pain Drugs' Transfer into Breast Milk.

There are widely accepted lists of safe pharmacological treatments based on the pharmacokinetics of transference between mother's plasma and breast milk, as well as information on drug safety in newborn babies. In the context of pain treatment, the transfer of drugs into breast milk is always an issue. Neonatal drug exposure is typically expressed as a relative infant dose (*RID*). The RID considers maternal and neonatal weights, and a cut-off RID of less than 10% is generally recommended for safety.

Additionally, the age of the infant should be considered. Premature babies' clear drugs poorly, but at the age of 7 months it becomes similar to adults. Additional strategies include alternating breast and bottle-feeding or adjusting the timing of drug administration relative to breast-feeding. The characteristics of drugs used for pain treatment regarding their pharmacological characteristics influencing plasma-milk transference are available [47, 48]. Due to slightly lower milk pH (7.2), basic drugs transfer more readily into breast milk and become trapped secondary to ionization. Milk at the end of a feed (hind milk), with a greater fatty content than foremilk, may concentrate liposoluble drugs. A summary of this information is shown in Table 1.

Analgesics such as paracetamol, ibuprofen, naproxen, and morphine are considered "*safe*" due to their low transfer into breast milk, high first-pass metabolism, and few problems with extensive usage. The latest revisions do not recommend the use of codeine, which in its metabolism is converted to morphine. Due to a variation in the liver enzyme CYP2D6, some people are ultra-rapid metabolizers, and may convert codeine to morphine more rapidly than other people. These people are more likely to have higher than normal levels of morphine in their breast milk, which in turn would lead to life-threatening or fatal side effects in nursing babies [49]. Controversy exists regarding oxycodone and meperidine newborn safety.

Table 1. Summary of the relevance of pain drugs transfer into breast milk.

Drug	Typically Used For	RID (%)	Recommendation	Caution
Aspirin	Acute pain	F/M = 1	Use with caution	Reyes syndrome, unknown effect on platelet function

(Table 1) cont.....

Drug	Typically Used For	RID (%)	Recommendation	Caution
Acetaminophen	Acute or chronic pain	1.3-6.4%	Compatible	Do not use the combined form with opioids (in order to diminish absolute opioid use) Use with caution in pre-term infants and liver pathology
nSAIDS	Acute or chronic pain	Ibuprophen: 0.1 -0.7% Ketorolac: 0.2-0.4%	Generally accepted Ibuprophen and Ketorolac has the lowest transfer	Isolated case reports on adverse effects with indomethacin and naproxen
Celecoxib	Acute or chronic pain	0.3%	Generally accepted	Use Ibuprophen when available, as there is more data
Metamizole	Acute or chronic pain	6-30%	Not recommended	Increased risk of acute lymphocytic leukaemia, agranulocytosis
Triptans	Chronic pain (migraine)	No data	No data	Only sumatriptan has been reviewed by AAP and considered safe
Gabapentin	Chronic pain	Adjuvant 1.3-6.5%	Maintain in chronic users, not routinely for acute pain treatment	Risk of neonatal sedation
Pregabalin	Chronic pain Adjuvant	No data	Compatible	Monitor drowsiness
Dexamethasone	Adjuvant	No data	Compatible	-
Ketamine	Acute pain	No data	Not recommended	Limit use

(Table 1) cont.....

	Drug	Typically Used For	RID (%)	Recommendation	Caution
OPIOIDS	Hydrocodone	Acute or chronic pain	1.6-3.7%	Not recommended by AAP Accepted by SOAP	Potential toxicity due to CYP2D6 metabolism No reports of neonatal sedation
	Oxycodone	Acute or chronic pain	1.5-8%	Not recommended by AAP Accepted by SOAP	Potential toxicity due to CYP2D6 metabolism No reports of neonatal sedation
	Morphine	Acute or chronic pain	5.8-10.7%	Compatible	High transfer, but low oral bioavailability in the infant Cases of neonatal sedation reported
	Hydromorphone	Acute or chronic pain	0.7%	Compatible	Low experience
	Tramadol	Acute or chronic pain	2.4-2.9%	Not recommended	Increased risk of neonatal apnea and death Fast CYP2D6 metabolism converts to morphine
	Fentanyl	Acute or chronic pain	0.9-3%	Compatible	Gold standard
	Methadone	Acute or chronic pain	F/M = 0.2	Compatible	-
	Remifentanil	Acute pain	F/M = 0,29-0,88	Compatible	High placental metabolism
	Meperidine	Acute or chronic pain	F/M = 0.35-1.6	Best to avoid	Sedation on the infant Active metabolites Recommended only for treatment of post-operative shivering
	Codeine	Acute or chronic pain	0.8-1.4%	Not recommended	Increased risk of neonatal apnea and death Fast CYP2D6 metabolism converts to morphine

(Table 1) cont.....

Drug	Typically Used For	RID (%)	Recommendation	Caution
Local Anesthetics	Acute pain Breakthrough pain	0.2-1.1%	Compatible	Commonly used for local techniques (wound infiltration) or treating breakthrough pain (TAP block) Ropivacaine is safer than Bupivacaine and Lidocaine (No real differences) Very low bioavailability

RID: relative infant dose. The RID takes into account maternal and neonatal weights, and an RID greater than 10% is generally considered a level of concern. When RID is unavailable. **F/M:** fetal/maternal ratio is referred. **AAP:** American Society of Pediatricians. **SOAP:** Society for Obstetric Anesthesia and Perinatology. **TAP:** Trans*versus* Abdominal Plane.

Although tramadol seems to have low transfer into breast milk, it's not recommended due to the same metabolic explanation, the rapid conversion to morphine in some patients [47 - 49]. Fentanyl and methadone are liposoluble drugs and have a higher pass from maternal plasma to milk, especially that at the end of each breastfeed. However, they are considered safe agents for pain treatment.

Most tricyclic antidepressants, fluoxetine, sertraline, and moclobemide (a reversible inhibitor of monoamine oxidase A), are compatible with breastfeeding due to low transfer into breast milk [50]. Gabapentin and pregabalin are extensively used for many CP conditions and they are frequently stopped in pregnant women because of fear of fetal malformations. In babies, gabapentin reaches plasma levels of about 6% of maternal plasma [13] and in the case of pregabalin, isolated reports found in the baby about 8% of mother's levels. Both drugs are associated with somnolence and lazy sucking in babies, and mothers treated with both these drugs should be warned to report any decrease in their babies' activity. At present, gabapentin is considered safer than other treatments for neonatal neurological irritability of different aetiologies, especially in preterm babies [50, 51] but there are no data about possible medium-long term adverse effects.

Treatment of Chronic Pain After Cesarean Section and Instrumentalized Vaginal Delivery

As with other postsurgical pain situations, CPCS presents the unique characteristic of knowing the exact moment in which CP mechanisms are triggered, that is, the surgical incision [5, 10]. Thus, several attempts to prevent CPCS incidence and severity have been made in the perioperative period [2].

One clinical trial has demonstrated that the addition of 150 microg of clonidine to intrathecal bupivacaine for CS is effective in decreasing postoperative secondary hyperalgesia, which has been demonstrated to be directly associated to persistent pain development [52]. In controlled studies, perioperative administration of gabapentin and pregabalin has not demonstrated benefit, either in postoperative acute pain intensity nor in CPCS incidence [3, 50, 53]. Although perioperative low doses of ketamine have been shown to reduce postoperative pain and opiate consumption, no evidence of effects in lowering the risk of CPCS has been demonstrated [54]. Although no adverse effects on the mother or newborn regarding perioperative administration of clonidine, gabapentin, pregabalin, or ketamine as analgesic adjuvants have been reported, they are rarely used by obstetric anaesthesiologists, even when risk factors for CPCS exist, due to their debatable benefits.

The most widely recommended and widely accepted strategy to decrease the CPCS risk is to optimize perioperative analgesia in order to control severe pain and its duration at rest and upon movement. This includes pain during labor and after CS, especially in women with the previously described risk factors for CP. Holland *et al.* have summarized this strategy as the combination of neuraxial anaesthesia-analgesia techniques, intrathecal morphine added to local anaesthetics, wound infiltration or parietal blocks after CS, postoperative multimodal analgesia with acetaminophen and Non-Steroidal Anti-Inflammatory Drugs (*NSAIDs*), and avoidance of systemic opioids [55].

Treatment for Other Types of Chronic Pain After Delivery

During pregnancy, NSAIDs as well as opiates are contraindicated. This is one of the reasons of poor pain control in pregnant women. However, after childbirth, these analgesics have been proven safe during breast feeding and most pain pharmacological protocols for different types of CP can be applied.

In chronic LBP, the most frequent CP condition after delivery, acetaminophen, NSAIDs, and weak opiates are the most commonly used drugs. Among non-pharmacological measures to decrease pain, psychological or emotional ones, such as hypnosis, relaxation, or music-therapy have very limited analgesic efficacy [55], but physical planned exercises performed regularly, as well as transcutaneous electrical nerve stimulation, are frequently considered effective in improving LBP during pregnancy and in the postpartum period [3, 32, 56] but a recent randomized study found conflicting results in this field [57].

For PGP, physical exercises are less useful than for LBP [36, 55] but pelvis floor manipulation techniques by specialized osteopathic physiotherapists have been proven useful [58]. A recent randomized trial has demonstrated that acupuncture associated with pelvic manipulation significantly increases PGP alleviation [59]. However, most articles on acupuncture to alleviate CP in the postpartum period are published in Chinese and are difficult to access.

Recently, the use of spinal cord stimulation (*SCS*) to treat neuropathic pain such as complex regional pain and failed back pain syndrome in 32 pregnant women has been published [60]. SCS demonstrated a significant improvement in pain intensity and the quality of life in pregnant patients without teratogenic or adverse effects during childbirth and lactation. Electrode displacement is frequent due to, among other factors, increased abdominal pressure during pregnancy and delivery, and SCS functioning should be checked early in postpartum.

Chronic migraine frequently improves during pregnancy and lactation. However, there is frequently a tensional headache in the first postpartum week in women without a previous history of migraines. When chronic migraine persists during pregnancy, women stop or switch medications and non-pharmacological measures, such as relaxation and antistress techniques, application of cold, avoidance of triggers, and biofeedback are initially used. Paracetamol is practically the only drug used for migraines during pregnancy, even if its fetal safety is not guaranteed [43]. As already mentioned, an intense headache appearing in late pregnancy or postpartum must be carefully evaluated to rule out underlying pathological conditions.

While keeping in mind drug safety during lactation, it is important to remember that good analgesia promotes successful breastfeeding and maternal-neonatal bonding and maternal recovery [61]. Uncontrolled pain may transform into maternal opioid misuse that will have consequences for mother and child during lactation [62]. Most CP treatments of neuropathic and musculoskeletal pain are safe during lactation. During pregnancy, non-pharmacological techniques for chronic migraines, vulvodynia or LBP are recommended [63], but after delivery pharmacological treatment should be evaluated.

CONCLUSION

Chronic postpartum pain is a relevant health problem as it affects a large population due to the number of births worldwide.

Obstetric pain management is considered an indicator of the quality of health organizations. However, pregnancy and the early postpartum period can turn into periods of suboptimal medical care due to the lack of treatment guidelines and the interruption of follow-up by chronic pain specialists.

Obstetric teams must be educated in chronic pain early detection and management, as well as have a closer relationship with pain clinics. The awareness that CPCS is associated with other CP conditions and psychological and emotional problems should be part of the education of the obstetric team. Also the prognosis of CPCS, like that of any other CP conditions, improves with the earliest reference to the pain clinic.

CONSENT FOR PUBLICATION

Not applicable.

CONFLICT OF INTEREST

The authors declare no conflict of interest, financial or otherwise.

ACKNOWLEDGEMENT

Declared none.

REFERENCES

[1]   Ray-Griffith S, Wendel M, Stowe Z, Magann E. Chronic pain during pregnancy: a review of the literature. Int J Womens Health 2018; 10: 153-64.
        [http://dx.doi.org/10.2147/IJWH.S151845] [PMID: 29692634]

[2]   Lavand'homme P. Postpartum chronic pain. Minerva Anestesiol 2019; 85(3): 320-4.
        [http://dx.doi.org/10.23736/S0375-9393.18.13060-4] [PMID: 30394066]

[3]   Komatsu R, Ando K, Flood PD. Factors associated with persistent pain after childbirth: a narrative review. Vol. 124, British Journal of Anaesthesia. Elsevier Ltd 2020; e117-30.

[4]   Lavand'homme P. Transition from acute to chronic pain after surgery. Pain 2017; 158(1) (Suppl. 1): S50-4.
        [http://dx.doi.org/10.1097/j.pain.0000000000000809] [PMID: 28134653]

[5]   Richebé P, Capdevila X, Rivat C. Persistent Postsurgical Pain. Anesthesiology 2018; 129(3): 590-607.
        [http://dx.doi.org/10.1097/ALN.0000000000002238] [PMID: 29738328]

[6]   Glare P, Aubrey KR, Myles PS. Transition from acute to chronic pain after surgery. Lancet Elsevier Ltd 2019; 393(10180): 1537-46.

[7]   Pozek JPJ, Beausang D, Baratta JL, Viscusi ER. The Acute to Chronic Pain Transition. Med Clin North Am 2016; 100(1): 17-30.
        [http://dx.doi.org/10.1016/j.mcna.2015.08.005] [PMID: 26614716]

[8]   Schnabel A. Acute neuropathic pain and the transition to chronic postsurgical pain. Pain Manag (Lond) 2018; 8(5): 317-9.
        [http://dx.doi.org/10.2217/pmt-2018-0026] [PMID: 30280642]

[9]   Masgoret P, Gomar C, Tena B, Taurá P, Ríos J, Coca M. Incidence of persistent postoperative pain after hepatectomies with 2 regimes of perioperative analgesia containing ketamine. 2017; 96: (15).

[10]   Masgoret P, de Soto I, Caballero Á, Ríos J, Gomar C. Incidence of contralateral neurosensitive changes and persistent postoperative pain 6 months after mastectomy. Medicine (Baltimore) 2020; 99(11): e19101.
[http://dx.doi.org/10.1097/MD.0000000000019101] [PMID: 32176037]

[11]   Boerma T, Ronsmans C, Melesse DY, *et al.* Global epidemiology of use of and disparities in caesarean sections. Lancet 2018; 392(10155): 1341-8.
[http://dx.doi.org/10.1016/S0140-6736(18)31928-7] [PMID: 30322584]

[12]   Gilron I, Vandenkerkhof E, Katz J, Kehlet H, Carley M. Evaluating the Association Between Acute and Chronic Pain After Surgery. Clin J Pain 2017; 33(7): 588-94.
[http://dx.doi.org/10.1097/AJP.0000000000000443] [PMID: 28145910]

[13]   Patorno E, Hernandez-Diaz S, Huybrechts KF, *et al.* Gabapentin in pregnancy and the risk of adverse neonatal and maternal outcomes: A population-based cohort study nested in the US Medicaid Analytic eXtract dataset. PLoS Med 2020; 17(9): e1003322.
[http://dx.doi.org/10.1371/journal.pmed.1003322] [PMID: 32870921]

[14]   Yimer H, Woldie H. Incidence and Associated Factors of Chronic Pain After Cesarean Section: A Systematic Review. J Obstet Gynaecol Canada [Internet]. Elsevier Inc.; 2019;41(6):840–54. Available from:
[http://dx.doi.org/10.1016/j.jogc.2018.04.006]

[15]   Weibel S, Neubert K, Jelting Y, *et al.* Incidence and severity of chronic pain after caesarean section. Eur J Anaesthesiol 2016; 33(11): 853-65.
[http://dx.doi.org/10.1097/EJA.0000000000000535] [PMID: 27635953]

[16]   Jin J, Peng L, Chen Q, *et al.* Prevalence and risk factors for chronic pain following cesarean section: a prospective study. BMC Anesthesiol 2016; 16(1): 99.
[http://dx.doi.org/10.1186/s12871-016-0270-6] [PMID: 27756207]

[17]   Nugraha B, Gutenbrunner C, Barke A, *et al.* The IASP classification of chronic pain for ICD-11: functioning properties of chronic pain. Pain 2019; 160(1): 88-94.
[http://dx.doi.org/10.1097/j.pain.0000000000001433] [PMID: 30586076]

[18]   Carrico JA, Mahoney K, Raymond KM, *et al.* Predicting opioid use following discharge after cesarean delivery. Ann Fam Med 2020; 18(2): 118-26.
[http://dx.doi.org/10.1370/afm.2493] [PMID: 32152015]

[19]   Kainu JP, Halmesmäki E, Korttila KT, Sarvela PJ. Persistent pain after cesarean delivery and vaginal delivery: A prospective cohort study. Anesth Analg 2016; 123(6): 1535-45.
[http://dx.doi.org/10.1213/ANE.0000000000001619] [PMID: 27870738]

[20]   Bijl RC, Freeman LM, Weijenborg PTM, Middeldorp JM, Dahan A, van Dorp ELA. A retrospective study on persistent pain after childbirth in the Netherlands. J Pain Res 2016; 9: 1-8.
[PMID: 26834496]

[21]   Turmo M, Echevarria M, Rubio P, Almeida C. Cronificación del dolor tras episiotomía. Rev Esp Anestesiol Reanim 2015; 62(8): 436-42.
[http://dx.doi.org/10.1016/j.redar.2014.10.008] [PMID: 25555717]

[22]   Schug SA, Bruce J. Risk stratification for the development of chronic postsurgical pain. Schmerz 2018; 32(6): 471-6.
[http://dx.doi.org/10.1007/s00482-018-0332-4] [PMID: 30324317]

[23]   Brandsborg B, Nikolajsen L. Chronic pain after hysterectomy. Curr Opin Anaesthesiol 2018; 31(3): 268-73.
[http://dx.doi.org/10.1097/ACO.0000000000000586] [PMID: 29474214]

[24]   Weinstein EJ, Levene JL, Cohen MS, Andreae DA, Chao JY, Johnson M, *et al.* Local anaesthetics and regional anaesthesia *versus* conventional analgesia for preventing persistent postoperative pain in adults and children. Cochrane Database Syst Rev 2018; 2018: 4.

[25] Ma G, Yang J, Zhao B, Huang C, Wang R. Correlation between CCL2, CALCA, and CX3CL1 gene polymorphisms and chronic pain after cesarean section in Chinese Han women A case control study. Med. 2019; 98: 34.

[26] Rosen SF, Ham B, Drouin S, *et al.* T-cell mediation of pregnancy analgesia affecting chronic pain in mice. J Neurosci 2017; 37(41): 9819-27.
[http://dx.doi.org/10.1523/JNEUROSCI.2053-17.2017] [PMID: 28877966]

[27] Breivik H, Stubhaug A. Management of acute postoperative pain: Still a long way to go! Pain 2008; 137(2): 233-4.
[http://dx.doi.org/10.1016/j.pain.2008.04.014] [PMID: 18479824]

[28] Liddle SD, Pennick V. Interventions for preventing and treating low-back and pelvic pain during pregnancy. Cochrane Libr 2015; 2015(9): CD001139.
[http://dx.doi.org/10.1002/14651858.CD001139.pub4] [PMID: 26422811]

[29] Virgara R, Maher C, Van Kessel G. The comorbidity of low back pelvic pain and risk of depression and anxiety in pregnancy in primiparous women. BMC Pregnancy Childbirth 2018; 18(1): 288.
[http://dx.doi.org/10.1186/s12884-018-1929-4] [PMID: 29291732]

[30] Kovacs FM, Garcia E, Royuela A, González L, Abraira V. Prevalence and factors associated with low back pain and pelvic girdle pain during pregnancy: a multicenter study conducted in the Spanish National Health Service. Spine 2012; 37(17): 1516-33.
[http://dx.doi.org/10.1097/BRS.0b013e31824dcb74] [PMID: 22333958]

[31] Bergström C, Persson M, Mogren I. Psychosocial and behavioural characteristics in women with pregnancy-related lumbopelvic pain 12 years postpartum. Chiropr Man Therap 2019; 27(1): 34.
[http://dx.doi.org/10.1186/s12998-019-0257-8]

[32] Manyozo S, Nesto T, Bonongwe P, Muula AS. Low back pain during pregnancy: Prevalence, risk factors and association with daily activities among pregnant women in urban Blantyre, Malawi. Malawi Med J 2019; 31(1): 71-6.
[http://dx.doi.org/10.4314/mmj.v31i1.12] [PMID: 31143400]

[33] Bryndal A, Majchrzycki M, Grochulska A, Glowinski S, Seremak-Mrozikiewicz A. Risk factors associated with low back pain among a group of 1510 pregnant women. J Pers Med 2020; 10(2): 51.
[http://dx.doi.org/10.3390/jpm10020051] [PMID: 32549306]

[34] Lindgren A, Kristiansson P. Finger joint laxity, number of previous pregnancies and pregnancy induced back pain in a cohort study. BMC Pregnancy Childbirth 2014; 14(1): 61. [Internet]. [Available from: BMC Pregnancy and Childbirth].
[http://dx.doi.org/10.1186/1471-2393-14-61]

[35] Passavanti MB, Pota V, Sansone P, Aurilio C, De Nardis L, Pace MC. Chronic Pelvic Pain: Assessment, evaluation, and objectivation. Pain Res Treat. Hindawi; 2017; 2017.

[36] Bjelland EK, Owe KM, Pingel R, Kristiansson P, Vangen S, Eberhard-Gran M. Pelvic pain after childbirth. Pain 2016; 157(3): 710-6.
[http://dx.doi.org/10.1097/j.pain.0000000000000427] [PMID: 26588694]

[37] Wuytack F, Begley C, Daly D. Risk factors for pregnancy-related pelvic girdle pain: a scoping review. BMC Pregnancy Childbirth 2020; 20(1): 739.
[http://dx.doi.org/10.1186/s12884-020-03442-5] [PMID: 33246422]

[38] Elden H, Gutke A, Kjellby-Wendt G, Fagevik-Olsen M, Ostgaard HC. Predictors and consequences of long-term pregnancy-related pelvic girdle pain: a longitudinal follow-up study. BMC Musculoskelet Disord 2016; 17(1): 276.
[http://dx.doi.org/10.1186/s12891-016-1154-0]

[39] Torstensson T, Butler S, Lindgren A, *et al.* Anatomical landmarks of the intra-pelvic side-wall as sources of pain in women with and without pregnancy-related chronic pelvic pain after childbirth: a descriptive study. BMC Womens Health 2018; 18(1): 54.

[http://dx.doi.org/10.1186/s12905-018-0542-z] [PMID: 29291721]

[40] Sakamoto A, Gamada K. Altered musculoskeletal mechanics as risk factors for postpartum pelvic girdle pain: a literature review. J Phys Ther Sci 2019; 31(10): 831-8.
[http://dx.doi.org/10.1589/jpts.31.831] [PMID: 31645815]

[41] Gausel AM, Malmqvist S, Andersen K, *et al.* Subjective recovery from pregnancy-related pelvic girdle pain the first 6 weeks after delivery: a prospective longitudinal cohort study. Eur Spine J 2020; 29(3): 556-63.
[http://dx.doi.org/10.1007/s00586-020-06288-9] [PMID: 32363562]

[42] Mackenzie J, Murray E, Lusher J. Women's experiences of pregnancy related pelvic girdle pain: A systematic review. Midwifery 2018; 56: 102-11.
[http://dx.doi.org/10.1016/j.midw.2017.10.011] [PMID: 29096278]

[43] Harris GME, Wood M, Eberhard-Gran M, Lundqvist C, Nordeng H. Patterns and predictors of analgesic use in pregnancy: a longitudinal drug utilization study with special focus on women with migraine. BMC Pregnancy Childbirth 2017; 17(1): 224.
[http://dx.doi.org/10.1186/s12884-017-1399-0] [PMID: 28049520]

[44] Urits I, Cai V, Aner M, *et al.* post dural puncture headache, managed with epidural blood patch, is associated with subsequent chronic low back pain in patients: a pilot study. Curr pain headache rep 2020; 24(1): 1-5.
[http://dx.doi.org/10.1007/s11916-020-0834-5] [PMID: 31916041]

[45] Falsetta ML, Foster DC, Bonham AD, Phipps RP. A review of the available clinical therapies for vulvodynia management and new data implicating proinflammatory mediators in pain elicitation. BJOG 2017; 124(2): 210-8.
[http://dx.doi.org/10.1111/1471-0528.14157] [PMID: 27312009]

[46] Johnson NS, Harwood EM, Nguyen RHN. "You have to go through it and have your children": reproductive experiences among women with vulvodynia. BMC Pregnancy Childbirth 2015; 15(1): 114.
[http://dx.doi.org/10.1186/s12884-015-0544-x]

[47] Anderson PO. Drugs in Lactation. Pharm Res 2018; 35(3): 45.
[http://dx.doi.org/10.1007/s11095-017-2287-z] [PMID: 29411152]

[48] Wang J, Johnson T, Sahin L, *et al.* evaluation of the safety of drugs and biological products used during lactation: workshop summary. Clin pharmacol ther 2017; 101(6): 736-44.
[http://dx.doi.org/10.1002/cpt.676] [PMID: 28510297]

[49] Halder S, Russell R, Quinlan J. Codeine and breast-feeding mothers 2015.
[http://dx.doi.org/10.1016/j.ijoa.2014.12.003]

[50] Ansari J, Carvalho B, Shafer SL, Flood P. pharmacokinetics and pharmacodynamics of drugs commonly used in pregnancy and parturition. Anesth analg 2016; 122(3): 786-804.
[http://dx.doi.org/10.1213/ANE.0000000000001143] [PMID: 26891392]

[51] Burnsed JC, Heinan K, Letzkus L, Zanelli S. Gabapentin for pain, movement disorders, and irritability in neonates and infants. Dev Med Child Neurol 2020; 62(3): 386-9.
[http://dx.doi.org/10.1111/dmcn.14324] [PMID: 31343730]

[52] Lavand'homme PM, Roelants F, Waterloos H, Collet V, De Kock MF. An evaluation of the postoperative antihyperalgesic and analgesic effects of intrathecal clonidine administered during elective cesarean delivery. Anesth Analg 2008; 107(3): 948-55.
[http://dx.doi.org/10.1213/ane.0b013e31817f1595] [PMID: 18713912]

[53] Sutton CD, Carvalho B. Optimal Pain Management After Cesarean Delivery. Anesthesiol Clin 2017; 35(1): 107-24.
[http://dx.doi.org/10.1016/j.anclin.2016.09.010] [PMID: 28131114]

[54] Heesen M, Böhmer J, Brinck ECV, *et al.* Intravenous ketamine during spinal and general anaesthesia

for caesarean section: systematic review and meta-analysis. Acta Anaesthesiol Scand 2015; 59(4): 414-26.
[http://dx.doi.org/10.1111/aas.12468] [PMID: 25789942]

[55] Holland E, Sudhof LS, Zera C. Optimal pain management for cesarean delivery. Int Anesthesiol Clin 2020; 58(2): 42-9.
[http://dx.doi.org/10.1097/AIA.0000000000000272] [PMID: 32039926]

[56] Morino S, Ishihara M, Umezaki F, *et al.* Low back pain and causative movements in pregnancy: a prospective cohort study. BMC Musculoskelet Disord 2017; 18(1): 416.
[http://dx.doi.org/10.1186/s12891-017-1776-x] [PMID: 28052768]

[57] Haakstad L, Bø K. Effect of a regular exercise programme on pelvic girdle and low back pain in previously inactive pregnant women: A randomized controlled trial. J Rehabil Med 2015; 47(3): 229-34.
[http://dx.doi.org/10.2340/16501977-1906] [PMID: 25385408]

[58] Franke H, Franke JD, Belz S, Fryer G. Osteopathic manipulative treatment for low back and pelvic girdle pain during and after pregnancy: A systematic review and meta-analysis. J Bodyw Mov Ther [Internet]. Elsevier Ltd; 2017; 21(4): 752-62.

[59] Wu J-M, Zhuo Y-Y, Qin X-L, Yu X-Y, Hu S, Ning Y. Pelvic-sacral tendon-regulation needling technique of acupuncture combined with manipulative reduction in treatment of postpartum pelvic girdle pain: a randomized controlled trial. Zhongguo Zhenjiu 2020; 40(3): 262-6.
[PMID: 32270638]

[60] Camporeze B, Simm R, Maldaun MC, Pires de Aguiar P. Spinal cord stimulation in pregnant patients: Current perspectives of indications, complications, and results in pain control: A systematic review. Asian J Neurosurg 2019; 14(2): 343-55.
[http://dx.doi.org/10.4103/ajns.AJNS_7_18] [PMID: 31143246]

[61] Benhamou D, Kfoury T. Enhanced recovery after caesarean delivery: Potent analgesia and adequate practice patterns are at the heart of successful management. Anaesth Crit Care Pain Med 2016; 35(6): 373-5.
[http://dx.doi.org/10.1016/j.accpm.2016.11.001] [PMID: 27989284]

[62] Hemsing N, Greaves L, Poole N, Schmidt R. Misuse of prescription opioid medication among women: A scoping review. Pain Res Manag. Hindawi Publishing Corporation 2016.

[63] Rosen NO, Dawson SJ, Brooks M, Kellogg-Spadt S. Treatment of Vulvodynia: Pharmacological and Non-Pharmacological Approaches. Drugs 2019; 79(5): 483-93.
[http://dx.doi.org/10.1007/s40265-019-01085-1] [PMID: 30847806]

CHAPTER 18

Anesthesia for Assisted Reproduction

Montserrat Franco Cabrera[1,2,3,4,*], Daniel Vieyra Cortés[5], Aniza S. González Lumbreras[6] and Luis Humberto García Lorant[6]

[1] *Hospital Angeles Lomas, 52763 Méx., Mexico*

[2] *Hospital Ángeles Pedregal, 05370 Ciudad de México, CDMX, Mexico*

[3] *Hospital Español de México, 11520 Ciudad de México, CDMX, Mexico*

[4] *The American British Cowdray Medical Center (ABC), 05370 Ciudad de México, CDMX, Mexico*

[5] *Genesis Reproductive Medicine, Hospital Ángeles del Pedregal, 10700 Ciudad de México, CDMX, Mexico*

[6] *Hospital Angeles Lomas, 52763 Méx., Mexico*

Abstract: Infertility is a common aspect globally affecting couples to 15%, and it is frequently increasing the need for anesthesiologists' participation in assisted reproductive techniques.

Currently, the procedures used to assist reproduction are unable to fully cover the detrimental effects of age. During anesthesia-analgesia in oocyte retrieval, the role of the anesthesiologist is to provide the patient with adequate anxiolysis, analgesia, and sedation as the key to success in the procedure. An adequate pre-anesthetic assessment is required to identify derivative diseases and take the appropriate care of each patient. Modern anesthetic techniques for oocyte retrieval include conscious sedation, general anesthesia, regional anesthesia, and other alternative techniques, such as electroacupuncture, or even a combination of these.

In this chapter, the main characteristics of these techniques will be exposed, as well as their complications and the recommendations so that anesthetic procedures are safe not only for the patient, but also for the whole process' success.

Keywords: Acupuncture, Anesthesia for Assisted Reproduction, Ambulatory Gynecological Procedures, Assisted Reproductive Technique/Technology, Infertility, Oocyte Retrieval, Sedation.

---

* **Corresponding author Montserrat Franco Cabrera:** Hospital Angeles Lomas, 52763 Méx., Mexico;
E-mail: monfran89@gmail.com

Eugenio Daniel Martinez-Hurtado, Monica Sanjuan-Alvarez & Marta Chacon-Castillo (Eds.)
All rights reserved-© 2022 Bentham Science Publishers

INTRODUCTION

Infertility is a common aspect globally affecting 15% couples, as shown by the statistics of the US National Survey of Family Growth (*NSFG*) reporting an infertility prevalence of 12.1% in women between 15 and 44 years during the period between 2010 and 2015. The primary infertility rate by age group was: 9% in 15- to 34-year-old women and 16% in 35- to 44-year-old women [1].

A woman under the age of 30 has a possibility of pregnancy per cycle of between 12 to 15% and over 40 years less than 5%, causing an increase in the demand for fertility clinics' services.

Currently, the procedures used to assist reproduction are unable to fully cover the detrimental effects of age. The average success rate of reproductive techniques is 41% in 35-year-old women and 4% after the age of 42 [1, 2].

BACKGROUND

The fusion of a human egg and sperm out of the woman and the subsequent transfer of the resulting embryo back to a uterus is relatively recent. The first reports of a successful implantation and pregnancy after this procedure's implementation in humans were published during the 1970s. From that time to date, *in vitro* fertilization (*IVF*) techniques have led to new knowledge about gamete interaction and early embryonic development, as well as the advent of thousands of normal pregnancies [3].

Ovarian Hyperstimulation

Ovulation induction involves homogeneous growth of a follicular cohort to produce a higher number of good-quality oocytes, *i.e.*, achieving the growth of more than one follicle per cycle using different treatment schemes [4]. Ovarian hyperstimulation is the first step in the assisted reproductive process. Multiple follicular development can be achieved by the proper selection of specific medications. Each with its advantages and indications, and the dose based on a woman's age, ovarian reserve, previous stimulation response, and body mass index. Some examples of such medications include gonadotropins (urinary or recombinant), gonadotropin releasing hormone analogues (agonists or antagonists), and recombinant or urinary human chorionic gonadotropin (*hCG*).

Follicular Puncture

Follicular puncture for oocytes retrieval is performed 34 to 36 hours after the administration of the above-mentioned medications. Transvaginal ultrasound-guided aspiration is performed under sedation or local anesthesia, which will depend on the location and access to the ovaries, the surgeon's experience, the patient's pain threshold, the medical site's availability, among other facts [5, 6].

Fertilization Techniques

In Vitro Fertilization

In vitro fertilization (*IVF*) is defined as an assisted reproductive technique involving extracorporeal fertilization. IVF is the most common procedure within assisted reproduction. In general terms, this technique initially consists of ovarian stimulation controlled by medications applied subcutaneously or intramuscularly. Its purpose is to obtain multiple follicles, which contain the oocytes that will then be vaginally aspirated under ultrasound guidance. These oocytes will be fertilized (*in vitro*) in the laboratory and subsequently, those which are fertilized and properly progress to embryos, either in day 3 or 5, will be transferred to the uterine cavity. This procedure generally taking about 2 weeks is called an IVF cycle [4].

IVF was initially developed for the treatment of tubular infertility, although it is currently used for many other indications [7]:

- Tubal factor.
- Endometriosis.
- Artificial insemination failure.
- Male factor (total motile sperm count (*TMSC*) less than 3 million).
- Infertility of unknown origin.
- Premature ovarian insufficiency.
- Decreased ovarian reserve.
- Cryopreservation of oocytes in cancer patients or with medical disease.
- Fertility preservation.

Intracytoplasmic Sperm Injection

It refers to a technique in which a single sperm is injected directly into the cytoplasm of a mature oocyte. This procedure is performed as part of an IVF cycle and provides an effective method to aid fertilization in men with altered semen parameters or who experienced null or low fertilization rates after conventional IVF. The efficiency of this technique has made it the most successful treatment for male infertility since 2016. The use of Intracytoplasmic Sperm Injection (*ICSI*) in male infertility increased from 84% in 2003 to 93% in 2012 [8].

ICSI is mainly indicated for the treatment of male factor infertility [9]:

- Oligozoospermia.
- Asthenozoospermia.
- Teratozoospermia.
- Anti-sperm antibodies.
- Absence of vas deferens.
- All alterations at the epididymal level.

It can also be useful in the following clinical conditions: failed fertilization in a previous IVF cycle, preimplantation genetic diagnosis, fertilization of previously cryopreserved oocytes, and *in vitro* maturation of oocytes.

The Practice Committees of the American Society for Reproductive Medicine (*ASRM*) and the Society for Assisted Reproductive Technology (*SART*) concluded that the existing evidence does not support the use of ICSI as a routine procedure to improve clinical pregnancy rates in couples with unexplained infertility, with low ovarian reserve or advanced maternal age [7].

Embryo Culture and Embryo Transfer

Embryo transfer can be carried out 3 to 5 days after the oocytes are fertilized and is currently carried out at stage 5 (blastocyst) since it allows a better embryo selection, and therefore an increase in the clinical pregnancy rate [10, 11].

ANESTHETIC CONSIDERATIONS

During anesthesia-analgesia in oocyte retrieval, the role of the anesthesiologist is to provide the patient with adequate anxiolysis, analgesia, and sedation as the key to success in the procedure.

An adequate pre-anesthetic assessment is required to identify derivative diseases and take the appropriate care of each patient. During the assessment, it is crucial to explain to the patients the anesthetic technique to be used and its possible complications, as well as to obtain their informed consent. One of the most common pathologies today is obesity, which is related to menstrual disorders, hyperandrogenism, and polycystic ovary syndrome (*PCOS*), and therefore with a high incidence of infertility. Other frequent comorbidities are cancer and autoimmune diseases, since they are found in patients who undergo treatments that can cause infertility [12, 13].

The purpose of the procedure is to retrieve the largest number of oocytes after the patient hormonal preparation. Such a procedure requires vaginal and ovarian capsule perforation, resulting in the potential risk of injury to surrounding organs due to the gynecologist's necessary manipulation. Hence the importance of adequate analgesia and patient control since it is a stressful and painful procedure [14].

Modern anesthetic techniques for oocyte retrieval include conscious sedation, general anesthesia (*GA*), regional anesthesia (paracervical block [*PCB*], preovarian block [*POB*], epidural block, subarachnoid block), and other alternative techniques, such as electroacupuncture, or even a combination of these [15 - 17]. However, the technique to be chosen must be individualized, depending on the patient's background, the medical team that will perform the procedure, and the resources of the medical site where it will be carried out. Prevailing evidence does not give preference to any of the aforementioned techniques, as neither has shown a higher pregnancy rate over the others. The combination of several of them (sedation with acupuncture or sedation with PCB) has indeed shown better pain control [17]. The use of PCB as the only method is not recommended, since the patients have undergone greater pain and less satisfaction [17, 18].

Regardless of the anesthetic technique chosen by the anesthesiologist, it is eminent to mention that the lowest possible doses should be implemented, as well as the shortest possible exposure time, as the anesthetics used can be found in different concentrations in the follicular fluid [14, 15]. The longer the anesthetic time (especially in GA), the greater the suppression of gonadotropin-releasing hormone (*GnRH*) secretion and the greater the stimulation of prolactin, which affects the luteal phase and the endometrium development [19].

The quintessential technique is sedation, which is used in 84% of oocyte retrievals in the United Kingdom and in 95% of cases in the United States [14].

The procedure will require an intravenous line, in addition to non-invasive monitoring (non-invasive blood pressure, pulse oximetry, electrocardiography, and, if possible, bispectral index or any other anesthetic depth monitor) [14]. It is essential to have complete respiratory support, since among the main complications in this technique are respiratory depression and the need for assisted ventilation.

Regarding pharmacological alternatives, benzodiazepines, such as midazolam, can be used in doses for anxiolysis (maximum 50 mcg/kg), finding it in extremely low or null doses in the follicular fluid, without interfering with fertilization and embryonic development [20, 21]. The use of midazolam in these techniques, in combination with propofol and opioids, is common and considered safe [14].

Propofol is the most widely used endovenous anesthetic agent [14, 22] as it is highly lipophilic with a rapid onset of action and predictable duration, due to its fast penetration of the brain-blood barrier and its distribution into the central nervous system, in addition to conferring an antiemetic effect and rapid recovery time [14]. The ideal way to infuse propofol is *via* Target Controlled Infusion (*TCI*) to keep plasma concentrations constant and in site-effect, and thus greater predictability. The Schnider model is the most used since it includes variables such as age, weight, size, and lean mass.

Opioids, such as alfentanil, sufentanil, fentanyl or remifentanil, can also be used, while the latter is often the first choice due to its plasma metabolism and ultra-short half-life [23]. Due to its very short context-sensitive half-life, it is required to be administered as an infusion using the pharmacokinetic model of Minto (*TCI*) (which is the most validated) reaching site-effect concentration according to the age, weight, size, and sex of the patient. It can be used at a concentration of 2 ng/ml with a progressive increase to 1 ng/ml at the time until providing the proper analgesia, considering the respiratory rate, as well as oxygen saturation in order to avoid excessive sedation, and therefore cause oxygen desaturation and hypopnea (respiratory rate of less than 8 breaths per minute). The infusion should be suspended at the time of removal of the last follicle.

In 2011, Demet Coskum *et al.* conducted a study at Gazi University in Ankara, Turkey, comparing the use of three different concentrations of TCI (Minto) remifentanil plus TCI (Schnider) propofol. They observed that patients under TCI remifentanil administration with a concentration of Ce 1.5 or 2 ng/ml plus propofol at 1.5 mcg/ml had better outcomes, gaining a faster recovery time, compared to patients under remifentanil administration with a concentration of Ce 2.5 ng/ml plus propofol at the same concentration [24]. No harmful effects have been found on reproductive outcomes after the combination of remifentanil and propofol [25].

Nitrous oxide was widely used in the 1980s and was correlated with low pregnancy rates compared to peridural blockage or sedation [26]; nevertheless, in 2002, Hadimiouglu showed that nitrous oxide increased success rates in IVF techniques [27]. Otherwise, nitrous oxide is known to inactivate methionine synthase by decreasing the amount of thymidine available for DNA synthesis in cell division [28]. Due to all these outcomes, its use is controversial and presently unattractive, after considering there are drugs with better tolerated profiles for patients and embryos, such as remifentanil and propofol [29].

The etomidate interferes with the ovary endocrine function, observing a decrease in plasma concentration of 17 beta-estradiol, progesterone, 17-hydroxyprogesterone, and testosterone 10 minutes after induction (at doses of 0.25 mg/kg), followed by a gradual recovery of baseline levels [30]. It is not widely used in assisted reproductive methods.

Multiple studies have demonstrated harmful effects of halogenated agents in IVF techniques; however, they were carried out from 1987 to 1996 and only conducted in mice, while currently there has been scarce research in this regard [31 - 35]. Matt *et al.* observed that the combination of isoflurane plus nitrous oxide in oocyte retrieval had no effect on pregnancy rates [30]. Ben-Shlomo *et al.* conducted a prospective randomized study on 50 patients, in which they observed that, using general anesthesia with fentanyl, propofol, and isoflurane, similar pregnancy rates were obtained compared to sedation with midazolam and ketamine [36]. In 2016, Piroli *et al.* also confirmed the superiority of sevoflurane use against other implemented techniques in mice [37]. In view of the little evidence in this matter, the use of halogenates is at the discretion of the leading anesthesiologist.

Lastly, regional anesthesia has been used with various blocking methodologies, such as PCB, in which local anesthetic is injected into 2-6 sites at a depth of 3-7 mm in the vaginal portion of the uterine cervix in the fornix. Another newer technique is the POB, in which the local anesthetic is infiltrated under ultrasound guidance between the vaginal wall and the peritoneal surface near the ovary. Finally, other well-known alternatives are epidural or spinal blocks, which have shown no adverse effects in oocyte retrieval, but their use has been limited in the face of longer anesthetic recovery times and patient discharge delays [14].

After conducting a comprehensive review of anesthetic techniques for oocyte retrieval, it is concluded that due to the countless randomized studies where these techniques are compared, individually used or combined, as well as the use of multiple drugs in different doses, there is no ideal anesthetic technique. Due to the extensive heterogeneity in all the randomized clinical trials contemplated in systematic reviews and meta-analyses, the results and conclusions have low or very low-quality evidence, without really being able to reach any conclusions [17, 38].

This inconclusiveness represents a great challenge for the anesthesiologist, since he has the responsibility of having extensive knowledge of these techniques, as well as the pharmacokinetics and pharmacodynamics of each of the drugs, and on the other hand, he must consider the comorbidities of the patients. The anesthesiologist must be able to tailor the use of each technique with the available information in order to reassure the patient, as well as to provide an adequate anesthetic depth so that the gynecologist can easily perform the procedure and the retrieval is successful.

ACUPUNCTURE AND ASSISTED REPRODUCTION

The use of acupuncture during the process of assisted reproductive techniques has been very controversial, especially in the Western world. However, according to a meta-analysis carried out by Cochrane in 2018 [39], it has been accepted that the use of acupuncture combined with intravenous sedation is convenient for reducing pain during egg collection (oocyte retrieval) and immediately post-surgery. It was even concluded that this combined technique is better compared to the use of sedation alone. Therefore, it is important that we learn more about this practice.

Acupuncture is based on the hypothesis that human physiology is controlled by Yin and Yang channels, which allow Qi to flow throughout the body through 12 meridians. The blockage of these channels is the cause of pain and disease, therefore, when inserting intramuscular needles in specific places within the body (365 points in the body, 15-25 mm deep) for 20 to 30 minutes prior to egg retrieval [40], the channels are unblocked, and the Qi can flow again [39, 41 - 44]. Manual acupuncture only uses needles, while in electroacupuncture a small current is added to these needles [40, 45, 46].

Experimental studies have shown that acupuncture has an effect due to changes in the autonomous nervous system, as well as the stimulation of neuropeptides (β-endorphin, dynorphin, oxytocin, neuropeptide Y, substance P) and neurotransmitters (catecholamines, glutamate, acetylcholine, GABA, and serotonin) [42, 44, 46 - 51]. Western studies have shown changes in functional MRIs after using acupuncture [52 - 64]. When inserting the needles, C and A-δ nerve fibers are activated [44, 46].

Electroacupuncture involves different theories for the choice of the frequencies administered during egg retrieval. There is currently no official consensus on which would be the best choice, since combinations of high and low frequencies (80-100 Hz and 2-4 Hz) or fixed frequencies (20 Hz) have been used [40, 65]. Three studies concluded that analgesia is greater with mixed frequencies [40, 65, 66].

During egg retrieval, the blood becomes stagnant in the Ren Mai, Chong Mai, and triple burner meridians, causing abdominal pain, nausea, and vomiting. Therefore, the most commonly used acupuncture points in egg retrieval are the following: CV4, CA1, BL23, BL32, LI4, and PC6 [67].

Three acupuncture points are of particular interest: the PC6, CV4, and LI4. Some meta-analyses demonstrated PC6 effectiveness for nausea and vomiting reduction, resulting in decreasing use of rescue antiemetics [43, 68, 69]. PC6 was compared to various antiemetics such as metoclopramide, cyclizine, prochlorperazine, droperidol, ondansetron, and dexamethasone. The authors concluded that there is no difference between PC6 stimulation and the administration of said drugs, *i.e.,* they are equally effective. It was also established that the combination of PC6 with the use of antiemetics is better than the sole administration of antiemetics [43].

Otherwise, it was shown that after electroacupuncture stimulation at CV4, signal deactivation occurred in the anterior cingulate cortex and infer medial prefrontal cortex, both important in the processing of emotions and pain, as well as attention and the autonomous nervous system [70].

Finally, it was concluded that after stimulation at LI4 acupoint, the signal was deactivated in the area of the limbic system in functional MRI, therefore, a lower perception of pain can be inferred [54]. Hence, it has also been used in other scopes, such as in dysmenorrhea and cystitis treatment [71, 72].

The purpose of this chapter is simply to present other options that might be within our reach, as the integration of some of these techniques with Western medicine may be possible. However, it should be noted that acupuncture is not shown to improve the final outcomes; that is, there are no higher rates of pregnancies or live births, nor fewer abortions when it is compared to the use of other anesthetic techniques [73]. Neither does it mean that acupuncture is better itself compared to the available anesthesia types, but it is simply mentioned that combining sedation with acupuncture showed improvement in pain and nausea [39].

OVARIAN HYPERSTIMULATION SYNDROME

As previously mentioned, assisted reproductive technology involves ovarian stimulation by means of exogenous use of hormones. Gonadotropin-releasing hormone (*GnRH*) antagonists or agonists are used to prevent premature ovulation by suppressing the hypothalamic-hypophyseal axis. Ovulation is subsequently induced to perform follicle aspiration by administering human chorionic gonadotropin (*hCG*), GnRH antagonists or agonists [74].

Ovarian stimulation may produce ovarian hyperstimulation syndrome (*OHSS*), an iatrogenic complication with high morbidity and mortality, generated by an excessive ovarian response [74, 75]. Its incidence varies from 0.1% to 2% in severe, 3% to 8% in moderate and 20% to 30% in mild cases [75, 76].

This syndrome does not have a clear physiopathology; however, it has been linked to arterial dilation with increased capillary permeability and hence, leakage of intravascular volume into the interstitial space. The association of hCG use with OHSS has been documented, as it increases levels of vascular endothelial growth factor (*VEGF*), which causes increased vascular permeability and angiogenesis [74, 75]. The ovarian renin-angiotensin system and prostaglandins (through angiotensin II synthesis) have also been linked to increased vascular permeability

[75]. There is also ovarian growth due to hyperstimulation, causing overproduction and release of vasoactive and pro-inflammatory cytokines (IL-1, IL-4, IL-6, IL-8, and TNF-α) and contributing in the same way to their physiopathology [74, 75].

Increased volume leakage into the interstitial space creates characteristic clinical conditions of OHSS, such as peripheral oedema, ascites, pleural or pericardial effusion, hypotension and oliguria, renal and respiratory failure with the high risk of thromboembolism due to severe hemoconcentration [75, 77].

Some risk factors that have been frequently associated with this syndrome include age under 35, low body mass index, asthenic habitus, polycystic ovary syndrome, atopy history, previous OHSS episode, high or repeated doses of exogenous hCG, protocol with GnRH agonists, use of clomiphene citrate, >35 developing follicles, >14 retrieved oocytes, and elevated serum estradiol >2500 pg/ml [78].

According to clinical, laboratory, and imaging parameters, the ASRM has classified OHSS in four stages. The mild stage is characterized by abdominal distension, nausea, vomiting, diarrhea, and enlarged ovaries. The moderate stage includes the same criteria as the mild stage plus ultrasonographic evidence of ascites, hematocrit >41%, and leukocytes >25,000/microL. The severe stage includes the presence of hydrothorax, clinical evidence of ascites, uncontrolled vomiting, severe dyspnea, oliguria/anuria, hematocrit >55%, leukocytes >25,000/microL, serum creatinine >1.6 mg/dl, creatinine clearance <50ml/min, Na+ <135mEq/L, K+ >5 mEq/L, elevated liver enzymes, as well as moderate stage criteria. Finally, the critical stage comprehends the presence of severe stage criteria plus pleural and/or pericardial effusion, low central blood and venous pressure, weight gain >1kg in 24 hours, syncope, arterial thrombosis, arrhythmias, acute renal failure, massive hydrothorax, sepsis, and acute respiratory distress syndrome [79].

In recent years, different ways to prevent OHSS have been studied and proposed [76]. The following has been recommended: 1. Use of GnRH antagonists instead of GnRH agonists to suppress the ovulatory period with the same pregnancy success rate and lower incidence of OHSS [76, 80]. 2. Dose reduction of hCG since it is the main stimulator of VEGF in granulosa cells [81]. 3. Use of metformin in patients with PCOS [76]. 4. Use of GnRH agonists as an ovulation trigger in donor patients [76]. 5. Use of low doses of aspirin as a preventive treatment, probably as it is a platelet aggregation inhibitor [81]. 6. Dopamine agonists, such as cabergoline, as VEGF 2 receptor inhibitors, have been shown to reduce the incidence of OHSS in women at high risk [82].

Despite preventive measures, there is a risk of developing this syndrome whose management depends on its severity. In general, it is a condition that is usually self-limiting as hGC levels decrease. In the case of mild-moderate OHSS, it can be treated on an outpatient basis with close monitoring, including fluid intake control, early thromboprophylaxis, and nephrotoxic medication prevention [75 - 83].

Severe OHSS treatment aims to hinder the development of multiple organ failure [75 - 84]. Crystalloids are usually the first choice to achieve adequate tissue perfusion; however, the use of albumin is justified to expand plasma volume in the presence of hemoconcentration, hypoalbuminemia or ascites. Furthermore, electrolyte disturbances should also be identified and corrected [84, 85].

Ultrasound-guided paracentesis is indicated in patients with ascites and an intra-abdominal pressure greater than 20 mmHg or spontaneous bacterial peritonitis. It is recommended not to extract large ascites volumes for the risk of rapid reaccumulation of peritoneal fluid. Nonetheless, the need to perform several paracentesis procedures in a single hospitalization has been reported [75 - 84].

CONCLUSION

The recent increase in the demand for assisted reproductive techniques represents a challenge for the anesthesiologist. As previously mentioned, it is not yet known the gold standard for the anesthetic choice. We must also be prepared to recognize the complications involved at any time in the process. In addition, we should learn other options like acupuncture to improve our management.

CONSENT FOR PUBLICATION

Not applicable.

CONFLICT OF INTEREST

The authors declare no conflict of interest, financial or otherwise.

ACKNOWLEDGEMENT

Declared none.

REFERENCES

[1]   Centers for Disease Control and Prevention, National Center for Health Statistics, Division of Vital Statistics. Key Statistics from the National Survey of Family Growth www.cdc.gov/nchs/nsfg/key_statistics/i.htm2019.

[2]   Chandra A, Copen CE, Stephen EH. 2. Chandra A, Copen CE, Stephen EH. Infertility and impaired fecundity in the United States, 1982–2010: Data from the National Survey of Family Growth. National health statistics reports; no 67 2013.

[3]   Eskew AM, Jungheim ES. A History of Developments to Improve *in vitro* Fertilization. Mo Med 2017; 114(3): 156-9.
[PMID: 30228571]

[4]   Van Voorhis BJ, Voorhis V. Clinical practice. *in vitro* fertilization. N Engl J Med 2007; 356(4): 379-86.
[http://dx.doi.org/10.1056/NEJMcp065743] [PMID: 17251534]

[5]   Alper MM, Fauser BC. Ovarian stimulation protocols for IVF: is more better than less? Reprod Biomed Online 2017; 34(4): 345-53.
[http://dx.doi.org/10.1016/j.rbmo.2017.01.010] [PMID: 28169189]

[6]   Speroff L, Fritz M. Técnicas de reproducción asistida en endocrinología ginecológica clínica y esterilidad. 8 ed. Madrid: lippincott Williams & Wilkins 2015; 12.

[7]   Bosch E, Broer S, Griesinger G, *et al.* ESHRE guideline: ovarian stimulation for IVF/ICSI†. Hum Reprod Open 2020; 2020(2): hoaa009.
[http://dx.doi.org/10.1093/hropen/hoaa009] [PMID: 32395637]

[8]   Zhang W, Xiao X, Zhang J, *et al.* Clinical outcomes of frozen embryo *versus* fresh embryo transfer following *in vitro* fertilization: a meta-analysis of randomized controlled trials. Arch Gynecol Obstet 2018; 298(2): 259-72.
[http://dx.doi.org/10.1007/s00404-018-4786-5] [PMID: 29881888]

[9]   Tannus S, Son WY, Gilman A, Younes G, Shavit T, Dahan MH. The role of intracytoplasmic sperm injection in non-male factor infertility in advanced maternal age. Hum Reprod 2017; 32(1): 119-24.
[PMID: 27852688]

[10]   Yang L, Cai S, Zhang S, *et al.* Single embryo transfer by Day 3 time-lapse selection *versus* Day 5 conventional morphological selection: a randomized, open-label, non-inferiority trial. Hum Reprod 2018; 33(5): 869-76.
[http://dx.doi.org/10.1093/humrep/dey047] [PMID: 29546361]

[11]   Shi Y, Sun Y, Hao C, *et al.* transfer of fresh *versus* frozen embryos in ovulatory women. N engl J med 2018; 378(2): 126-36.
[http://dx.doi.org/10.1056/NEJMoa1705334] [PMID: 29320646]

[12]   Egan B, Racowsky C, Hornstein MD, Martin R, Tsen LC. Anesthetic impact of body mass index in patients undergoing assisted reproductive technologies. J Clin Anesth 2008; 20(5): 356-63.
[http://dx.doi.org/10.1016/j.jclinane.2008.03.003] [PMID: 18761244]

[13]   Trikha A, Sharma A, Borle A. Anesthesia for *in vitro* fertilization. J Obstet Anaesth Crit Care 2015; 5(2): 62-72.
[http://dx.doi.org/10.4103/2249-4472.165132]

[14]   Guasch E, Gómez R, Brogly N, Gilsanz F. Anesthesia and analgesia for transvaginal oocyte retrieval. Should we recommend or avoid any anesthetic drug or technique? Curr Opin Anaesthesiol 2019; 32(3): 285-90.
[http://dx.doi.org/10.1097/ACO.0000000000000715] [PMID: 31045635]

[15]   Vlahos NF, Giannakikou I, Vlachos A, Vitoratos N. Analgesia and anesthesia for assisted reproductive technologies. Int J Gynaecol Obstet 2009; 105(3): 201-5.
[http://dx.doi.org/10.1016/j.ijgo.2009.01.017] [PMID: 19249049]

[16]   Tsen LC, Vincent RD. *in vitro* Fertilization ana other assited Reproductive Technology. 2009.

[17]   Kwan BS, Knox F, Mcneil A. Conscious Sedation ana analgeisa for Oocyte Retrieval During *in vitro* Fertilizaton Procedures: a Cochrane review. Hum Reprod 2006; 21: 1672-9.
[http://dx.doi.org/10.1093/humrep/del002] [PMID: 16818961]

[18]   Oliveira Júnior GL, Serralheiro FC, Fonseca FLA, *et al.* Randomized double-blind clinical trial comparing two anesthetic techniques for ultrasound-guided transvaginal follicular puncture. Einstein

(Sao Paulo) 2016; 14(3): 305-10.
[http://dx.doi.org/10.1590/S1679-45082016AO3714] [PMID: 27759816]

[19]　Hayes MF, Sacco AG, Savoy-Moore RT, Magyar DM, Endler GC, Moghissi KS. Effect of general anesthesia on fertilization and cleavage of human oocytes *in vitro*. Fertil Steril 1987; 48(6): 975-81.
[http://dx.doi.org/10.1016/S0015-0282(16)59594-6] [PMID: 2960566]

[20]　Soussis I, Boyd O, Paraschos T, *et al.* Follicular fluid levels of midazolam, fentanyl, and alfentanil during transvaginal oocyte retrieval Supported by Roche Products Ltd., Welwyn Garden City, United Kingdom.†Presented at the Annual Meeting of the British Fertility Society, Oxford, England, December 17, 1993. Fertil Steril 1995; 64(5): 1003-7.
[http://dx.doi.org/10.1016/S0015-0282(16)57919-9] [PMID: 7589618]

[21]　Casati A, Valentini G, Zangrillo A, *et al.* Anaesthesia for ultrasound guided oocyte retrieval: midazolam/remifentanil *versus* propofol/fentanyl regimens. Eur J Anaesthesiol 1999; 16(11): 773-8.
[http://dx.doi.org/10.1046/j.1365-2346.1999.00584.x] [PMID: 10713871]

[22]　Goutziomitrou E, Kolibianakis EM, Venetis CA, *et al.* The use of pentothal for anesthesia during oocyte retrieval is associated with decreased pregnancy rates as compared to propofol: a randomised controlled trial. Hum Reprod 2011; 26: i96.

[23]　Hossein M, Davare R, Reza H, *et al.* Remifentanyl *versus* Fentanyl for assisted reproductive Technologies: effect on hemodynamic recovery from anesthesia and outcome at ART cycles. Int J Fertil Steril 2011; 1(5): 86-9.

[24]　Coskun D, Gunaydin B, Tas A, Inan G, Celebi H, Kaya K. A comparison of three different target-controlled remifentanil infusion rates during target-controlled propofol infusion for oocyte retrieval. Clinics (São Paulo) 2011; 66(5): 811-5.
[http://dx.doi.org/10.1590/S1807-59322011000500017] [PMID: 21789385]

[25]　Wilhelm W, Hammadeh ME, White PF, Georg T, Fleser R, Biedler A. General anesthesia *versus* monitored anesthesia care with remifentanil for assisted reproductive technologies: effect on pregnancy rate. J Clin Anesth 2002; 14(1): 1-5.
[http://dx.doi.org/10.1016/S0952-8180(01)00331-2] [PMID: 11880013]

[26]　Hadimioglu N, Aydogdu Titiz T, Dosemeci L, Erman M. Comparison of various sedation regimens for transvaginal oocyte retrieval. Fertil Steril 2002; 78(3): 648-9.
[http://dx.doi.org/10.1016/S0015-0282(02)03274-0] [PMID: 12215353]

[27]　Elstein D, Ioscovich A, Rivilis A, Weitman M, Altarescu G, Eldar-Geva T. Anesthetic management for oocyte retrieval: An exploratory analysis comparing outcome in *in vitro* fertilization cycles with and without pre-implantation genetic diagnosis. J Hum Reprod Sci 2013; 6(4): 263-6.
[http://dx.doi.org/10.4103/0974-1208.126303] [PMID: 24672167]

[28]　Gonen O, Shulman A, Ghetler Y, *et al.* The impact of different types of anesthesia on *in vitro* fertilization-embryo transfer treatment outcome. J Assist Reprod Genet 1995; 12(10): 678-82.
[http://dx.doi.org/10.1007/BF02212892] [PMID: 8624422]

[29]　Heytens L, Devroey P, Camu F, Van Steirteghem AC. Effects of etomidate on ovarian steroidogenesis. Hum Reprod 1987; 2(2): 85-90.
[http://dx.doi.org/10.1093/oxfordjournals.humrep.a136506] [PMID: 3108307]

[30]　Matt DW, Steingold KA, Dastvan CM, James CA, Dunwiddie W. Effects of sera from patients given various anesthetics on preimplantation mouse embryo development *in vitro*. J *in vitro* Fert Embryo Tranf 1991; 191-7.

[31]　Jennings JC, Moreland K, Peterson CM. *in vitro* fertilisation. A review of drug therapy and clinical management. Drugs 1996; 52(3): 313-43.
[http://dx.doi.org/10.2165/00003495-199652030-00002] [PMID: 8875126]

[32]　Matt DW, Steingold KA, Dastvan CM, James CA, Dunwiddie W. Effects of sera from patients given various anesthetics on preimplantation mouse embryo development *in vitro*. J in vitro Fert Embryo

Transf 1991; 8(4): 191-7.
[http://dx.doi.org/10.1007/BF01130803] [PMID: 1753163]

[33] Chetkowski RJ, Nass TE. Isofluorane inhibits early mouse embryo development *in vitro*. Fertil Steril 1988; 49(1): 171-3.
[http://dx.doi.org/10.1016/S0015-0282(16)59673-3] [PMID: 3335266]

[34] Fishel S, Webster J, Faratian B, Jackson P. General anesthesia for intrauterine placement of human conceptuses after *in vitro* fertilization. J in vitro Fert Embryo Transf 1987; 4(5): 260-4.
[http://dx.doi.org/10.1007/BF01555200] [PMID: 3320229]

[35] Naito Y, Tamai S, Fukata J, *et al.* Comparison of endocrinological stress response associated with transvaginal ultrasound-guided oocyte pick-up under halothane anaesthesia and neuroleptanaesthesia. Can J Anaesth 1989; 36(6): 633-6.
[http://dx.doi.org/10.1007/BF03005413] [PMID: 2555076]

[36] Ben-Shlomo I, Moskovich R, Katz Y, Shalev E. Midazolam/ketamine sedative combination compared with fentanyl/propofol/isoflurane anaesthesia for oocyte retrieval. Hum Reprod 1999; 14(7): 1757-9.
[http://dx.doi.org/10.1093/humrep/14.7.1757] [PMID: 10402383]

[37] Norton WB, Scavizzi F, Smith CN, Dong W, Raspa M, Parker-Thornburg JV. Refinements for embryo implantation surgery in the mouse: comparison of injectable and inhalant anesthesias – tribromoethanol, ketamine and isoflurane – on pregnancy and pup survival. Lab Anim 2016; 50(5): 335-43.
[http://dx.doi.org/10.1177/0023677215616530] [PMID: 26566637]

[38] Kwan I, Bhattacharya S, Knox F, McNeil A. Pain relief for women undergoing oocyte retrieval for assisted reproduction. Cochrane Collaboration Syst Rev. 2013; (11): CD004829.

[39] Kwan I, Wang R, Pearce E, Bhattacharya S. Pain relief for women undergoing oocyte retrieval for assisted reproduction. Cochrane Libr 2018; 2018(5): CD004829.
[http://dx.doi.org/10.1002/14651858.CD004829.pub4] [PMID: 29761478]

[40] Humaidan P, Stener-Victorin E. Pain relief during oocyte retrieval with a new short duration electro-acupuncture technique--an alternative to conventional analgesic methods. Hum Reprod 2004; 19(6): 1367-72.
[http://dx.doi.org/10.1093/humrep/deh229] [PMID: 15105387]

[41] Han JS. Acupuncture analgesia: Areas of consensus and controversy. Pain 2011; 152(3) (Suppl.): S41-8.
[http://dx.doi.org/10.1016/j.pain.2010.10.012] [PMID: 21078546]

[42] Guo XL, Li X, Wei W, *et al.* Acupuncture for pain relief of women undergoing transvaginal oocyte retrieval. Medicine (Baltimore) 2020; 99(39): e22383.
[http://dx.doi.org/10.1097/MD.0000000000022383] [PMID: 32991459]

[43] Lee A, Chan SKC, Fan LTY. Stimulation of the wrist acupuncture point PC6 for preventing postoperative nausea and vomiting. Cochrane Libr 2015; 2016(6): CD003281.
[http://dx.doi.org/10.1002/14651858.CD003281.pub4] [PMID: 26522652]

[44] Leung L. Neurophysiological basis of acupuncture-induced analgesia--an updated review. J Acupunct Meridian Stud 2012; 5(6): 261-70.
[http://dx.doi.org/10.1016/j.jams.2012.07.017] [PMID: 23265077]

[45] Zhao ZQ. Neural mechanism underlying acupuncture analgesia. Prog Neurobiol 2008; 85(4): 355-75.
[http://dx.doi.org/10.1016/j.pneurobio.2008.05.004] [PMID: 18582529]

[46] Franconi G, Manni L, Aloe L, *et al.* Acupuncture in clinical and experimental reproductive medicine: A review. J. Endocrinol. Invest 2011; 34: 307-11.
[http://dx.doi.org/10.3275/7500]

[47] Zijlstra FJ, van den Berg-de Lange I, Huygen FJPM, Klein J. Anti-inflammatory actions of acupuncture. Mediators Inflamm 2003; 12(2): 59-69.

[http://dx.doi.org/10.1080/0962935031000114943] [PMID: 12775355]

[48] Stener-Victorin E, Waldenström U, Nilsson L, Wikland M, Janson PO. A prospective randomized study of electro-acupuncture *versus* alfentanil as anaesthesia during oocyte aspiration in in-vitro fertilization. Hum Reprod 1999; 14(10): 2480-4.
[http://dx.doi.org/10.1093/humrep/14.10.2480] [PMID: 10527973]

[49] Andersson S, Lundeberg T. Acupuncture — from empiricism to science: Functional background to acupuncture effects in pain and disease Pain and disease. Med Hypotheses 1995; 45(3): 271-81.
[http://dx.doi.org/10.1016/0306-9877(95)90117-5] [PMID: 8569551]

[50] Chen S, Wang S, Rong P, *et al.* Acupuncture for visceral pain: neural substrates and potential mechanisms. Evid Based Complement Alternat Med 2014; 2014: 1-12.
[http://dx.doi.org/10.1155/2014/609594] [PMID: 25614752]

[51] Chou LW, Kao MJ, Lin JG. Probable mechanisms of needling therapies for myofascial pain control. Evid Based Complement Alternat Med 2012; 2012: 1-11.
[http://dx.doi.org/10.1155/2012/705327] [PMID: 23346211]

[52] Cho HZ, *et al.* Functional magnetic resonance of the brain in the investigation of acupuncture. In: Stux G, Hammerschlag R, Eds. Clinical acupuncture Scientific basis 2001; 83-95.
[http://dx.doi.org/10.1007/978-3-642-56732-2_5]

[53] Yoo SS, Kerr CE, Park M, *et al.* Neural activities in human somatosensory cortical areas evoked by acupuncture stimulation. Complement Ther Med 2007; 15(4): 247-54.
[http://dx.doi.org/10.1016/j.ctim.2007.01.010] [PMID: 18054726]

[54] Wang W, Liu L, Zhi X, *et al.* Study on the regulatory effect of electro-acupuncture on Hegu point (LI4) in cerebral response with functional magnetic resonance imaging. Chin J Integr Med 2007; 13(1): 10-6.
[http://dx.doi.org/10.1007/s11655-007-0010-3] [PMID: 17578311]

[55] Hui KK, Liu J, Makris N, *et al.* Acupuncture modulates the limbic system and subcortical gray structures of the human brain: evidence from fMRI studies in normal subjects. Hum Brain Mapp 2000; 9(1): 13-25.
[http://dx.doi.org/10.1002/(SICI)1097-0193(2000)9:1<13::AID-HBM2>3.0.CO;2-F] [PMID: 10643726]

[56] Kong J, Ma L, Gollub RL, *et al.* A pilot study of functional magnetic resonance imaging of the brain during manual and electroacupuncture stimulation of acupuncture point (LI-4 Hegu) in normal subjects reveals differential brain activation between methods. J Altern Complement Med 2002; 8(4): 411-9.
[http://dx.doi.org/10.1089/107555302760253603] [PMID: 12230901]

[57] Krings T, Weidemann J, Meister IG, Thron A, Fang JL. Functional MRI in healthy subjects during acupuncture: different effects of needle rotation in real and false acupoints. Neuroradiology 2004; 46(5): 359-62.
[http://dx.doi.org/10.1007/s00234-003-1125-7] [PMID: 15103431]

[58] Napadow V, Makris N, Liu J, Kettner NW, Kwong KK, Hui KKS. Effects of electroacupuncture *versus* manual acupuncture on the human brain as measured by fMRI. Hum Brain Mapp 2005; 24(3): 193-205.
[http://dx.doi.org/10.1002/hbm.20081] [PMID: 15499576]

[59] Fang J, Jin Z, Wang Y, *et al.* The salient characteristics of the central effects of acupuncture needling: Limbic-paralimbic-neocortical network modulation. Hum Brain Mapp 2009; 30(4): 1196-206.
[http://dx.doi.org/10.1002/hbm.20583] [PMID: 18571795]

[60] Dhond RP, Yeh C, Park K, Kettner N, Napadow V. Acupuncture modulates resting state connectivity in default and sensorimotor brain networks. Pain 2008; 136(3): 407-18.
[http://dx.doi.org/10.1016/j.pain.2008.01.011] [PMID: 18337009]

[61] Bai L, Qin W, Tian J, *et al.* Acupuncture modulates spontaneous activities in the anticorrelated resting brain networks. Brain Res 2009; 1279(C): 37-49.
[http://dx.doi.org/10.1016/j.brainres.2009.04.056] [PMID: 19427842]

[62] Hui KK, Marina O, Claunch JD, *et al.* Acupuncture mobilizes the brain's default mode and its anti-correlated network in healthy subjects. Brain Research. 2009; 1287: 84-103.

[63] Wu MT, Hsieh JC, Xiong J, *et al.* Central nervous pathway for acupuncture stimulation: localization of processing with functional MR imaging of the brain--preliminary experience. Radiology 1999; 212(1): 133-41.
[http://dx.doi.org/10.1148/radiology.212.1.r99jl04133] [PMID: 10405732]

[64] Cho ZH, Chung SC, Jones JP, *et al.* New findings of the correlation between acupoints and corresponding brain cortices using functional MRI. Proc Natl Acad Sci USA 1998; 95(5): 2670-3.
[http://dx.doi.org/10.1073/pnas.95.5.2670] [PMID: 9482945]

[65] Humaidan P, Brock K, Bungum L, Stener-Victorin E. Pain relief during oocyte retrieval — exploring the role of different frequencies of electro-acupuncture. Reprod Biomed Online 2006; 13(1): 120-5.
[http://dx.doi.org/10.1016/S1472-6483(10)62025-1] [PMID: 16820123]

[66] Han JS. Acupuncture: neuropeptide release produced by electrical stimulation of different frequencies. Trends Neurosci 2003; 26(1): 17-22.
[http://dx.doi.org/10.1016/S0166-2236(02)00006-1] [PMID: 12495858]

[67] Cui SL, Yu CY, Tee YW, Ho LM, Seah CN, Yu SL. *Retracted:* Acupuncture Compared to Conscious Sedation for Pain Relief During *In-Vitro* Fertilization Oocyte Retrieval. Med Acupunct 2020; 32(6): e411-8.
[http://dx.doi.org/10.1089/acu.2020.1416]

[68] Vickers AJ. Can acupuncture have specific effects on health? A systematic review of acupuncture antiemesis trials. J R Soc Med 1996; 89(6): 303-11.
[http://dx.doi.org/10.1177/014107689608900602] [PMID: 8758186]

[69] Lee A, Done ML. The use of nonpharmacologic techniques to prevent postoperative nausea and vomiting: a meta-analysis. Anesth Analg 1999; 88(6): 1362-9.
[http://dx.doi.org/10.1213/00000539-199906000-00031] [PMID: 10357346]

[70] Fang J, Wang X, Liu H, *et al.* The Limbic-Prefrontal Network Modulated by Electroacupuncture at CV4 and CV121 2012.
[http://dx.doi.org/10.1155/2012/515893]

[71] Wu l *et al.* Effects of Noninvasive Electroacupuncture at Hegu (LI4) and Sanyinjiao (SP6) Acupoints on Dysmenorrhea. The Journal Of Alternative And Complementary Medicine 2012; 18(2): 137-42.

[72] Alraek T, Baerheim A, Birch S. Acupuncture points used in the prophylaxis against recurrent uncomplicated cystitis, patterns identified and their possible relationship to physiological measurements. Chin J Integr Med 2016; 22(7): 510-7.
[http://dx.doi.org/10.1007/s11655-014-1988-y] [PMID: 25491541]

[73] Cheong YC, Dix S, Hung Yu Ng E, Ledger WL, Farquhar C. Acupuncture and assisted reproductive technology. Cochrane Database Syst Rev 2013; (7): CD006920.
[PMID: 23888428]

[74] Blumenfeld Z. The Ovarian Hyperstimulation Syndrome. Vitam Horm 2018; 107: 423-51.
[http://dx.doi.org/10.1016/bs.vh.2018.01.018] [PMID: 29544639]

[75] Timmons D, Montrief T, Koyfman A, Long B. Ovarian hyperstimulation syndrome: A review for emergency clinicians. Am J Emerg Med 2019; 37(8): 1577-84.
[http://dx.doi.org/10.1016/j.ajem.2019.05.018] [PMID: 31097257]

[76] Mourad S, Brown J, Farquhar C. Interventions for the prevention of OHSS in ART cycles: an overview of Cochrane reviews. Cochrane Libr 2017; 2017(1): CD012103.

[http://dx.doi.org/10.1002/14651858.CD012103.pub2] [PMID: 28111738]

[77] Kwik M, Maxwell E. Pathophysiology, treatment and prevention of ovarian hyperstimulation syndrome. Curr Opin Obstet Gynecol 2016; 28(4): 236-41.
[http://dx.doi.org/10.1097/GCO.0000000000000284] [PMID: 27273307]

[78] Namavar Jahromi B, Parsanezhad ME, Shomali Z, *et al.* Ovarian Hyperstimulation Syndrome: A Narrative Review of Its Pathophysiology, Risk Factors, Prevention, Classification, and Management. Iran J Med Sci 2018; 43(3): 248-60.
[PMID: 29892142]

[79] Pfeifer S, Butts S, Dumesic D, *et al.* Prevention and treatment of moderate and severe ovarian hyperstimulation syndrome: a guideline. Fertil Steril 2016; 106(7): 1634-47.
[http://dx.doi.org/10.1016/j.fertnstert.2016.08.048] [PMID: 27678032]

[80] Toftager M, Bogstad J, Bryndorf T, *et al.* Risk of severe ovarian hyperstimulation syndrome in GnRH antagonist *versus* GnRH agonist protocol: RCT including 1050 first IVF/ICSI cycles. Hum Reprod 2016; 31(6): 1253-64.
[http://dx.doi.org/10.1093/humrep/dew051] [PMID: 27060174]

[81] Meldrum DR. Preventing severe OHSS has many different facets. Fertil Steril 2012; 97(3): 536-8.
[http://dx.doi.org/10.1016/j.fertnstert.2012.01.095] [PMID: 22265035]

[82] Tang H, Mourad S, Zhai SD, Hart RJ. Dopamine agonists for preventing ovarian hyperstimulation syndrome. Cochrane Libr 2016; 11(11): CD008605.
[http://dx.doi.org/10.1002/14651858.CD008605.pub3] [PMID: 27901279]

[83] Nelson SM. Prevention and management of ovarian hyperstimulation syndrome. Thromb Res 2017; 151 (Suppl. 1): S61-4.
[http://dx.doi.org/10.1016/S0049-3848(17)30070-1] [PMID: 28262238]

[84] Aboulghar M, Evers JH, Al-Inany H. Intra-venous albumin for preventing severe ovarian hyperstimulation syndrome. Cochrane Database Syst Rev 2002; 2(2): CD001302.
[PMID: 12076404]

[85] Franco-Cabrera M, Lambertinez-Juarez NA, Olavarría-Guadarrama MY. Consideraciones anestésicas en las técnicas de reproducción asistida. Acta Med Grupo Ángeles 2019; 17(1): 38-46.

CHAPTER 19

Anesthetic Management for External Cephalic Version

María Luz Serrano Rodriguez[1,*], **Sara Hervilla Ezquerra**[1], **Laura Fernandez Tellez**[1], **Andrea Alejandra Rodriguez Esteve**[1] and **Marta Chacon Castillo**[2]

[1] *Department of Anaesthesiology, Hospital Universitario Fundación Alcórcon, Madrid, Spain*

[2] *Department of Anaesthesiology, Hospital Universitario Severo Ochoa, Leganés, Madrid, Spain*

Abstract: Approximately 3% to 4% of term fetuses are in breech presentation, and this is a common indication for cesarean delivery. Twenty percent of elective cesarean sections are due to breech position.

External cephalic version (*ECV*) is an obstetric maneuver that applies external pressure to the fetal posture through the maternal abdomen, to convert a breech presentation to a vertex presentation. Since the risk of adverse events after an ECV is small, the possibility of ECV should be offered in all pregnancies with breech presentation, provided that there is no contraindication.

A standardized protocol, an experienced gynecologist and adequate analgesia can facilitate the maneuver and improve the success rate, turning the ECV into a maneuver with an excellent safety profile which is an interesting option to avoid a cesarean section.

Keywords: Analgesia, Anesthesia, Anesthesia, Breech Presentation, Breech Delivey, Cesarean Section, External Cephalic Version, Epidural Anesthesia, Inhalational Anesthesia, Intravenous Anesthesia, Neuraxial Anesthesia, Remifentanyl, Spinal Anesthesia, Tocolytics.

BACKGROUND

In recent years, WHO has highlighted in several reports the substantial increase in caesarean birth rates, exceeding the recommended rate to ensure optimal maternal and neonatal outcomes.

This situation, which occurs in both developed and developing countries, is concerning, because caesarean section is associated with an increase in maternal

* **Corresponding author María Luz Serrano Rodriguez:** Department of Anaesthesiology, Hospital Universitario Fundacion Alcorcon, Madrid, Spain; E-mail: marialuz.serrano@salud.madrid.org

Eugenio Daniel Martinez-Hurtado, Monica Sanjuan-Alvarez & Marta Chacon-Castillo (Eds.)
All rights reserved-© 2022 Bentham Science Publishers

morbidity and mortality, and a higher cost of healthcare compared to vaginal delivery. Therefore, there is considerable interest in the obstetric community in identifying and implementing strategies to reduce the need for caesarean delivery.

Approximately 3% to 4% of term fetuses are in breech presentation, and this is a common indication for cesarean delivery. Twenty percent of elective cesarean sections are due to breech position.

EXTERNAL CEPHALIC VERSION

The external cephalic version (*ECV*) is a maneuver that applies external pressure to the fetal posture through the maternal abdomen, to turn a breech or transverse fetal position into a vertex presentation, allowing for a vaginal delivery.

The Term Breech Trial (Hannah, 2000) [1] concluded that elective caesarean section was associated with a lower risk of perinatal morbidity and mortality than scheduled breech delivery, thereby increasing the rate of elective caesarean sections in this type of presentation.

A subsequent study conducted in 2003 [2] concluded that, following Hannah's study, 92.5% of hospitals stopped performing vaginal breech deliveries and adopted elective caesarean section in breech presentations.

Subsequent analyses showed clear methodological deficiencies in this study, but there had already been a definite change in clinical practice in developed countries, with an increase in the rate of scheduled caesarean section in breech presentation, and with a reduction in breech delivery training and experience in obstetricians.

The obstetric experience needed to safely assist a breech delivery has disappeared and this, coupled with an effort to reduce the frequency of caesarean sections, has led to a resurgence of ECV, and anesthesia to increase its success.

Morbidity and mortality associated with elective caesarean section are three times higher compared to vaginal delivery [3]. In addition, there is a greater likelihood of caesarean sections in future pregnancies. The presence of a uterine scar increases the risk of complications such as ectopic pregnancy, placenta previa or accretion, placental abruption and uterine rupture.

The external cephalic version is a safe technique. The frequency of complications is very low. Severe complications, such as placental abruption and emergent cesarean section due to fetal distress, appear in less than 1% of procedures.

ECV is not associated with increased perinatal morbidity or mortality. Interesting in this regard, in a recent observational study [4], the authors compared perinatal outcomes among women with breech presentation at term who underwent an attempt at ECV with those who were treated expectantly. They did not find greater perinatal morbidity or mortality associated with attempted EVS compared to expectant management. In addition, although success can be difficult to predict for sure, an attempt at ECV reduces the chance of caesarean section compared to expectant follow-up.

In addition, it is an effective technique. Although the heterogeneity of studies does not allow for precise statistics, the success rate of ECV is 40-70%, managing to significantly decrease the number of caesarean sections for breech presentation from 9-16%. Spontaneous reversion to the breech position after successful ECV is less than 5%.

Currently, scientific societies recommend ECV due to the low risks to both the pregnant woman and the fetus [5 - 7].

Factors that Predict a Successful ECV

Among the factors associated with successful ECV are: the use of tocolysis, posterior insertion of the placenta, complete breech or transverse presentation, amniotic fluid index higher than 10 cm and maternal weight under 65 kg. Success rate is also higher in multiparous than in primiparous women and if the obstetrician who performs the ECV has experience in the technique.

Contraindications

The evidence on contraindications is limited, but according to the opinion of experts, there are situations that would contraindicate the ECV:

- Placenta previa or placental abruption.
- Severe oligoamnios or premature rupture of membranes.
- Fetal monitoring indicating risk of loss of fetal well-being.
- Severe fetal malformation.
- Uterine anomalies.
- Multiple gestation. In this scenario, ECV is contraindicated before delivery, but it can be performed for the extraction of the second fetus.
- Relative contraindications: maternal hypertension, maternal obesity.

UPDATED RECOMMENDATIONS ACCORDING TO SCIENTIFIC SOCIETIES

Recommendation with a High Level of Evidence (Level A)

Since the risk of adverse events following ECV is small and the caesarean section rate is lower in women who have successfully undergone ECV, all women with breech presentation should be offered the possibility of ECV, provided there is no contraindication.

The use of tocolysis increases the success rate of ECV. A 2015 Cochrane review concluded that betamimetics are the best-studied tocolytics, and that when they are used in ECV, there is an increase in cephalic presentation at labor (RR 1.68, 95% CI 1.14-2.48) and a reduction in the number of caesarean sections (RR 0.77; 95% CI 0.67 to 0.88). The effect was demonstrated in both multiparous and nulliparous women.

Recommendation with Limited Scientific Evidence Level (Level B)

ECV should preferably be offered from 36-37 weeks of gestation, when the amount of amniotic liquid allows the performance of the technique and the number of spontaneous reversions after success is low.

Women should be informed that, with appropriate precautions, ECV has a very low rate of complications. They also must be warned that labor after ECV is associated with a slightly higher rate of caesarean section and instrumental delivery compared to spontaneous cephalic labor.

In a systematic review of three cohort studies and eight case-control studies, Hundt et al. [7] concluded that even after successful ECV, women continued to have an increased risk of cesarean delivery for both arrested labor (OR 2.2; 95% CI 1.6 to 3.0) and fetal distress (OR 2.2; 95% CI 1.6 to 2.9). There is also an increased risk of instrumental vaginal delivery (OR 1.4; 95% CI: 1.1–1.7).

Neuraxial analgesia in combination with tocolytic therapy can be considered a reasonable intervention to increase the EVC success rate.

Evidence Level C Recommendations

Although most women tolerate EVC, they should be informed that EVC may be a painful procedure.

Women should be informed that performing ECV after a previous caesarean section does not seem to carry a higher risk of complications than in an intact uterus.

For the practice of an ECV in women who are RhD negative, anti-D immunoglobulin administration is recommended unless the baby is also D negative.

ANESTHESIA IN THE EXTERNAL CEPHALIC VERSION

Data from current guidelines from the American College of Obstetricians and Gynecologists (*ACOG*), the Society for Obstetric Anesthesia and Perinatology (*SOAP*), and the Royal College of Obstetricians & Gynaecologists (*BJOG*) are insufficient to conclusively evaluate neuraxial analgesia without a tocolytic. However neuraxial analgesia in combination with tocolytic therapy can be considered a reasonable intervention to increase the ECV success rate.

Clinical experience based on scientific evidence [8, 11] demonstrates that adequate neuraxial or systemic anesthetic management increases the success rate of ECV and improves the perinatal outcome associated with ECV.

Neuraxial, intravenous and inhalational anesthesia have all been evaluated to reduce discomfort caused by abdominal manipulation during ECV, and to increase the success rate of ECV.

NEURAXIAL ANESTHESIA

Although neither the type of neuraxial anesthesia nor the optimal dose has been determined, its role in the success of ECV must not be ignored, as it can increase both its safety and efficacy.

Neuraxial anesthesia (spinal, combined spinal-epidural and epidural) together with tocolytics, significantly increases the success rate of ECV, compared to the use of tocolytics alone [8].

The use of regional anesthesia for ECV is not associated with a higher incidence of emergency caesarean section due to serious adverse events.

The realization of combined techniques allows to titrate the anesthetic doses to minimize side effects, such as arterial hypotension. The anesthetic effects can be maintained with complementary doses for better analgesia or even to perform a cesarean section, if necessary, during the ECV.

Some scientific societies have developed ECV protocols that recommend the combined spinal-epidural technique, such as the Protocol proposed by the Obstetric Anesthesia Section of the Spanish Society of Anesthesiology, Resuscitation and Pain Therapy (*SEDAR*) 3rd Edition, 2021. Epidural spinal is combined with anesthesia (Combined Spinal-Epidural anesthesia [*CSE*]), with a spinal dose of 5-7.5 mg hyperbaric bupivacaine + 20 mcgr fentanyl, and epidural catheter placement. In case of emergency caesarean section, analgesia is reinforced with 2% lidocaine (15-20 ml) through the epidural catheter.

Although the role of neuraxial anesthesia in facilitating the external cephalic version is well established, the dosing has not been fully elucidated. The study of Chalifoux *et al.* [9] demonstrates that several neuraxial dosing regimens can be used to help facilitate the external cephalic version and improve the likelihood of a successful version.

The optimal regimen should probably be adjusted to the specific clinical context. If the patient will be discharged regardless of the success/failure of the external cephalic version, the most logical indication would be the lowest dose (*e.g.*, 2.5 mg bupivacaine plus 15 µg fentanyl). The authors found that the time to discharge was increased by 60 min (range, 16 to 116 min) with a dose higher than 7.5 mg of bupivacaine compared to 2.5 mg ($P = 0.004$).

However, if the plan is to perform delivery by caesarean section, if the external cephalic version is not successful or to immediately start the induction of labor, if the external cephalic version is successful, then a higher dose can be justified. Larger spinal doses (*e.g.*, 10 mg of bupivacaine) would facilitate delivery by caesarean section under neuraxial anesthesia, due to the failure of version or in case of emergency during the ECV.

Chalifoux *et al.* conclude that increasing the dose of the local intrathecal anesthetic to achieve greater density of motor and sensory block does not increase the success rate of external cephalic version, nor does it reduce the rate of deliveries by cesarean section. Unsurprisingly, they note that increased intrathecal bupivacaine dose results in better analgesia, as well as a higher incidence of hypotension and prolonged stay.

Neuraxial anesthesia is associated with a high incidence of arterial hypotension (30-50%). Maternal hemodynamic instability has been suggested as a cause of a higher number of caesarean sections. However, no statistical association has been found between neuraxial anesthesia for ECV and fetal monitoring findings that warrant an emergency cesarean section.

Administration of vasopressors, such as phenylephrine infusion, and the use of low spinal doses are recommended preventive strategies to avoid hypotension when performing the neuraxial technique.

Although the administration of neuraxial anesthesia seems to reduce significantly the rate of caesarean sections, more studies are needed, as there are still conflicting results in the current literature, possibly due to limitations and methodological differences in extracting objective data [10 - 12].

REMIFENTANIL

Intravenous anesthesia with remifentanil is an alternative to neuraxial anesthesia. It can be an alternative approach so that the woman tolerates ECV more comfortably, followed by the use of regional anesthesia in selected women in whom the first attempt at ECV has failed.

Remifentanil is an ultra-short μ-opioid receptor-antagonist, with a rapid onset and cessation of effect. Remifentanil readily crosses the placenta, but it is quickly metabolized by nonspecific esterases with a half-life of 3 to 4 minutes.

Comparative studies show [13] that patients in the IV remifentanil group have less pain compared to the control group without anesthesia, but it does not increase the odds of successful ECV, and it shows a significantly higher patient satisfaction compared with neuraxial anesthesia. The incidence of fetal bradycardia requiring emergency caesarean section is similar to the control group without anesthesia. IV analgesia may have advantages over regional analgesia in terms of complications of dural puncture such as PDPH. Intravenous anesthesia may be a good option when regional anesthesia is contraindicated, such as in coagulation disorders, or in pregnant women who refuse neuraxial techniques. It may also be an option if the financial and personnel resources of the health institution are limited and regional anesthesia is not available [14].

INHALATIONAL ANESTHESIA

There is little literature regarding the use of inhalational anesthesia.

Sevoflurane has sedative and uterine relaxation effects, which would facilitate ECV and increase its success rate.

The most important pharmacokinetic characteristic of sevoflurane is its low blood-gas partition coefficient that allows rapid induction and anesthetic recovery. At the same time, this low blood solubility allows for a more precise control of the anesthetic depth plane while maintaining spontaneous breathing throughout the procedure.

So far, there is a single study, by Piñel Pérez, C.S. *et al.* [15], with 101 patients comparing two groups. A group of 57 patients received inhalational anesthesia with sevoflurane and the second group of 44 women received spinal anesthesia. The inhalational procedure starts with 100% oxygen preoxygenation for 3 minutes, followed by 1% sevoflurane in a mixture of oxygen and air (FiO$_2$ 0.5) using an adjusted face mask with a gas flow of 6 L/min.

The intervention will stop if the woman reports severe pain, if the version is not easily achieved or if sustained fetal bradycardia, uterine haemorrhage or placental abruption appears.

The results in terms of success rate, vaginal delivery rate, complications and cost are similar. No statistically significant differences between both anesthetic procedures were found. No maternal or fetal complications were reported and the authors consider it a safe and less invasive technique.

Nitrous oxide has not shown differences in pain, anxiety, and patient satisfaction scores between patients receiving nitrous oxide *versus* oxygen as a placebo during ECV [16, 17].

OTHER ANALGESIC OPTIONS

Women should be warned that there is no evidence of postural management alone promoting a spontaneous version to cephalic presentation.

Women may want to consider the use of moxibustion for breech presentation at 33–35 weeks of gestation.

A small non-randomised study suggested that clinical hypnosis combined with tocolysis before ECV may increase success rates [18].

CONCLUSION

ECV is an intervention that decreases the number of caesarean sections in pregnancies with breech presentation and, avoiding the first cesarean section, reduces complications in subsequent pregnancies due to uterine scars.

External cephalic versions should be performed by experienced personnel and only in environments where monitoring and immediate delivery are readily available.

The existence of a standardized hospital protocol and the collaboration of the anesthesiologist with the obstetrician are essential to achieve optimal quality standards in maternal-fetal care.

Each case should be individualized and the procedure explained to the patient, as well as the alternatives, if they exist. An informed consent form must be signed by the patient.

Analgesia, and especially neuraxial anesthesia, together with tocolytics, significantly increase the success rate of ECV.

Cost-effectiveness studies carried out in the US and Europe show a reduction in the healthcare cost with the realization of ECV when compared to an elective caesarean section for breech presentation.

It is also likely that neuraxial anesthesia is cost-effective, as it increases the success rate of ECV with the consequent reduction in the rate of caesarean sections. This compensates for the costs of providing anesthesia to facilitate the external cephalic version [19].

CONSENT FOR PUBLICATION

Not applicable.

CONFLICT OF INTEREST

The authors declare no conflict of interest, financial or otherwise.

ACKNOWLEDGEMENT

Declared none.

REFERENCES

[1]   Hannah ME, Hannah WJ, Hewson SA, Hodnett ED, Saigal S, Willan AR. Planned caesarean section *versus* planned vaginal birth for breech presentation at term: a randomised multicentre trial. Lancet 2000; 356(9239): 1375-83.
        [http://dx.doi.org/10.1016/S0140-6736(00)02840-3] [PMID: 11052579]

[2]   Hogle KL, Kilburn L, Hewson S, Gafni A, Wall R, Hannah ME. Impact of the international term breech trial on clinical practice and concerns: a survey of centre collaborators. J Obstet Gynaecol Can 2003; 25(1): 14-6.
        [http://dx.doi.org/10.1016/S1701-2163(16)31077-5] [PMID: 12548320]

[3]   de Hundt M, Velzel J, de Groot CJ, Mol BW, Kok M. Mode of delivery after successful external cephalic version: a systematic review and meta-analysis. Obstet Gynecol 2014; 123(6): 1327-34.
        [http://dx.doi.org/10.1097/AOG.0000000000000295] [PMID: 24807332]

[4]   Son M, Roy A, Grobman WA, Miller ES. association between attempted external cephalic version and perinatal morbidity and mortality. obstet gynecol 2018; 132(2): 365-70.
        [http://dx.doi.org/10.1097/AOG.0000000000002699] [PMID: 29995733]

[5]   American College of Obstetricians and Gynecologists External Cephalic Version. Obstet Gynecol 2020; 135(5): e203-12.
        [http://dx.doi.org/10.1097/AOG.0000000000003837] [PMID: 32332415]

[6]   American College of Obstetricians and Gynecologists. ACOG Committee Opinion No. 745 Mode of term singleton breech delivery. Obstet Gynecol 2018; 132(2): e60-3.
[http://dx.doi.org/10.1097/AOG.0000000000002755] [PMID: 30045211]

[7]   Royal College of Obstetrician & Gynaecologists. Guideline No. 20a. External Cephalic Version and reducing the Incidence of Breech Presentation BJOG 2017; 124: e178-e192. 2021.

[8]   Magro-Malosso ER, Saccone G, Di Tommaso M, Mele M, Berghella V. Neuraxial analgesia to increase the success rate of external cephalic version: a systematic review and meta-analysis of randomized controlled trials. Am J Obstet Gynecol 2016; 215(3): 276-86.
[http://dx.doi.org/10.1016/j.ajog.2016.04.036] [PMID: 27131581]

[9]   Chalifoux LA, Bauchat JR, Higgins N, *et al*. Effect of intrathecal bupivacaine dose on the success of external cephalic version for breech presentation: A prospective, randomized, blinded clinical trial. Anesthesiology 2017; 127(4): 625-32.
[http://dx.doi.org/10.1097/ALN.0000000000001796] [PMID: 28723831]

[10]   Carvalho B, Bateman BT. Not Too Little, Not Too Much. Anesthesiology 2017; 127(4): 596-8.
[http://dx.doi.org/10.1097/ALN.0000000000001839] [PMID: 28799953]

[11]   Weiniger CF. Analgesia/anesthesia for external cephalic version. Curr Opin Anaesthesiol 2013; 26(3): 278-87.
[http://dx.doi.org/10.1097/ACO.0b013e328360f64e] [PMID: 23614959]

[12]   Khaw KS, Lee SWY, Ngan Kee WD, *et al*. Randomized trial of anaesthetic interventions in external cephalic version for breech presentation. Br J Anaesth 2015; 114(6): 944-50.
[http://dx.doi.org/10.1093/bja/aev107] [PMID: 25962611]

[13]   Hao Q, Hu Y, Zhang L, *et al*. A systematic review and Meta-analysis of clinical trials of neuraxial, intravenous, and inhalational anesthesia for external cephalic version. Anesth Analg 2020; 131(6): 1800-11.
[http://dx.doi.org/10.1213/ANE.0000000000004795] [PMID: 32282385]

[14]   Muñoz H, Guerra S, Perez-Vaquero P, Valero Martinez C, Aizpuru F, Lopez-Picado A. Remifentanil *versus* placebo for analgesia during external cephalic version: a randomised clinical trial. Int J Obstet Anesth 2014; 23(1): 52-7.
[http://dx.doi.org/10.1016/j.ijoa.2013.07.006] [PMID: 24388737]

[15]   Piñel Pérez CS, Herencia Rivero A, Gómez-Roso Jareño MJ, Solis Ruiz A. Gómez-Roso Jareño MJ, Solis Ruiz A.I, Izquierdo Méndez N, Herráiz Martínez MA. Sevoflurane versus spinal anesthesia for external cephalic version. Journal of Perinatal Medicine 2015 43 SUPPL. 1

[16]   Straube LE, Fardelmann KL, Penwarden AA, *et al*. Nitrous oxide analgesia for external cephalic version: A randomized controlled trial. J Clin Anesth 2021; 68110073
[http://dx.doi.org/10.1016/j.jclinane.2020.110073] [PMID: 33017784]

[17]   Burgos J, Cobos P, Osuna C, *et al*. Nitrous oxide for analgesia in external cephalic version at term: prospective comparative studya. J Perinat Med 2013; 41(6): 719-23.
[http://dx.doi.org/10.1515/jpm-2013-0046] [PMID: 23924521]

[18]   Reinhard J, Heinrich TM, Reitter A, Herrmann E, Smart W, Louwen F. Clinical hypnosis before external cephalic version. Am J Clin Hypn 2012; 55(2): 184-92.
[http://dx.doi.org/10.1080/00029157.2012.665399] [PMID: 23189523]

[19] Carvalho B, Tan JM, Macario A, El-Sayed YY, Sultan P. Brief report: a cost analysis of neuraxial anesthesia to facilitate external cephalic version for breech fetal presentation. Anesth Analg 2013; 117(1): 155-9.
[http://dx.doi.org/10.1213/ANE.0b013e31828e5bc7] [PMID: 23592608]

CHAPTER 20

Mindfulness-Based Interventions during Pregnancy and Labour

Míriam Sánchez Merchante[1,*] and **Eugenio D. Martinez Hurtado**[2]

[1] *Department of Anesthesiology and Crtical Care, Hospital Universitario Fundación Alcorcón, Madrid, Spain*

[2] *Department of Anaesthesiology and Intensive Care, Hospital Universitario Infanta Leonor, Madrid, Spain*

Abstract: During pregnancy, events occur that can negatively affect a woman's mental health, such as vaginal bleeding, concern for the health of the fetus, decreased fetal movements, ultrasound results, or fear of childbirth itself. Pregnant women must be able to cope with these stressful events, as perinatal mental health problems can have adverse consequences for both parents and babies.

Psychological disturbances in the mother during pregnancy can adversely affect the development of the fetus, leading to long-term negative effects on the health of the child. It is therefore important to identify prenatal interventions that can reduce this maternal distress, and one possible approach to address these perinatal mental health difficulties is mindfulness-based interventions.

Keywords: Acceptance-Based Coping, Adverse Events, Antidepressant Drugs, Anxiety, Behavioural Intervention, Child Health Outcomes, CBT, Cognitive Behavioural Therapy, CBT-I, Cognitive Behavioural Therapy for Insomnia, Comorbidity, Compassion, Childbirth, Depression, Emotion Regulation, Fetal Programming, Fear, Iatrogenic, Labour, Maternal Mindfulness, Maternal Anxiety, Mindfulness, Mindfulness-Based Interventions, Mindfulness-Based Cognitive Therapy, Mindfulness Yoga, Mindful Motherhood Training, MMT, Mindfulness Mom Training, Noradrenaline, Obesity, Pregnancy, Perceived Stress, Perinatal Depression, Postpartum Depression, Pain, Reuptake Inhibitors, Self-Regulation, Stress, Safety, Serotonin, Side Effects, Temperament, TAU, Treatment As Usual, Tolerability, Tricyclic.

---

* **Corresponding author Míriam Sánchez Merchante:** Department of Anesthesiology and Crtical Care, Hospital Universitario Fundación Alcorcón, Madrid, Spain; Email: msmerchante@hotmail.com

Eugenio Daniel Martinez-Hurtado, Monica Sanjuan-Alvarez & Marta Chacon-Castillo (Eds.)
All rights reserved-© 2022 Bentham Science Publishers

INTRODUCTION

One in four women will develop a perinatal mental disorder, with depression being the most frequent complication [1]. In fact, anxiety multiplies the risk of depression threefold and its presence is a factor that can maintain and/or aggravate the depressive state [2].

Pregnancy-specific anxiety and stress reflect specific emotional concepts [3 - 6]. Postpartum depression (*PPD*) is diagnosed in up to 20% of women during the first 6 months after childbirth. Depressive symptomatology (maternity or baby blues) has a prevalence of 50-85% [7], and these rates are higher when there has been depression in other periods of life or in a previous pregnancy [8].

It has been observed that this symptomatology worsens in the first postpartum week and begins to improve days later, with the exception of cases that progress to PPD. Generalized anxiety disorder (*GAD*) in the perinatal stage has a prevalence of 8.5-10.5% [9]. Similarly, anxious symptomatology in pregnant women is higher, reaching up to 39% [10]. PPD and GAD, usually diagnosed in the postpartum period, may be a consequence of depressive and anxious symptomatology already initiated during pregnancy [11].

There are few studies analysing outcomes associated with postpartum anxiety. In the mother, this condition may be associated with negative effects on factors that will establish the mother-infant relationship (*e.g.*, maternal parenting behaviours, mother-infant interaction, bonding). In the infant, there may also be negative effects (*e.g.*, crying, distress at novelty, social and physiological responses), which may increase the risk of behavioural problems and be a source of infant psychopathology [10, 12, 13].

Perinatal stress, anxiety and depression do not only affect parents. In the long term, as these disorders can also affect the mental and physical health of the child [14, 15]. ring pregnancy, stress levels or negative effects of the mother have a direct impact on the fetus, being risk factors for disorders as they grow [16, 17].

Once born, the attachment between mother and baby plays an important role in the child's cognitive and emotional development, as well as in his or her later mental health [18]. If parents are depressed or distressed, they may not be able to recognize the infant's cues, and this may result in an inappropriate attachment style. Thus, an insecure attachment style in childhood increases the risk of anxiety and behavioural disorders later in life [19].

Considering the crucial role that parental mental health plays in the future mental health of children, and considering the increasing mental health problems in today's society, we understand the importance of research in this area [13].

The Developmental Origins of Behaviour, Health, and Disease (*DOBHD*) analysed the short- and long-term effects of an individual's experiences during the perinatal period on later phenotypic variations in health and disease [20]. They found that the magnitude of these effects was clinically relevant, estimating that the risk on emotional and behavioural problems in childhood attributable to prenatal anxiety was approximately 10-15%. Thus, given the negative impact of prenatal exposure to maternal anxiety, anxious women and their infants may benefit from processes that support maternal well-being during pregnancy. Unfortunately, emotional care is often poorly monitored [21].

MENTAL DISSORDES EXPERIENCED BY PREGNANT AND POSTPARTUM WOMEN

Pregnancy and childbirth represent a time of great vulnerability during which women experience many physiological and psychosocial changes. These changes put pregnant and postpartum women at increased risk of mental health problems. This risk is higher in low- and lower-middle-income countries (*LMIC*) [22] than in high-income countries (*HIC*) [23].

The most common mental health problems in pregnant and postpartum women are anxiety, perinatal depression, and postpartum depression [24, 25]. These conditions can hinder the mother's ability to care for herself, but also for her newborn, jeopardizing the establishment of a positive bond between the mother and her baby [26].

In addition, mental illness can contribute to adverse outcomes in the child during pregnancy and in the neonatal period [27 - 29], such as a small for gestational age baby [30], lower head circumference, retarded growth, delays in child development [31], poor mother-infant interaction [32], lower neonatal test scores (*e.g.* lower APGAR) [33 - 37], erratic sleep, irritability, excessive crying, and in the medium/long term emotional and behavioural difficulties [38], negative affect in the infant [39], infant cognitive developmental problems [40], delayed motor development [41], and affective disorders, attention-deficit or hyperactivity disorder (*ADHD*) in children [42].

Maternal anxiety during pregnancy can produce, in addition to problems during childbirth, alterations in socioemotional, behavioural and early neurocognitive development, and even mental health problems in adolescence and early adulthood [20, 43, 44].

All of these mental health problems can be associated with other serious problems for parents and children. Thus, severe postpartum psychiatric disorders are associated with high rates of maternal suicide, with up to 70 times the risk of suicide in the first postpartum year compared with age-specific rates for the general female population [25, 45]. There are also data suggesting that these perinatal mental health problems are associated with worse pregnancy outcomes [46] and long-lasting emotional, social, and cognitive difficulties in children, which appear to be mediated by troubled early interactions between parent and child [13].

Studies suggest that there are also important economic implications, with women with postpartum depression incurring higher health care expenditures. This cost overrun can be up to 90% higher than in non-depressed postpartum women in some studies [47]. In the UK, perinatal depression, anxiety and psychosis account for a total long-term cost of up to £8.1 billion per year [48].

Traditionally, anxiety disorders in the perinatal period have received less attention than depression. This is despite the fact that several studies have shown that up to 13% of pregnant or postpartum women suffer from anxiety disorders [1]. Studies indicate that adolescents whose mothers were depressed during pregnancy were up to 4.7 times more likely to be depressed at age 16 than those whose mothers did not experience depression during pregnancy [49].

Regarding fathers, about 10% of fathers also suffer from depression in the perinatal period [50 - 53] compared with a 12-month prevalence rate of depression of 4.8% in the male population as a whole [54].

PHYSIOLOGY OF MATERNAL DISTRESS DURING PREGNANCY

Pregnant women often experience stress secondary to factors specific to their situation, such as prenatal examinations [55, 56], concern for the baby's health and development [55 - 57], or having an unwanted pregnancy [58]. Stress during pregnancy can be classified as acute or chronic, with each type of stress presenting different degrees of severity. Depression and anxiety are relatively common mood disorders during pregnancy [59]. Repeated or chronic stress is considered to be risk factors and a similar alteration of the underlying physiological stress response [60, 61]. This stress response will be coordinated by the neuroendocrine, vascular and immune systems [62].

A number of physiological alterations occur during pregnancy (Fig. **1**), and in the presence of a stressor, a complex interaction can occur between this altered internal maternal physiological environment and the changes induced by the stress response [63]. All these physiological changes that occur in response to stress can have significant adverse effects on the intrauterine environment in which the fetus is developing.

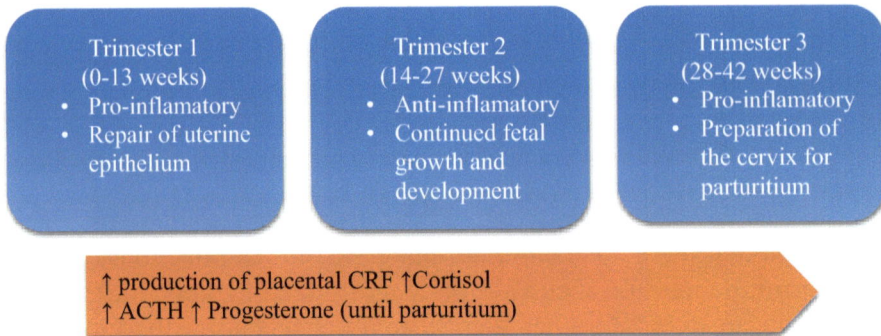

Fig 1. Pregnancy consists of three stages characterized by distinct physiological conditions. Physiological changes during pregnancy.

POSSIBLE PHYSIOLOGICAL MEDIATORS OF THE EFFECTS OF MATERNAL PSYCHOLOGICAL DISTRESS ON BIRTH AND HEALTH OUTCOMES

In view of the relationship between high levels of maternal psychological distress in pregnancy and subsequent poor outcomes for the child, research has investigated how maternal distress reaches the body of the growing fetus to subsequently influence the child's development.

One theory is fetal programming, which suggests that changes in the fetal environment brought about by hormonal changes can alter the structure and function of the developing biological systems of the fetus. There are several possible mediators. One of these is the maternal hypothalamic-pituitary-adrenal (*HPA*) axis, which is a primary pathway linking psychological and physiological experiences.

It is possible that increased plasma cortisol, as well as the increased levels of catecholamines frequently observed in depressed patients, which by decreasing uterine blood flow may affect placental function [64].

Psychological states such as maternal depression, anxiety and stress have been associated with alterations in maternal HPA function too, with changes in glucocorticoid levels implicated in the transmission pathways between maternal distress and infant development [65 - 69].

Thus, fetal basal corticosteroid levels are increased by exposure to maternal stress, and there is an increased corticosterone response to stress in the infant, which could affect long-term HPA functioning, as well as the regulation of psychological and physiological responses to stressful events [70]. Exposure to elevated maternal cortisol levels from maternal psychological distress [71 - 74] leads to alterations in infant outcomes [75].

Cardiovascular stress reactivity is another possible mechanism linking maternal psychological distress during pregnancy to negative obstetric outcomes. Reactivity to cardiovascular stress decreases physiologically as pregnancy progresses [72, 76] as an adaptive process that reduces the risk of experiencing gestational hypertension [77, 78]. Nevertheless, there is a lower response to cardiovascular stress among those pregnant women who report elevated levels of distress.

In fact, women with high levels of psychological distress during pregnancy have been shown to have a greater magnitude and duration of physiological reactivity to psychological distress, significantly increasing the risk of vasoconstriction [79]. This increased vasoconstriction during pregnancy may affect uteroplacental blood flow, reducing the volume of oxygen and nutrients delivered to the fetus [80, 81].

Psychological distress is also associated with alterations in physiological recovery processes, such as subjective and objective measures of sleep [82 - 85].

Thus, women who experience high levels of psychological distress in pregnancy report poorer sleep quality, with greater disturbances and greater daytime dysfunction relative to those who do not experience distress [82]. Poor subjective sleep quality, in addition to objective measures such as short sleep duration, are also associated with other physiological markers of stress such as cortisol and inflammation [72, 86, 87], as well as negative obstetric outcomes such as increased pain perception and discomfort during labour, prolonged labour, and increased likelihood of requiring caesarean section [88, 89].

Finally, lack of sleep during pregnancy may be another pathway linking maternal psychological distress and poor obstetric and infant outcomes. Thus, these sleep disturbances are also associated with negative birth outcomes, such as preterm birth and low birth weight [90].

PERINATAL DEPRESSION AND POSTPARTUM DEPRESSION

Perinatal Depression

As already discussed, perinatal depression (*PD*) is one of the most common illnesses that can occur during pregnancy and postpartum, and includes minor and major depressive episodes during pregnancy and/or in the first 12 months after delivery [91] . The prevalence of this disease is around 10%-15% in rich countries and 20% in developing countries [25, 91 - 93].

According to various studies, risk factors for perinatal depression include a history of depression, adverse life events, poor social support, marital disagreements and unwanted pregnancies [94, 95] (Table 1). Psychosocial factors, such as low socioeconomic status, poor employment status, low educational level, lack of access to prenatal care, drug abuse and conflicts with partners also contribute to stress during pregnancy [96].

Table 1. Risk factors for perinatal depression.

- History of depression, especially perinatal. - Unwanted pregnancy. - Conflict in the couple's relationship. - Absence of a partner. - Psychosocial stress. - Low socio-economic status. - Poor social support.

The disease pattern of depression in pregnancy is similar to that of depressive episodes at other times of life. In addition to the cardinal symptoms of depression, symptoms including distress, irritability and lack of concentration often appear.

They may feel rejection of the pregnancy, anger or even ambivalence, especially when the pregnancy was unplanned. There may also be anxiety about the responsibility of assuming the role of mother, or feelings of guilt for not contributing to the baby's well-being.

According to the definition of the American Psychiatric Association, the diagnosis of major depression requires, among other clinical characteristics, that the depressed mood lasts at least two weeks. Therefore, early diagnosis of major depressive episodes is essential (Table 2) [25, 97]. To minimize the risk of false positives, it is recommended to systematically analyse those psychological symptoms typical of major depression, especially anhedonia, feelings of guilt, hopelessness and suicidal ideation.

Table 2. Symptoms of major depression.

- Depressed mood most of the time, almost every day for two weeks, and/or - Loss of interest in, or ability to enjoy, activities that the person usually enjoys.
Other symptoms that may occur:

(Table 2) cont.....

- Fatigue or lack of energy.
- Restlessness or a feeling of slowing down.
- Feelings of guilt or disability.
- Difficulties in concentrating.
- Sleep disturbances.
- Recurrent thoughts of death or suicide.

Until the fourth version of its classification of mental disorders (DSM-IV), the American Psychiatric Association stipulated that a specifier for the onset of depression called "*postpartum*" could be included [98]. In its most recent version (DSM-V) in 2013, this specifier was renamed "*peripartum*" and can be applied to any depressive episode that begins in pregnancy or within four weeks of delivery [97]. This change was made after finding that 50% of postpartum depressive episodes actually began during pregnancy, and since the last revision, depressive disorders that begin during pregnancy or appear up to one year after delivery are referred to as perinatal depression, as experts consider the criterion of limiting depression to the first four weeks of the puerperium to be too restrictive. It should also be borne in mind that there is no evidence of a specific etiology or clearly distinct psychopathology. Still, the term is justified by the specific needs of depressed pregnant/postpartum women.

Several scales are available for the detection of depression during pregnancy [95, 99]. However, the most widely used instrument for the diagnosis of prenatal depression worldwide is the **Edinburgh Postnatal Depression Scale** (*EPDS*) [100, 101], validated in pregnancy [100, 102]. It consists of a 10 item self-administered scale, in which the woman is asked to answer how she has felt in the last seven days. Each question is scored from 0-3 (Tables **3 - 5**).

Table 3. Edinburgh Perinatal/Postnatal Depression Scale (EPDS) [100, 101].

For use between 28–32 weeks in all pregnancies and 6–8 weeks postpartum		
Name:	Date:	Gestation in Weeks:
As you are having a baby, we would like to know how you are feeling. Please mark "X" in the box next to the answer which comes closest to how you have felt in the past 7 days–not just how you feel today. **In the past 7 days:**		
1. I have been able to laugh and see the funny side of things • As much as I always could • 1 Not quite so much now 2 Definitely not so much now 3 Not at all	6. Things have been getting on top of me • Yes, most of the time I haven't been able to cope • Yes, sometimes I haven't been coping as well as usual • No, most of the time I have coped quite well • No, I have been coping as well as ever	

(Table 3) cont.....

	7. I have been so unhappy that I have had difficulty sleeping 3 Yes, most of the time 2 Yes, sometimes 1 Not very often • No, not at all
2. I have looked forward with enjoyment to things • As much as I ever did 1 Rather less than I used to 2 Definitely less than I used to 3 Hardly at all	
3. I have blamed myself unnecessarily when things went wrong 3 Yes, most of the time 2 Yes, some of the time 1 Not very often • No, never	8. I have felt sad or miserable 3 Yes, most of the time 2 Yes, quite often 1 Not very often • No, not at all
4. I have been anxious or worried for no good reason • No, not at all 1 Hardly ever 2 Yes, sometimes 3 Yes, very often	9. I have been so unhappy that I have been crying 3 Yes, most of the time 2 Yes, quite often 1 Only occasionally • No, never
5. I have felt scared or panicky for no very good reason 3 Yes, quite a lot 2 Yes, sometimes 1 No, not much • No, not at all	10. The thought of harming myself has occurred to me 3 Yes, quite often 2 Sometimes 1 Hardly ever • Never
Total Score	
Talk about your answers to the above questions with your health care provider.	

Table 4. Edinburgh Perinatal/Postnatal Depression Scale (*EPDS*) [100, 101].

SCORING GUIDE	
1. I have been able to laugh and see the funny side of things 0 As much as I always could 1 Not quite so much now 2 Definitely not so much now 3 Not at all	6. Things have been getting on top of me 3 Yes, most of the time I haven't been able to cope 2 Yes, sometimes I haven't been coping as well as usual 1 No, most of the time I have coped quite well 0 No, I have been coping as well as ever
2. I have looked forward with enjoyment to things 0 As much as I ever did 1 Rather less than I used to 2 Definitely less than I used to 3 Hardly at all	7. I have been so unhappy that I have had difficulty sleeping 3 Yes, most of the time 2 Yes, sometimes 1 Not very often 0 No, not at all

(Table 4) cont.....

3. I have blamed myself unnecessarily when things went wrong 3 Yes, most of the time 2 Yes, some of the time 1 Not very often 0 No, never	8. I have felt sad or miserable 3 Yes, most of the time 2 Yes, quite often 1 Not very often 0 No, not at all
4. I have been anxious or worried for no good reason 0 No, not at all 1 Hardly ever 2 Yes, sometimes 3 Yes, very often	9. I have been so unhappy that I have been crying 3 Yes, most of the time 2 Yes, quite often 1 Only occasionally 0 No, never
5. I have felt scared or panicky for no very good reason 3 Yes, quite a lot 2 Yes, sometimes 1 No, not much 0 No, not at all	10. The thought of harming myself has occurred to me 3 Yes, quite often 2 Sometimes 1 Hardly ever 0 Never

Table 5. EPDS Score interpretation and action [100, 101].

EPDS Score	Interpretation	Action
Less than 8	Depression not likely.	Continue support.
9–11	Depression possible.	Support, re-screen in 2–4 weeks. Consider referral to primary care provider (PCP).
12–13	Fairly high possibility of depression	Monitor, support and offer education. Refer to PCP.
14 and higher (positive screen)	Probable depression.	Diagnostic assessment and treatment by PCP and/or specialist.
Positive score (1, 2 or 3) on question 10 (suicidality risk)		Immediate discussion required. Refer to PCP ± mental health specialist or emergency resource for further assessment and intervention as appropriate. Urgency of referral will depend on several factors including: whether the suicidal ideation is accompanied by a plan, whether there has been a history of suicide attempts, whether symptoms of a psychotic disorder are present and/or there is concern about harm to the baby.

As an alternative to using the EPDS in pregnancy, in the UK, the National Institute for Health and Clinical Excellence (*NICE*) guidance [103] recommends that health professionals routinely ask the so-called Whooley Questions [104] at all pre- and postnatal check-ups:

1. *Have you often felt discouraged, depressed or hopeless in the last month?*
2. In the last month, have you often felt that you have little interest or enjoyment in things?

If the woman answers "Yes" to either question, a third question will be asked: In relation *"to this, do you feel that you need or want help?"*. The limitation of the Whooley questions is that their sensitivity and specificity have not been established, and it doesn´t ask about infrequent thoughts that potentially involve life-threatening thoughts, such as thoughts of self-harm or thoughts of harming the baby.

Postpartum Depression

Postpartum depression (*PPD*) is a disorder whose symptomatology use to be similar to major depressive episodes occurring at other times of life (Table **2**) [25, 97, 98]. Indeed, motherhood influences the presentation of symptoms and so, for example, ideas of guilt and worthlessness often found in depressed people are translated here into feelings of inability to assume the role of mother and reluctance to take on the care of the child. There may be fantasies or fear of harming the baby, or indifference, but rarely rejection. The mother-child bond may suffer. Mothers may become less involved or, conversely, over-stimulating. Children may be less responsive, less prone to interaction and generally display more negative emotions.

Frequently, cases of PPD occurs in the first month of the postpartum period or shortly afterwards, and symptoms are usually at their peak between 8 and 12 weeks after the woman has given birth.

"Postpartum blues" (postpartum dysphoria) is a very common transient disorder, occurring in approximately 40-60% of postpartum women [105]. It appears in the first few days postpartum, typically around the third day, lasting only a few hours and at most a day or two. It is a state marked by anxiety, emotional lability and sometimes depressed mood, all of which are very transient symptoms and therefore do not require treatment.

Postpartum psychosis, on the other hand, has an incidence of 0.1 to 0.2% [106]. The clinical picture is dramatic in presentation and represents a psychiatric emergency. It usually begins during the first two weeks postpartum, sometimes 48 to 72 hours after delivery. It usually begins with symptoms such as sleep disturbances, agitation or irritability. The progression of puerperal psychosis is usually rapid, with symptoms including emotional lability, depressed or exalted mood, behavioural disturbances, and delusions and hallucinations. It is still debated whether postpartum psychosis is a separate diagnostic entity or whether it is a rapidly evolving affective psychosis (mood disorder).

The most commonly used screening instrument to detect probable cases of PPD is the Edinburgh Postpartum Depression Scale (*EPDS*) (Tables **3** - **5**) [100, 101].

TREATMENT OF DEPRESSION DURING PREGNANCY

Prenatal depression (*PD*) is often under-diagnosed and under-treated, when not undiagnosed and untreated. This implies a major risk factor for postpartum depression (*PPD*), which have a global prevalence at 17.7% [107 - 109].

Other risk factors for postpartum depression are the mother's youth, a history of previous depression, and the presence of previous postpartum blues (a transient mood disorder characterized by mild depressive symptoms that is common in first-time mothers) [7, 110 - 115].

Because of the prevalence of PD and the adverse effects that this disorder presents to women, children, and families [116 - 118], the development and implementation of cost-effective programs and interventions have important health implications. The common treatments for PD include counselling, psychotherapy, and antidepressant medication. Nonetheless, the risks to both the fetus and infants limit the use of antidepressants [91, 119 - 124], and in pregnant women exposure to these drugs during pregnancy may increase susceptibility to disorders such as hypertension [125, 126].

Treatment of acute major depressive disorders of pregnancy is relatively often untreated or undertreated [119, 120, 122, 127, 128], even if the diagnosis is made during pregnancy [127, 129].

The goal of treating depression in the pregnant woman is to improve her mood while minimizing the risks to the developing embryo or fetus. This begins with general strategies, such as recommending cessation of caffeine, nicotine and alcohol, or trying to maximize rest times.

Many patients with mild to moderate depression can be treated exclusively with psychotherapy, relaxation techniques and environmental management measures may be beneficial, and recent studies have shown that physical exercise can be effective in treating depression during pregnancy [130, 131].

Regarding treatment of postpartum depression, postpartum dysphoria does not require treatment because the mood disturbance is mild and self-limiting. However, it is useful to explain to the mother that what is happening is normal, attributable to the hormonal changes she is experiencing, and that it will cease without treatment.

Psychoses, on the other hand, given their characteristics (behavioural disturbances, delusions and/or hallucinations), are usually referred to a psychiatrist. They are treated in the same way as any other affective psychosis that occurs at another time in life.

Both psychotherapeutic strategies and pharmacological treatments should be considered in the treatment of non-psychotic postpartum depression.

Pharmacotherapy

In general, their use would be indicated in pregnant women with moderate to severe depression, in pregnant women who have not responded to other treatments, or in those patients in whom there is a high probability of relapse.

For obvious ethical reasons, it has not been possible to carry out studies on the efficacy of antidepressants in the treatment of depression in pregnant women. However, there is no reason to believe that the therapeutic response to them in these patients may be different from that observed in non-pregnant women.

Therefore, a series of guidelines have been established for the pharmacological treatment of depression during pregnancy [132 - 134].

According to the risk classification of drugs for the fetus according to the Food and Drug Administration (*FDA*) of the United States, it is still recommended to avoid the use of psychotropic drugs during the first 12 weeks of gestation due to the risk of malformations during the period of organogenesis (Table **6**) [135 - 139].

Table 6. Degree of risk posed to the fetus by the use of drugs during pregnancy according to the US Food and Drug Administration (*FDA*).

Category	Interpretation
A	Controlled studies show no foetal risk
B	No evidence of risk in humans
C	Possible foetal risk cannot be excluded.
D	There is positive evidence of risk, although the potential benefits may outweigh any risks.
X	Absolute contraindication in pregnancy

The categorization for each drug of the risk posed by its use during pregnancy has, however, significant limitations. Thus, in 1992, the American Teratology

Society noted that only about 20 drugs were recognized as teratogenic in humans, while in the FDA manuals of that year, about 140 drugs appeared with a D or X classification (those with the highest risk). Subsequently, some authors warned that in the US, wanted pregnancies were unnecessarily terminated by closely following FDA classifications.

A recent study looking at antidepressant use in women before conception and those who continued taking them during pregnancy found that discontinuing these drugs led to a relapse rate of up to 68%, compared to a relapse rate of only 25% in pregnant women who continued taking them [140].

The largest evidence related to antidepressants and pregnancy is for the use of Selective Serotonin Reuptake Inhibitors (*SSRIs*) (fluoxetine, sertraline, paroxetine and citalopram). Overall, the data show little evidence of teratogenesis or adverse effects associated with exposure during lactation [141 - 145].

It can be concluded that SSRIs, except maybe paroxetine, are a good therapeutic option and are often preferred during pregnancy/postpartum; they represent a safe alternative, even during the first trimester of pregnancy.

In relation to the puerperal stage, experts agree that an alternative to SSRIs are secondary amines (*e.g.* desipramine and nortriptyline), as they produce fewer anticholinergic effects and hypotension compared to tricyclic antidepressants.

The available data on most atypical antidepressants, other than SSRIs and tricyclics (including duloxetine, mirtazapine and venlafaxine), are limited and do not appear to suggest an increased risk of teratogenesis or adverse obstetric or neonatal effects associated with its use during pregnancy [146 - 150]. Nevertheless, the administration of bupropion during the first trimester has been associated with the development of cardiac malformations in the fetus, which is why it is not recommended for use in pregnant [151].

The decision whether or not to use an antidepressant during breastfeeding will be based on a rigorous risk-benefit analysis given the known benefits of breastfeeding for both mother and child.

All drugs pass into the infant through breast milk and that, in general, only 1-2% of the maternal dose of any drug will appear in the milk. This transfer is significantly less than in the intrauterine situation and, in practice, as far as antidepressants are concerned, does not result in clinical problems for the neonate in the vast majority of cases [152 - 154]. However, if an infant develops abnormal symptoms and it is suspected to be related to the mother's intake of the antidepressant, breastfeeding should be interrupted immediately.

Optimal duration of antidepressant treatment of PPD is unknown. However, the usual recommendation is to maintain therapy for at least 12 months. If for some reason it is desired to shorten the treatment period, it is advisable to extend it until after other hormonal changes (*e.g.* return of menstrual cycles) have occurred.

Up to 70% of women who have had an episode of puerperal psychosis suffer another episode in the subsequent postpartum period [155]. Women with a history of postpartum depression are at increased risk, with up to 50% of postpartum relapses [156], while the risk of recurrence of bipolar postpartum depression ranges from 30-50% [94].

The decision whether or not to use psychotropic drugs during the postpartum/pregnancy period should always be individualised, based on a careful analysis of the risk/benefit ratio.

Refraining from prescribing an antidepressant to a pregnant woman who is depressed, or at high risk of relapse, may pose a risk to the woman and the fetus that is more serious than that derived from exposure to the medication, and this is something to keep in mind.

In cases where there is a history of pre/postpartum depression, general (*e.g.* psychoeducational, logistical, *etc.*) and/or specific (psychotherapeutic and pharmacological) measures should be taken to minimize the risk of a new episode.

Risks of not Treating Maternal Depression during Pregnancy

It has been shown that depressed pregnant women neglect their pregnancies more, are more likely to neglect prenatal check-ups and often do not follow medical advice, or do so incorrectly. Increased use of tobacco, alcohol and drugs, all of which have deleterious effects on obstetric outcome, has also been seen. In addition, some symptoms of depression, such as anorexia, can alter aspects of pregnancy, such as weight gain, contributing to an increase in adverse pregnancy outcomes.

Several adverse effects associated with PPD have negative consequences on the establishment of the maternal-infant bond and on the subsequent development of the child in all areas (emotional, behavioural and cognitive) [113, 157, 158], reason why PD that is not adequately treated has a devastating effect on women, babies and their families [116, 159, 160].

But pregnant women are reluctant to take psychotropic medicines such as antidepressants and benzodiazepines because of the potential risks to the fetus [161]. That is why the National Institute for Health and Clinical Excellence

(*NICE*) recommends: "*There are risks associated with taking psychotropic medicines in pregnancy and during breastfeeding*" [111].

In this context, the potential risks associated with the use of psychotropic medication in pregnant and lactating women, added to the preferences that women express for non-pharmacological interventions, suggest that evidence should be sought on the use of behavioural and cognitive therapies that are safe and acceptable for health in the perinatal period. One of these possible non-pharmacological interventions is mindfulness training.

All of these non-pharmacological interventions are inexpensive and approach pregnancy from a holistic perspective that promotes the mental, emotional and physical health of both the woman and the child. So they improve self-efficacy and help women feel more empowered and aware of the processes that will shape their future motherhood.

SLEEP PROBLEMS DURING PREGNANCY

Sleep is fundamental to life, and it has been shown that sleep of low duration, lack of continuity, or poor quality is associated with an increased risk of diseases, such as diabetes, cardiovascular disease, depression, and anxiety [162 - 167]. Sleep is an important regulator of psychophysiological and impulsive behaviour [168 - 172], both key mediators of normal adaptation to stress [173 - 176].

During pregnancy, women experience a number of sleep disturbances that may increase the risk of developing long-term insomnia [177, 178]. Up to 78% complained of sleep disturbances during the third trimester of pregnancy, according to results of the 2007 National Sleep Foundation's Women and Sleep Survey [179, 180], with alterations in the duration [181, 182], quality [183, 184], and sleep pattern [184 - 186] during all gestation, not just during late pregnancy [187 - 189].

Sleep is a predictor of increased levels of stress during pregnancy, which may be associated to a cascade of negative consequences for the birth, the mother and the child. Poor sleep quality during pregnancy is a prospective risk factor for depression during the prenatal and postpartum period [164, 190, 191]. Sleep disturbances are associated with adverse pregnancy outcomes, including intrauterine growth restriction, preterm birth, higher risk of caesarean birth and longer labour [88, 192 - 197].

It has been shown that poor sleep quality can be associated with feelings of high levels of stress experienced, two processes that are associated with endocrinologic and immunologic problems, as well as with increased morbidity for patients [198

- 200]. The treatment proposed for insomnia by European and American guidelines is cognitive behavioural therapy for insomnia (*CBT-I*) [201 - 203], a first-line treatment that also serves for insomnia-related problems.

CBT-I therapy has demonstrated beneficial effects on comorbidities [163 - 166, 204 - 207], so it could prevent negative health outcomes [204, 205, 208, 209] and could be effective and easy to implement in standard patient care [201].

As stated, sleep disorders pose a critical risk factor for the development of depression and mental disorders during pregnancy. This represents a field of research that will try to improve the nocturnal and diurnal symptoms of pregnant women, as well as for the preventive effects of sleep disorders.

MATERNAL MENTAL HEALTH MANAGEMENT

Decreasing perinatal psychological distress, stress, depression and anxiety during pregnancy and in the first postpartum year should be a goal to be pursued by public health [210, 211] taking advantage of the fact that pregnancy is a good time to establish health interventions [110, 212].

Treatments initially offered were based on psychopharmacology. However, pregnant women often prefer not to resort to medication for fear of the potential risk to their baby's development [1]. Psychological interventions are a good alternative to the use of medication. Cognitive behavioural therapy (*CBT*) is a well-established and empirically validated first-line therapy for anxiety and depressive disorders. In the perinatal stage, CBT has been successfully applied in depression, but less used in the case of anxiety [1, 9].

Symptoms such as irritability, lack of interest, appetite or sleep disorders, and feelings of sadness, guilt or hopelessness can begin at any time during the perinatal period. All these symptoms have repercussions on the health of the mother-child binomial, presenting greater use and abuse of alcohol and tobacco, a greater number of medical consultations and obstetric complications, shorter gestations and children with low birth weight. Therefore, they are a risk factor for delay in the mental, motor and emotional neurodevelopment of children.

Therefore, cognitive-behavioural therapies constitute a safe and acceptable strategy to improve health during the perinatal period. Mindfulness training is one such therapy.

Mindfulness is defined as "*the awareness that arises from paying attention to a purpose, in the present moment, and without judgment of the unfolding moment-to-moment experience*" [213].

Mindfulness-based interventions (*MBIs*) have shown beneficial physiological changes in patients. Derived from Buddhist practice, these interventions focus on cultivating non-judgmental awareness of present moment experiences [214]. When performed in healthy populations, they have also shown decreased levels of inflammation, with a decrease in circulating proinflammatory proteins, and a lower cortisol response to social stressors [215 - 218]. MBIs also reduce psychological and physiological arousal due to stress [218 - 220], reduce blood pressure (*BP*) improve heart rate variability (*HRV*) [221 - 224], and improve the subjective quality of sleep [225, 226].

There are several psychological methods within MBI that include mindfulness-based cognitive therapy (*MBCT*), mindfulness based stress reduction (*MBSR*) and integrated mindfulness yoga practices, that can reduce mental health difficulties seen during pregnancy and perinatal care [227, 228].

Data support that these therapies are an effective approach to reducing psychological stress [111, 229 - 231] as well as effective in reducing levels of stress [112, 232 - 234], anxiety [112, 228, 232, 233, 235 - 240], and in the occurrence of depression [29, 232, 234, 237, 238] during pregnancy, with studies suggesting that the effects obtained by MBIs persist up to 4-6 weeks after delivery [28, 29, 232, 233, 241].

Mindfulness is a state of mind that focuses attention on the present moment without judgment and without engaging irrelevant thoughts or movements [242]. The objective of the training is to fully perceive each thought, sensation, or emotion that arises, and then "*let go*" distractions by focusing attention on an object, such as the breath [219].

When applied to the reduction of perceived stress, anxiety and depression, MBIs have proved to have good outcomes [243, 244], and appear useful in reducing maternal distress during pregnancy. The first of the mindfulness development interventions, the Mindfulness-Based Stress Reduction (*MBSR*) program, was developed in the 1980s. It was later integrated with cognitive therapy in a program called Mindfulness-Based Cognitive Therapy (*MBCT*) for the prevention of depression relapse.

In view of the good results observed in the reduction of anxiety and depression in the general population demonstrated with both therapies, both programs have begun to be applied in the perinatal stage with promising results so far.

MINDFULNESS-BASED INTERVENTIONS IN PREGNANCY

As discussed above, Mindfulness is a state of mind that focuses attention on the present moment without judgment and without engaging irrelevant thoughts or movements [242], with the objective of training perception in every thought, sensation, or emotion that arises, and then "let go" distractions by focusing attention to the breath [219].

These mindfulness-based interventions began to be applied in healthcare after Kabat-Zinn's pioneering research on mindfulness-based stress reduction (*MBSR*). By conducting eight-session interventions in the form of a hospital course, he demonstrated benefits for patients with chronic pain, hypertension or heart disease, as well as psychological problems such as anxiety and stress [214].

With Kabat-Zinn's research as a reference, a group of psychologists combined MBSR with cognitive therapy, creating Mindfulness-Based Cognitive Therapy (*MBCT*). Several studies have been conducted on its effect on the relapse rate of depression, finding very positive results for the treatment of anxiety, bipolar disorder, as well as for the prevention of suicidal depression.

At the same time, Nancy Bardacke developed prenatal classes for both parents using MBSR. Her goal was to reverse the negative impact that elevated stress levels and fear have on maternal and neonatal outcomes. Her studies led to mindfulness-based childbirth and parenting (*MBCP*) [238].

The use of mindfulness applied to pregnant women has shown a generalized positive impact on maternal well-being, with a decrease in negative affect, anxiety and stress, thus confirming the potential of mindfulness in these patients [236]. The components of mindfulness, which are derived from Zen, are [213, 245 - 248]:

1. *Attention to the present moment*: stop thinking about the past (ruminations) or about the future (expectations, desires and fears), focusing on the present moment. While meditating, one can attend to one's own inner processes and, in daily life, focus on the task at hand.

2. *Openness to experience*: ability to observe experience without the filter of one's own beliefs. That is, observing the present experience as if for the first time. This is called "*beginner's mind*".

3. *Acceptance*: defined as experiencing events fully and without defences, as they are. It can also be defined as not fighting against the flow of life.

4. *Letting go*: this is letting go, detaching oneself from something to which one clings. Nothing in the material world is stable for long, everything persists for a certain time and then disappears.

5. *Intention*: this is what each person pursues when practising mindfulness. This may sound contradictory to one of the attitudes of mindfulness, which is not to strive for any purpose. When you are meditating you should not try to achieve any immediate purpose, you should simply engage in full awareness of what you are doing. However, you must also have a purpose, a personal goal that motivates movement towards that purpose.

Mindfulness-based interventions (*MBI*) are based on ancient Buddhist practices, updated and adapted to the occidental context. They have been included among the third generation therapies that revolve around the concept of acceptance, and have been proven to be useful in the treatment of various physical and psychological problems in addition to increasing well-being [249].

These interventions are based on attending to the quality of attention, with the aim of becoming aware of the automatisms and learned psychological processes that contribute to emotional imbalance and dysfunctional behaviour. The central premise of MBI is based on the idea that the active metacognitive monitoring state of mind promoted by such practice is capable of altering the automatic circuits created by repetitive thinking over time [250].

MBIs have been widely used in healthcare settings demonstrating a reduction in the risk of relapse in depression, relief of chronic pain, reduction of anxiety and improvement of health problems secondary to stress [251 - 253].

Several studies have demonstrated the efficacy and acceptability of MBIs in pregnant women who had reported elevated levels of pregnancy-related anxiety (*PRA*) and who do not currently report psychological distress. The data obtained in these studies suggest that Mindfulness-Based Cognitive Therapy (MBCT) during pregnancy has been shown in several studies to reduce fear, anxiety and comorbid symptoms of depression in pregnant women with clinically elevated symptoms of generalized anxiety disorder (*GAD*) [161]. In addition, several studies have shown that MBCT has been shown to increase positive affect, decreasing symptoms of perceived stress, PRA and depression [232, 233, 236, 238, 254].

A recent study conducted with a modified version of MBCT adapted for prevention of perinatal depression (*MBCT-PD*) on pregnant women with a history of depression found significant improvement in depressive symptoms [254].

A randomized controlled trial of MBCT- PD found a reduction in depressive symptoms and depressive relapses in those women who received this intervention compared with those who received treatment as usual (*TAU*) [255].

A recent systematic review examining the impact of mindfulness and perinatal mental health concluded that there was "*insufficient evidence from high-quality research*" to make recommendations on the use of mindfulness to improve mental health during pregnancy despite the fact that MBIs, specifically MBCT, appear to hold promise for the treatment and prevention of perinatal mood disorders [256].

However, and although a recent study was able to demonstrate the efficacy of MBCT-PD in reducing postpartum depression in a population of women with a history of depression [255], no studies have demonstrated the efficacy of MBCT when performed on a population with a broader range of diagnoses, including high levels of pregnancy-related anxiety and stress, and none have examined if exists positive impact over physiological function.

Mindfulness Interventions to Reduce Maternal Prenatal Stress

Mindfulness improves attention control, emotion regulation, and self-awareness [244], thus having an effect on cognitive appraisal of stressors.

It has been shown that following mindfulness interventions, there is a reduction in the grey matter of the amygdala [244, 257] as well as in the functional connectivity between the different brain regions that drive stress reactivity with the amygdala [172, 244, 258 - 264].

Mindfulness interventions increase parasympathetic nervous system activation in the face of stressors, which counteracts the sympathetic fight response [118, 244]. It has also been shown that these interventions can normalize diurnal cortisol secretion [244], especially if levels are chronically elevated.

Mindfulness practice decreases the cognitive aspects of anxiety by decreasing the frequency of negative automatic thoughts [265] or by acting on the physiological arousal itself. Preliminary results from several studies also suggest that MBIs promote sleep quality in pregnant women [226]. As anxious arousal in the perinatal period may be linked to over-activity of the Hypothalamic – Pituitary – Adrenal axis (*HPA*) [266], it is possible that the decrease in anxiety that would be achieved through MBIs and the reduction in maternal distress may lead to a better regulation of maternal HPA arousal, which would have a lower reactivity to stress, with benefits to the child, as fetal exposure to glucocorticoids would be reduced. A decrease in BP and BP reactivity to stress would also be observed, and there would be an improvement in sleep quality, changes that would translate into a more favourable intrauterine environment for fetal development [267].

Efficacy of Mindfulness and Yoga Interventions

We have already mentioned that mindfulness intervention is derived from meditation techniques in which individuals present thoughts and sensations with acceptance and without judgment [268, 269]. The strategies carried out in MBIs reduce stress by seeking to regulate emotional reactivity, and also attenuates cognitive and somatic arousal associated with insomnia [269 - 272]. In addition, there is growing evidence that they may also improve well-being during pregnancy [226, 273 - 275].

On the other hand, intervention studies applying a prenatal yoga intervention have shown a significant improvement in sleep quality [276 - 280], also demonstrating in the treatment group when compared to controls a significantly lower incidence of adverse perinatal outcomes.

MINDFULNESS-BASED PROGRAMS

In studies conducted to test the reduction of stress in pregnant women in which they carried out interventions derived from the practice of mindfulness meditation, it was seen that many of these studies included approaches similar to the relaxation program developed by Kabat-Zinn (*MBSR*) [58, 281, 282], and mindfulness-based cognitive therapy with the aim of preventing relapse in individuals with depression developed by Segal et al. [58, 161, 254, 283 - 287].

Several interventions have been developed that incorporate yoga practices with exercises geared specifically for pregnant women. Other studies have focused on pregnant women with psychological disorders such as anxiety, depression or bipolar disorder. All of these interventions are typically 6 and 12 weeks in duration, with weekly sessions and home practice.

Mindfulness-based programs (*MBPs*) are courses that seek to train the mind through the practice of meditation, so as to reach a non-judgmental awareness focused on the present moment [288].

Their joint mind-body approach has been shown to be beneficial for people with symptoms of depression and other mental disorders [244, 289], and its application during pregnancy appears to improve not only the mother's depressive symptoms, but also the baby's weight at birth [221].

Therefore, it is quite possible that incorporating these mindfulness and compassion interventions into childbirth education programs may offer these patients and their partners, who are at risk for or have PD, alternative strategies for addressing mood disorders without the stigma usually associated with psychotherapy, nor the risks that antidepressant medication may pose to mother and baby [29]. It may also offer a preventive strategy accessible to all pregnant women, as PD can arise without prior risk factors [29], and offer a preventive strategy that is accessible to all pregnant women [290].

There are many mindfulness-based intervention programs that have been targeted for pregnancy, childbirth and the postpartum period, such as Mindful Motherhood [236], Mindfulness Based Childbirth Education (*MBCE*) [241], Mind Baby Body [237], and the Mindfulness-Based Childbirth and Parenting (*MBCP*) program [238]. MBCP protocol has been specifically adapted and shown to decrease fear of childbirth [291] with significant mental health benefits for mothers, improving childbirth-related assessments and prevention of postpartum depression symptoms [29]. Other programs adapted from Mindfulness-Based Cognitive Therapy (*MBCT*) and aimed at pregnant women suffering from anxiety and depression have also shown promising results [161, 255, 285].

The most widely accessible and researched MBIs are Mindfulness-based stress reduction (*MBSR*) and mindfulness-based cognitive therapy (*MBCT*), and they considered as the "*gold standard*", an 8-week intervention group [225, 292] which are conducted in group sessions of 2-3 hours per week plus an additional full day session. In other interventions such as MBSR and MBCT, group sessions of 30-40 minutes are conducted, followed by a teacher-led analysis. They also encourage daily mindfulness practice at home supported with audio recordings. These practices invite to focus attention with an attitude of curiosity and acceptance on the experiences of the present moment, such as breathing, body sensations, sounds and thoughts.

The intervention using MBCT achieved a 43% reduction in the relative risk of depression in healthy people with a history of relapse to depression of three or more episodes compared to the control group [293], which has led the UK national clinical guidelines to recommend MBCT in this population [294].

MBIs have been empirically shown to reduce current symptoms of depression, anxiety, and stress [111, 244, 295 - 298], suggesting that they may be useful when these pathologies arise. Data support that MBIs can reduce levels of rumination and, given that factors such as "*melancholic rumination*" may predict maintenance of depression in the perinatal period [1], which could make them particularly appropriate interventions.

Some researchers have also proposed that MBIs may improve early interactions between parents and infants by eliminating negative or self-critical parental thoughts, thereby increasing the ability to care for infants. It has also been suggested that they may improve the way women relate to pain, thereby reducing the anxiety associated with child birth. All this would support the therapeutic potential of MBIs in the perinatal period, both in the prevention of mental health problems and in alleviating them when they occur.

Beyond MBCT and MBSR, two interventions that are considered the "*gold standard*", various adaptations have been developed specifically for perinatal populations. Some of these are performed over a shorter period of time, others involve shorter practices, and/or require less practice at home.

Several MBIs based on MBSR and MBCT have been developed over time specifically for use in pregnancy. The most relevant are summarized further below:

8 week mindful motherhood programme (2 hours per week). Intervention developed in 3 approaches. Each one of these concepts constitutes approximately 1/3 of the intervention [236]:

1. Mindfulness of thoughts and feelings carried out through awareness of breathing and contemplation.

2. Attention to the body through hatha yoga, seeking guided body awareness meditation.

3. Acceptance and cultivation of an observing self to achieve exposure of psychological concepts.

- 7 week mindfulness-based yoga programme (1.25 hours weekly), combining it with MBSR [112].
- 10 sessions (*MBCP*) consisting of 9 (3 hours per week), with a 7-hour weekend silent retreat day between class 6 and class 7, and a face-to-face class 4 to 12 weeks after giving birth. These classes will be from 8 to 12 couples [238].
- An intervention combining mindfulness and yoga by adapting hatha yoga and MBSR, carried out in 10 weeks (*MYoga*) (1.5 hours/week) [299].
- MBCT-based mindful pregnancy and childbirth programme on 8-week. Modifications were made to the conscious movement component to adapt the intervention to pregnant women [232].
- Group intervention consisting of 6 mindfulness sessions developed specifically for pregnancy. Pregnant women are incorporated into an approach and strategies that include formal and informal practices, conscious movement and cognitive exercises, developing them face-to-face on weekdays [237].

- Coping with Anxiety through Mindful Living (*CALM*) is a program focused on mindful living during pregnancy consisting of 8 weekly group MBCT sessions lasting 2 hours. The intervention is carried out in 3 groups with 6 to 12 women in each group [161].
- Pilot randomised controlled trial for stress reduction during pregnancy of 6 weeks, with 2-hour group classes [233].
    The groups included mindfulness training tailored to pregnancy that sought to increase body awareness and provide a greater sense of peace and acceptance in the face of bodily changes, greater awareness of emotional patterns, and mental states specifically related to their pregnancy. All this by providing strategies that seek to improve understanding and compassion towards the participants themselves [28].
- Pilot study of childbirth education that applies mindfulness to the search for maternal self-efficacy and fear of childbirth. Conducted in 2.5 hours per week over 8 weeks. It is a childbirth education protocol developed specifically for this study, based on Mindfulness Based Childbirth Education (*MBCE*) derived from MBSR, with an empowerment model that includes the use of benefits, risks, alternatives, intuition, nothing (*BRAIN*) [241].
- An open trial of mindfulness-based cognitive therapy delivered in groups over 8 sessions, following standard MBCT treatment practices modified for the perinatal period [286].
- 8 cognitive therapy sessions that are based on the MBCT-PD perinatal depression intervention, itself based on the standard MBCT treatment modified for the pregnancy and postpartum environment [283]. We addressed the theory that when there is a history of previous depression, subjects are vulnerable during dysphoric states, since they present patterns of maladaptation in those previous episodes that can be reactivated, triggering the onset of new episodes [300].
- 5-week mindfulness meditation program, developed in 2 weekly sessions. In these sessions the techniques were explained, practiced and feedback on the techniques was provided. Subsequently, 30 minutes of daily practice are carried out at home. The development of this intervention is based on the guidelines provided by Kabat-Zinn with specific modifications for the patients participating in the study [301].

EXAMPLE OF A MINDFULNESS-BASED PROGRAMME

Based on the above, a mindfulness training program to be carried out in health centres in the context of prenatal mental health education for pregnant women could be as follows in Table 7.

Table 7. Mindfulness training programme during pregnancy.

Session	Activities	Duration
Week 1	Introduction to mindfulness and mindful motherhood training	15 minutes
	Introduce mindful movement	15 minutes
	Introduce mindful sitting meditation and awareness in breathing	15 minutes
	Body scanning. Introduce mindful mothers' check-in	15 minutes
	Informal practice teaching (moment-to-moment attention to everyday activities)	-
Week 2	Attention to breathing	5-10 minutes
	Mindful movements	20 minutes
	Mindful mothers' check-in and body scan (observing sell)	30 minutes
	Informal practice teaching (moment-to-moment attention to everyday activities)	-
Week 3	Attention to breathing	10 minutes
	Mindful walking exercise	20 minutes
	Mindful mothers' check-in and body scan (concentrating on the mother's belly, and on the baby's movements).	30 minutes
	Informal practice (observing the activities of mind, observing thoughts, paid heed to one pleasant event per day).	-
Week 4	Attention to breathing	10 minutes
	Mindful walking exercise	20 minutes
	Body scanning (concentrating on the mother's bell y, and on the baby's movements).	30 minutes
	Informal practice (observing the activities of mind, observing thoughts paid heed to an unpleasant event per day).	-
Week 5	Mindful mothers' check-in and body scan	10 minutes
	Sitting meditation (present movement focus)	30 minutes
	Loving kindness meditation	15 minutes
	Informal practice (identify mindful/unmindful moments)	-
Week 6	Sitting meditation	45 minutes
	Loving kindness meditation (loving-kindness will be sent to 15 minutes the baby)	15 minutes
Week 7	Sitting or walking meditation	30 minutes
	Mindful mothers' check-in and body scan	15 minutes
	Loving kindness meditation	15 minutes
Week 8	Sitting meditation and/or Body scan	30 minutes
	Mindful awareness as a refuse and source of strength	15 minutes
	Mindfulness in childbirth	15 minutes

The programme is mainly based on the 8-week programme developed by Jon Kabat-Zinn in 1990 [214], although other interventions have also been taken into account [232, 241, 275, 302, 303]. It consists of 8 sessions of 45-60 minutes during which the pregnant woman is taught techniques for the acquisition of serenity, as well as techniques for the development of a loving attitude towards the child.

Within the first half of the programme, you will develop self-awareness: of the body, feelings and thoughts. Body awareness will start in the first week, moving on to emotions in the second week and thoughts in the third week.

In the third week, the idea of dealing with the most difficult bodily sensations or feelings or thoughts, those that are unpleasant, will be introduced. This self-awareness is developed through both formal meditation practices and more informal Mindfulness of the present moment in daily life.

In the fourth week, the sensations of the womb and the movements of the foetus will begin to be explored.

From the fifth week onwards, awareness of other people and the immediate environment will be raised, broadening awareness in three ways. First, focus on being able to include and live one's own experience of sensations in the body within a broader perspective: for example, if there are any uncomfortable pregnancy symptoms, such as heartburn, one becomes aware of them, but within the broader perspective of the totality of the experience. Secondly, the environment is included, and thirdly other people.

Week seven is a week of practice and consolidation of what has already been learned. In week eight, in addition to concluding the course, you look to the future. You will assess whether you have managed to maintain a calm attitude during pregnancy, and you will establish how you will deal with childbirth and pain.

CONCLUSION

It teaches skills to enhance managing pain, stress, anxiety and other emotions during the transition to parenthood and everyday life. Participants learn to pay attention to present moment experiences (sensations, thoughts, feelings) deliberately and non-judgementally. Mindfulness helps participants to see more clearly the patterns of the mind, halting the escalation of negative thinking and the tendency to be on autopilot. Mindfulness Based Cognitive Therapy (*MBCP*) has the potential to reduce the risk of postnatal depression and increase *"availability"* of attention for the baby. Skills are applicable to pregnancy, childbirth and parenting and are transferrable life skills.

CONSENT FOR PUBLICATION

Not applicable.

CONFLICT OF INTEREST

The authors declare no conflict of interest, financial or otherwise.

ACKNOWLEDGEMENT

Declared none.

REFERENCES

[1]   Vesga-López O, Blanco C, Keyes K, Olfson M, Grant BF, Hasin DS. Psychiatric disorders in pregnant and postpartum women in the United States. Arch Gen Psychiatry 2008; 65(7): 805-15.
        [http://dx.doi.org/10.1001/archpsyc.65.7.805] [PMID: 18606953]

[2]   Mohamad Yusuff AS, Tang L, Binns CW, Lee AH. Prevalence and risk factors for postnatal depression in Sabah, Malaysia: A cohort study. Women Birth 2015; 28(1): 25-9.
        [http://dx.doi.org/10.1016/j.wombi.2014.11.002] [PMID: 25466643]

[3]   Roesch SC, Schetter CD, Woo G, Hobel CJ. Modeling the types and timing of stress in pregnancy. Anxiety Stress Coping 2004; 17(1): 87-102.
        [http://dx.doi.org/10.1080/1061580031000123667]

[4]   Redshaw M, Martin C, Rowe R, Hockley C. The Oxford Worries about Labour Scale: Women's experience and measurement characteristics of a measure of maternal concern about labour and birth. Psychol Health Med 2009; 14(3): 354-66.
        [http://dx.doi.org/10.1080/13548500802707159] [PMID: 19444713]

[5]   Yali AM, Lobel M. Coping and distress in pregnancy: An investigation of medically high risk women. J Psychosom Obstet Gynaecol 1999; 20(1): 39-52.
        [http://dx.doi.org/10.3109/01674829909075575] [PMID: 10212886]

[6]   Lobel M, Cannella DL, Graham JE, DeVincent C, Schneider J, Meyer BA. Pregnancy-specific stress, prenatal health behaviors, and birth outcomes. Health Psychol 2008; 27(5): 604-15.
        [http://dx.doi.org/10.1037/a0013242] [PMID: 18823187]

[7]   Norhayati MN, Nik Hazlina NH, Asrenee AR, Wan Emilin WMA. Magnitude and risk factors for postpartum symptoms: A literature review. J Affect Disord 2015; 175: 34-52.
        [http://dx.doi.org/10.1016/j.jad.2014.12.041] [PMID: 25590764]

[8]   Meltzer-Brody S. New insights into perinatal depression: pathogenesis and treatment during pregnancy and postpartum. Dialogues Clin Neurosci 2011; 13(1): 89-100.
        [http://dx.doi.org/10.31887/DCNS.2011.13.1/smbrody] [PMID: 21485749]

[9]   Green SM, Haber E, Frey BN, McCabe RE. Cognitive-behavioral group treatment for perinatal anxiety: a pilot study. Arch Women Ment Health 2015; 18(4): 631-8.
        [http://dx.doi.org/10.1007/s00737-015-0498-z] [PMID: 25652951]

[10]   Goodman JH, Watson GR, Stubbs B. Anxiety disorders in postpartum women: A systematic review and meta-analysis. J Affect Disord 2016; 203: 292-331.
        [http://dx.doi.org/10.1016/j.jad.2016.05.033] [PMID: 27317922]

[11]   Howard LM, Flach C, Mehay A, Sharp D, Tylee A. The prevalence of suicidal ideation identified by the Edinburgh Postnatal Depression Scale in postpartum women in primary care: findings from the RESPOND trial. BMC Pregnancy Childbirth 2011; 11(1): 57.
[http://dx.doi.org/10.1186/1471-2393-11-57] [PMID: 21812968]

[12]   Glasheen C, Richardson GA, Fabio A. A systematic review of the effects of postnatal maternal anxiety on children. Arch Women Ment Health 2010; 13(1): 61-74.
[http://dx.doi.org/10.1007/s00737-009-0109-y] [PMID: 19789953]

[13]   Stein A, Pearson RM, Goodman SH, *et al.* Effects of perinatal mental disorders on the fetus and child. Lancet 2014; 384(9956): 1800-19.
[http://dx.doi.org/10.1016/S0140-6736(14)61277-0] [PMID: 25455250]

[14]   Buss C, Davis EP, Hobel CJ, Sandman CA. Maternal pregnancy-specific anxiety is associated with child executive function at 6–9 years age. Stress 2011; 14(6): 665-76.
[http://dx.doi.org/10.3109/10253890.2011.623250] [PMID: 21995526]

[15]   Glover V, Bergman K, O'Connor TG. The effects of maternal stress, anxiety, and depression during pregnancy on the neurodevelopment of the child. Perinatal and postpartum mood disorders: Perspectives and treatment guide for the health care practitioner 2008; 3-15.

[16]   Entringer S, Buss C, Wadhwa PD. Prenatal stress and developmental programming of human health and disease risk: concepts and integration of empirical findings. Curr Opin Endocrinol Diabetes Obes 2010; 17(6): 507-16.
[http://dx.doi.org/10.1097/MED.0b013e3283405921] [PMID: 20962631]

[17]   Merlot E, Couret D, Otten W. Prenatal stress, fetal imprinting and immunity. Brain Behav Immun 2008; 22(1): 42-51.
[http://dx.doi.org/10.1016/j.bbi.2007.05.007] [PMID: 17716859]

[18]   Broberg A, Risholm Mothander P, Granqvist P, Ivarsson T. Anknytning i praktiken: Tillämpningar av anknytningsteorin [Internet]. Natur och Kultur, Stockholm; 2008 [citado 14 de agosto de 2021]. Disponible en: 2008.http://urn.kb.se/resolve?urn=urn:nbn:se:su:diva-15469

[19]   Chase-Brand J. Effects of maternal postpartum depression on the infant and older siblings. Perinatal and postpartum mood disorders: Perspectives and treatment guide for the health care practitioner 2008; 41-64.

[20]   Van Den Bergh BRH. Developmental programming of early brain and behaviour development and mental health: a conceptual framework. Dev Med Child Neurol 2011; 53(53) (Suppl. 4): 19-23.
[http://dx.doi.org/10.1111/j.1469-8749.2011.04057.x] [PMID: 21950389]

[21]   Glover V. Maternal depression, anxiety and stress during pregnancy and child outcome; what needs to be done. Best Pract Res Clin Obstet Gynaecol 2014; 28(1): 25-35.
[http://dx.doi.org/10.1016/j.bpobgyn.2013.08.017] [PMID: 24090740]

[22]   Fisher J, Cabral de Mello M, Patel V, *et al.* Prevalence and determinants of common perinatal mental disorders in women in low- and lower-middle-income countries: a systematic review. Bull World Health Organ 2012; 90(2): 139-149H.
[http://dx.doi.org/10.2471/BLT.11.091850] [PMID: 22423165]

[23]   Hendrick V, Altshuler L, Cohen L, Stowe Z. Evaluation of mental health and depression during pregnancy: position paper. Psychopharmacol Bull 1998; 34(3): 297-9.
[PMID: 9803758]

[24]   O'hara MW, Swain AM. Rates and risk of postpartum depression—a meta-analysis. Int Rev Psychiatry 1996; 8(1): 37-54.
[http://dx.doi.org/10.3109/09540269609037816]

[25]   Le Strat Y, Dubertret C, Le Foll B. Prevalence and correlates of major depressive episode in pregnant and postpartum women in the United States. J Affect Disord 2011; 135(1-3): 128-38.
[http://dx.doi.org/10.1016/j.jad.2011.07.004] [PMID: 21802737]

[26]   Murray L. The development of children of postnatally depressed mothers: Evidence from the Cambridge longitudinal study. Psychoanal Psychother 2009; 23(3): 185-99.
[http://dx.doi.org/10.1080/02668730903227289]

[27]   Grigoriadis S, VonderPorten EH, Mamisashvili L, *et al.* The impact of maternal depression during pregnancy on perinatal outcomes: a systematic review and meta-analysis. J Clin Psychiatry 2013; 74(4): e321-41.
[http://dx.doi.org/10.4088/JCP.12r07968] [PMID: 23656857]

[28]   Bowen A, Baetz M, Schwartz L, Balbuena L, Muhajarine N. Antenatal group therapy improves worry and depression symptoms. Isr J Psychiatry Relat Sci 2014; 51(3): 226-31.
[PMID: 25618288]

[29]   Duncan LG, Cohn MA, Chao MT, Cook JG, Riccobono J, Bardacke N. Benefits of preparing for childbirth with mindfulness training: a randomized controlled trial with active comparison. BMC Pregnancy Childbirth 2017; 17(1): 140.
[http://dx.doi.org/10.1186/s12884-017-1319-3] [PMID: 28499376]

[30]   Dejin-Karlsson E, Hanson BS, Ostergren PO, Lindgren A, Sjöberg NO, Marsal K. Association of a lack of psychosocial resources and the risk of giving birth to small for gestational age infants: a stress hypothesis. BJOG 2000; 107(1): 89-100.
[http://dx.doi.org/10.1111/j.1471-0528.2000.tb11584.x] [PMID: 10645867]

[31]   Bernard-Bonnin A-C. Maternal depression and child development. Paediatr Child Health 2004; 9(8): 575-83.
[http://dx.doi.org/10.1093/pch/9.8.575] [PMID: 19680490]

[32]   Cohn JF, Tronick E. Specificity of infants' response to mothers' affective behavior. J Am Acad Child Adolesc Psychiatry 1989; 28(2): 242-8.
[http://dx.doi.org/10.1097/00004583-198903000-00016] [PMID: 2925579]

[33]   Orr ST, Miller CA. Maternal depressive symptoms and the risk of poor pregnancy outcome. Review of the literature and preliminary findings. Epidemiol Rev 1995; 17(1): 165-71.
[http://dx.doi.org/10.1093/oxfordjournals.epirev.a036172] [PMID: 8521934]

[34]   Orr ST, James SA, Blackmore Prince C. Maternal prenatal depressive symptoms and spontaneous preterm births among African-American women in Baltimore, Maryland. Am J Epidemiol 2002; 156(9): 797-802.
[http://dx.doi.org/10.1093/aje/kwf131] [PMID: 12396996]

[35]   Dayan J, Creveuil C, Herlicoviez M, *et al.* Role of anxiety and depression in the onset of spontaneous preterm labor. Am J Epidemiol 2002; 155(4): 293-301.
[http://dx.doi.org/10.1093/aje/155.4.293] [PMID: 11836191]

[36]   Steer RA, Scholl TO, Hediger ML, Fischer RL. Self-reported depression and negative pregnancy outcomes. J Clin Epidemiol 1992; 45(10): 1093-9.
[http://dx.doi.org/10.1016/0895-4356(92)90149-H] [PMID: 1474405]

[37]   Zuckerman B, Bauchner H, Parker S, Cabral H. Maternal depressive symptoms during pregnancy, and newborn irritability. J Dev Behav Pediatr 1990; 11(4): 190-4.
[http://dx.doi.org/10.1097/00004703-199008000-00006] [PMID: 2212032]

[38]   Fishell A. Depression and anxiety in pregnancy. J Popul Ther Clin Pharmacol J Ther Popul Pharmacol Clin 2010; 17(3): e363-9.
[PMID: 21041870]

[39]   Tronick E, Reck C. Infants of depressed mothers. Harv Rev Psychiatry 2009; 17(2): 147-56.
[http://dx.doi.org/10.1080/10673220902899714] [PMID: 19373622]

[40]   Singer JM, Fagen JW. Negative affect, emotional expression, and forgetting in young infants. Dev Psychol 1992; 28(1): 48-57.
[http://dx.doi.org/10.1037/0012-1649.28.1.48]

[41] Huizink AC, Robles de Medina PG, Mulder EJH, Visser GHA, Buitelaar JK. Stress during pregnancy is associated with developmental outcome in infancy. J Child Psychol Psychiatry 2003; 44(6): 810-8.
[http://dx.doi.org/10.1111/1469-7610.00166] [PMID: 12959490]

[42] Lesesne CA, Visser SN, White CP. Attention-deficit/hyperactivity disorder in school-aged children: association with maternal mental health and use of health care resources. Pediatrics 2003; 111(5 Pt 2) (Suppl. 1): 1232-7.
[http://dx.doi.org/10.1542/peds.111.S1.1232] [PMID: 12728144]

[43] Graignic-Philippe R, Dayan J, Chokron S, Jacquet A-Y, Tordjman S. Effects of prenatal stress on fetal and child development: A critical literature review. Neurosci Biobehav Rev 2014; 43: 137-62.
[http://dx.doi.org/10.1016/j.neubiorev.2014.03.022] [PMID: 24747487]

[44] Mulder EJH, Robles de Medina PG, Huizink AC, Van den Bergh BRH, Buitelaar JK, Visser GHA. Prenatal maternal stress: effects on pregnancy and the (unborn) child. Early Hum Dev 2002; 70(1-2): 3-14.
[http://dx.doi.org/10.1016/S0378-3782(02)00075-0] [PMID: 12441200]

[45] Appleby L, Mortensen PB, Faragher EB. Suicide and other causes of mortality after post-partum psychiatric admission. Br J Psychiatry 1998; 173(3): 209-11.
[http://dx.doi.org/10.1192/bjp.173.3.209] [PMID: 9926095]

[46] Grote NK, Bridge JA, Gavin AR, Melville JL, Iyengar S, Katon WJ. A meta-analysis of depression during pregnancy and the risk of preterm birth, low birth weight, and intrauterine growth restriction. Arch Gen Psychiatry 2010; 67(10): 1012-24.
[http://dx.doi.org/10.1001/archgenpsychiatry.2010.111] [PMID: 20921117]

[47] Dagher RK, McGovern PM, Dowd BE, Gjerdingen DK. Postpartum depression and health services expenditures among employed women. J Occup Environ Med 2012; 54(2): 210-5.
[http://dx.doi.org/10.1097/JOM.0b013e31823fdf85] [PMID: 22267187]

[48] Bauer A, Parsonage M, Knapp M, Iemmi V, *et al.* The costs of perinatal mental health problems. :44

[49] Pawlby S, Hay DF, Sharp D, Waters CS, O'Keane V. Antenatal depression predicts depression in adolescent offspring: Prospective longitudinal community-based study. J Affect Disord 2009; 113(3): 236-43.
[http://dx.doi.org/10.1016/j.jad.2008.05.018] [PMID: 18602698]

[50] Paulson JF, Bazemore SD. Prenatal and postpartum depression in fathers and its association with maternal depression: a meta-analysis. JAMA 2010; 303(19): 1961-9.
[http://dx.doi.org/10.1001/jama.2010.605] [PMID: 20483973]

[51] Wang D, Li YL, Qiu D, Xiao SY. Factors Influencing Paternal Postpartum Depression: A Systematic Review and Meta-Analysis. J Affect Disord 2021; 293: 51-63.
[http://dx.doi.org/10.1016/j.jad.2021.05.088] [PMID: 34171611]

[52] Albicker J, Hölzel LP, Bengel J, *et al.* Prevalence, symptomatology, risk factors and healthcare services utilization regarding paternal depression in Germany: study protocol of a controlled cross-sectional epidemiological study. BMC Psychiatry 2019; 19(1): 289.
[http://dx.doi.org/10.1186/s12888-019-2280-7] [PMID: 31533685]

[53] Wang T, Xu Y, Li Z, Chen L. Prevalence of paternal postpartum depression in China and its association with maternal postpartum depression: A Meta-analysis. Zhong Nan Da Xue Xue Bao Yi Xue Ban 2016; 41(10): 1082-9.
[PMID: 27807332]

[54] Kessler RC, Berglund P, Demler O, *et al.* The epidemiology of major depressive disorder: results from the National Comorbidity Survey Replication (NCS-R). JAMA 2003; 289(23): 3095-105.
[http://dx.doi.org/10.1001/jama.289.23.3095] [PMID: 12813115]

[55] Coussons-Read ME, Lobel M, Carey JC, *et al.* The occurrence of preterm delivery is linked to pregnancy-specific distress and elevated inflammatory markers across gestation. Brain Behav Immun

2012; 26(4): 650-9.
[http://dx.doi.org/10.1016/j.bbi.2012.02.009] [PMID: 22426431]

[56]   Isgut M, Smith AK, Reimann ES, Kucuk O, Ryan J. The impact of psychological distress during pregnancy on the developing fetus: biological mechanisms and the potential benefits of mindfulness interventions. J Perinat Med [Internet]. 20 de diciembre de 2017 [citado 14 de agosto de 2017; 45(9)https://www.degruyter.com/document/doi/10.1515/jpm-2016-0189/html

[57]   Reynolds RM, Labad J, Buss C, Ghaemmaghami P, Räikkönen K. Transmitting biological effects of stress in utero: Implications for mother and offspring. Psychoneuroendocrinology 2013; 38(9): 1843-9.
[http://dx.doi.org/10.1016/j.psyneuen.2013.05.018] [PMID: 23810315]

[58]   Howerton CL, Bale TL. Prenatal programing: At the intersection of maternal stress and immune activation. Horm Behav 2012; 62(3): 237-42.
[http://dx.doi.org/10.1016/j.yhbeh.2012.03.007] [PMID: 22465455]

[59]   Lee AM, Lam SK, Sze Mun Lau SM, Chong CSY, Chui HW, Fong DYT. Prevalence, course, and risk factors for antenatal anxiety and depression. Obstet Gynecol 2007; 110(5): 1102-12.
[http://dx.doi.org/10.1097/01.AOG.0000287065.59491.70] [PMID: 17978126]

[60]   Powers SI, Laurent HK, Gunlicks-Stoessel M, Balaban S, Bent E. Depression and anxiety predict sex-specific cortisol responses to interpersonal stress. Psychoneuroendocrinology 2016; 69: 172-9.
[http://dx.doi.org/10.1016/j.psyneuen.2016.04.007] [PMID: 27107208]

[61]   Belvederi Murri M, Pariante C, Mondelli V, *et al*. HPA axis and aging in depression: Systematic review and meta-analysis. Psychoneuroendocrinology 2014; 41: 46-62.
[http://dx.doi.org/10.1016/j.psyneuen.2013.12.004] [PMID: 24495607]

[62]   Wadhwa PD, Culhane JF, Rauh V, Barve SS. Stress and preterm birth: neuroendocrine, immune/inflammatory, and vascular mechanisms. Matern Child Health J 2001; 5(2): 119-25.
[http://dx.doi.org/10.1023/A:1011353216619] [PMID: 11573837]

[63]   Mor G, Cardenas I, Abrahams V, Guller S. Inflammation and pregnancy: the role of the immune system at the implantation site. Ann N Y Acad Sci 2011; 1221(1): 80-7.
[http://dx.doi.org/10.1111/j.1749-6632.2010.05938.x] [PMID: 21401634]

[64]   Teixeira JMA, Fisk NM, Glover V. Association between maternal anxiety in pregnancy and increased uterine artery resistance index: cohort based study. BMJ 1999; 318(7177): 153-7.
[http://dx.doi.org/10.1136/bmj.318.7177.153] [PMID: 9888905]

[65]   Yong Ping E, Laplante DP, Elgbeili G, Jones SL, Brunet A, King S. Disaster-related prenatal maternal stress predicts HPA reactivity and psychopathology in adolescent offspring: Project Ice Storm. Psychoneuroendocrinology 2020; 117104697
[http://dx.doi.org/10.1016/j.psyneuen.2020.104697] [PMID: 32442863]

[66]   Kinsella MT, Monk C. Impact of maternal stress, depression and anxiety on fetal neurobehavioral development. Clin Obstet Gynecol 2009; 52(3): 425-40.
[http://dx.doi.org/10.1097/GRF.0b013e3181b52df1] [PMID: 19661759]

[67]   Newport DJ, Wilcox MM, Stowe ZN. Maternal depression: A child's first adverse life event. Semin Clin Neuropsychiatry 2002; 7(2): 113-9.
[http://dx.doi.org/10.1053/scnp.2002.31789] [PMID: 11953935]

[68]   Glynn LM, Davis EP, Sandman CA. New insights into the role of perinatal HPA-axis dysregulation in postpartum depression. Neuropeptides 2013; 47(6): 363-70.
[http://dx.doi.org/10.1016/j.npep.2013.10.007] [PMID: 24210135]

[69]   Dickens MJ, Pawluski JL. The hpa axis during the perinatal period: implications for perinatal depression. endocrinology 2018; 159(11): 3737-46.
[http://dx.doi.org/10.1210/en.2018-00677] [PMID: 30256957]

[70]   Schlotz W, Phillips DIW. Fetal origins of mental health: Evidence and mechanisms. Brain Behav Immun 2009; 23(7): 905-16.

[http://dx.doi.org/10.1016/j.bbi.2009.02.001] [PMID: 19217937]

[71] Giesbrecht GF, Campbell T, Letourneau N, Kooistra L, Kaplan B. Psychological distress and salivary cortisol covary within persons during pregnancy. Psychoneuroendocrinology 2012; 37(2): 270-9.
[http://dx.doi.org/10.1016/j.psyneuen.2011.06.011] [PMID: 21752548]

[72] Tollenaar MS, Beijers R, Jansen J, Riksen-Walraven JMA, de Weerth C. Maternal prenatal stress and cortisol reactivity to stressors in human infants. Stress 2011; 14(1): 53-65.
[http://dx.doi.org/10.3109/10253890.2010.499485] [PMID: 20666659]

[73] Giesbrecht GF, Poole JC, Letourneau N, Campbell T, Kaplan BJ. The buffering effect of social support on hypothalamic-pituitary-adrenal axis function during pregnancy. Psychosom Med 2013; 75(9): 856-62.
[http://dx.doi.org/10.1097/PSY.0000000000000004] [PMID: 24163383]

[74] Kane HS, Dunkel Schetter C, Glynn LM, Hobel CJ, Sandman CA. Pregnancy anxiety and prenatal cortisol trajectories. Biol Psychol 2014; 100: 13-9.
[http://dx.doi.org/10.1016/j.biopsycho.2014.04.003] [PMID: 24769094]

[75] Baibazarova E, van de Beek C, Cohen-Kettenis PT, Buitelaar J, Shelton KH, van Goozen SHM. Influence of prenatal maternal stress, maternal plasma cortisol and cortisol in the amniotic fluid on birth outcomes and child temperament at 3 months. Psychoneuroendocrinology 2013; 38(6): 907-15.
[http://dx.doi.org/10.1016/j.psyneuen.2012.09.015] [PMID: 23046825]

[76] Entringer S, Buss C, Shirtcliff EA, *et al.* Attenuation of maternal psychophysiological stress responses and the maternal cortisol awakening response over the course of human pregnancy. Stress 2010; 13(3): 258-68.
[http://dx.doi.org/10.3109/10253890903349501] [PMID: 20067400]

[77] Christian LM. Physiological reactivity to psychological stress in human pregnancy: Current knowledge and future directions. Prog Neurobiol 2012; 99(2): 106-16.
[http://dx.doi.org/10.1016/j.pneurobio.2012.07.003] [PMID: 22800930]

[78] Braeken MAKA, Jones A, Otte RA, *et al.* Anxious women do not show the expected decrease in cardiovascular stress responsiveness as pregnancy advances. Biol Psychol 2015; 111: 83-9.
[http://dx.doi.org/10.1016/j.biopsycho.2015.08.007] [PMID: 26316361]

[79] Monk C, Fifer WP, Myers MM, Sloan RP, Trien L, Hurtado A. Maternal stress responses and anxiety during pregnancy: Effects on fetal heart rate. Dev Psychobiol 2000; 36(1): 67-77.
[http://dx.doi.org/10.1002/(SICI)1098-2302(200001)36:1<67::AID-DEV7>3.0.CO;2-C]   [PMID: 10607362]

[80] McCubbin JA, Lawson EJ, Cox S, Sherman JJ, Norton JA, Read JA. Prenatal maternal blood pressure response to stress predicts birth weight and gestational age: A preliminary study. Am J Obstet Gynecol 1996; 175(3): 706-12.
[http://dx.doi.org/10.1053/ob.1996.v175.a74286] [PMID: 8828438]

[81] Hilmert CJ, Schetter CD, Dominguez TP, *et al.* Stress and blood pressure during pregnancy: racial differences and associations with birthweight. Psychosom Med 2008; 70(1): 57-64.
[http://dx.doi.org/10.1097/PSY.0b013e31815c6d96] [PMID: 18158373]

[82] Volkovich E, Tikotzky L, Manber R. Objective and subjective sleep during pregnancy: links with depressive and anxiety symptoms. Arch Women Ment Health 2016; 19(1): 173-81.
[http://dx.doi.org/10.1007/s00737-015-0554-8] [PMID: 26250541]

[83] Manber R, Steidtmann D, Chambers AS, Ganger W, Horwitz S, Connelly CD. Factors associated with clinically significant insomnia among pregnant low-income Latinas. J Womens Health 2002. agosto de 2013; 22(8): 694-701.

[84] Edinger JD, Fins AI, Glenn DM, *et al.* Insomnia and the eye of the beholder: Are there clinical markers of objective sleep disturbances among adults with and without insomnia complaints? J Consult Clin Psychol 2000; 68(4): 586-93.

[http://dx.doi.org/10.1037/0022-006X.68.4.586] [PMID: 10965634]

[85] Tollenaar MS, Beijers R, Jansen J, Riksen-Walraven JMA, de Weerth C. Solitary sleeping in young infants is associated with heightened cortisol reactivity to a bathing session but not to a vaccination. Psychoneuroendocrinology 2012; 37(2): 167-77.
[http://dx.doi.org/10.1016/j.psyneuen.2011.03.017] [PMID: 21530088]

[86] Omisade A, Buxton OM, Rusak B. Impact of acute sleep restriction on cortisol and leptin levels in young women. Physiol Behav. 19 de abril de 2010; 99(5): 651-.
[http://dx.doi.org/10.1016/j.physbeh.2010.01.028]

[87] Chang JJ, Pien GW, Duntley SP, Macones GA. Sleep deprivation during pregnancy and maternal and fetal outcomes: Is there a relationship? Sleep Med Rev 2010; 14(2): 107-14.
[http://dx.doi.org/10.1016/j.smrv.2009.05.001] [PMID: 19625199]

[88] Lee KA, Gay CL. Sleep in late pregnancy predicts length of labor and type of delivery. Am J Obstet Gynecol 2004; 191(6): 2041-6.
[http://dx.doi.org/10.1016/j.ajog.2004.05.086] [PMID: 15592289]

[89] Beebe KR, Lee KA. Sleep disturbance in late pregnancy and early labor. J Perinat Neonatal Nurs 2007; 21(2): 103-8.
[http://dx.doi.org/10.1097/01.JPN.0000270626.66369.26] [PMID: 17505229]

[90] Eberth J, Sedlmeier P. The Effects of Mindfulness Meditation: A Meta-Analysis. Mindfulness 2012; 3(3): 174-89.
[http://dx.doi.org/10.1007/s12671-012-0101-x]

[91] Gavin NI, Gaynes BN, Lohr KN, Meltzer-Brody S, Gartlehner G, Swinson T. Perinatal Depression. Obstet Gynecol 2005; 106(5, Part 1): 1071-83.
[http://dx.doi.org/10.1097/01.AOG.0000183597.31630.db] [PMID: 16260528]

[92] Pereira PK, Lima LA, Legay LF, de Cintra Santos JF, Lovisi GM. Maternal mental disorders in pregnancy and the puerperium and risks to infant health. World J Clin Pediatr 2012; 1(4): 20-3.
[http://dx.doi.org/10.5409/wjcp.v1.i4.20] [PMID: 25254163]

[93] Banti S, Mauri M, Oppo A, *et al.* From the third month of pregnancy to 1 year postpartum. Prevalence, incidence, recurrence, and new onset of depression. Results from the Perinatal Depression–Research & Screening Unit study. Compr Psychiatry 2011; 52(4): 343-51.
[http://dx.doi.org/10.1016/j.comppsych.2010.08.003] [PMID: 21683171]

[94] Alvarado R, Perucca E, Neves E, *et al.* Depressive disorders during pregnancy and associated factors. Rev Chil Obstet Ginecol 1993; 58(2): 135-41.
[PMID: 8209041]

[95] Jadresic E, Jara C, Araya R. [Depression in pregnancy and puerperium: study of risk factors]. Acta Psiquiatr Psicol Am Lat 1993; 39(1): 63-74.
[PMID: 8237436]

[96] Cardwell MS. Stress. Obstet Gynecol Surv 2013; 68(2): 119-29.
[http://dx.doi.org/10.1097/OGX.0b013e31827f2481] [PMID: 23417218]

[97] American Psychiatric Association. 2013. https://psychiatryonline.org/doi/book/10.1176/appi.books.9780890425596

[98] Guze SB. Diagnostic and Statistical Manual of Mental Disorders 1995.

[99] Gorman LL, O'Hara MW, Figueiredo B, *et al.* Adaptation of the Structured Clinical Interview for DSM-IV Disorders for assessing depression in women during pregnancy and post-partum across countries and cultures. Br J Psychiatry 2004; 184(S46): s17-23.
[http://dx.doi.org/10.1192/bjp.184.46.s17] [PMID: 14754814]

[100] Cox J. Use and misuse of the Edinburgh Postnatal Depression Scale (EPDS): a ten point 'survival analysis'. Arch Women Ment Health 2017; 20(6): 789-90.

[http://dx.doi.org/10.1007/s00737-017-0789-7] [PMID: 29101480]

[101] Cox JL, Holden JM, Sagovsky R. Detection of postnatal depression. Development of the 10-item Edinburgh Postnatal Depression Scale. Br J Psychiatry 1987; 150(6): 782-6.
[http://dx.doi.org/10.1192/bjp.150.6.782] [PMID: 3651732]

[102] Rubertsson C, Börjesson K, Berglund A, Josefsson A, Sydsjö G. The Swedish validation of Edinburgh Postnatal Depression Scale (EPDS) during pregnancy. Nord J Psychiatry 2011; 65(6): 414-8.
[http://dx.doi.org/10.3109/08039488.2011.590606] [PMID: 21728782]

[103] National Collaborating Centre for Mental Health (UK). Antenatal and Postnatal Mental Health: The NICE Guideline on Clinical Management and Service Guidance [Internet]. Leicester (UK): British Psychological Society; 2007 [citado 14 de agosto de 2021]. (National Institute for Health and Clinical Excellence: Guidance). http://www.ncbi.nlm.nih.gov/books/NBK54487/

[104] Whooley MA, Avins AL, Miranda J, Browner WS. Case-finding instruments for depression. J Gen Intern Med 1997; 12(7): 439-45.
[http://dx.doi.org/10.1046/j.1525-1497.1997.00076.x] [PMID: 9229283]

[105] Kendell RE, McGuire RJ, Connor Y, Cox JL. Mood changes in the first three weeks after childbirth. J Affect Disord 1981; 3(4): 317-26.
[http://dx.doi.org/10.1016/0165-0327(81)90001-X] [PMID: 6459348]

[106] O'hara MW. Post-partum 'blues,' depression, and psychosis: A review. J Psychosom Obstet Gynaecol 1987; 7(3): 205-27.
[http://dx.doi.org/10.3109/01674828709040280]

[107] Hahn-Holbrook J, Cornwell-Hinrichs T, Anaya I. economic and health predictors of national postpartum depression prevalence: A systematic review, meta-analysis, and meta-regression of 291 studies from 56 countries. front psychiatry 2018; 8: 248.
[http://dx.doi.org/10.3389/fpsyt.2017.00248] [PMID: 29449816]

[108] Özcan NK, Boyacıoğlu NE, Dinç H. Postpartum Depression Prevalence and Risk Factors in Turkey: A Systematic Review and Meta-Analysis. Arch Psychiatr Nurs 2017; 31(4): 420-8.
[http://dx.doi.org/10.1016/j.apnu.2017.04.006] [PMID: 28693880]

[109] Villegas L, McKay K, Dennis CL, Ross LE. Postpartum depression among rural women from developed and developing countries: a systematic review. J Rural Health 2011; 27(3): 278-88.
[http://dx.doi.org/10.1111/j.1748-0361.2010.00339.x] [PMID: 21729155]

[110] Cowan CP, Cowan PA. When partners become parents: the big life change for couples 1999.

[111] Lever Taylor B, Cavanagh K, Strauss C. The Effectiveness of Mindfulness-Based Interventions in the Perinatal Period: A Systematic Review and Meta-Analysis. PLoS One 2016; 11(5)e0155720
[http://dx.doi.org/10.1371/journal.pone.0155720] [PMID: 27182732]

[112] Beddoe AE, Paul Yang CP, Kennedy HP, Weiss SJ, Lee KA. The effects of mindfulness-based yoga during pregnancy on maternal psychological and physical distress. J Obstet Gynecol Neonatal Nurs 2009; 38(3): 310-9.
[http://dx.doi.org/10.1111/j.1552-6909.2009.01023.x] [PMID: 19538619]

[113] Tompkins A. Postpartum Mood Disorders. Midwifery Today Int Midwife 2017; (121): 38-9.
[PMID: 29912534]

[114] Zivoder I, Martic-Biocina S, Veronek J, Ursulin-Trstenjak N, Sajko M, Paukovic M. Mental disorders/difficulties in the postpartum period. Psychiatr Danub 2019; 31 (Suppl. 3): 338-44.
[PMID: 31488750]

[115] Brummelte S, Galea LAM. Postpartum depression: Etiology, treatment and consequences for maternal care. Horm Behav 2016; 77: 153-66.
[http://dx.doi.org/10.1016/j.yhbeh.2015.08.008] [PMID: 26319224]

[116] Committee Opinion No. 630. Obstet Gynecol 2015; 125(5): 1268-71.

[http://dx.doi.org/10.1097/01.AOG.0000465192.34779.dc] [PMID: 25932866]

[117]   Staneva AA, Bogossian F, Wittkowski A. The experience of psychological distress, depression, and anxiety during pregnancy: A meta-synthesis of qualitative research. Midwifery 2015; 31(6): 563-73.
[http://dx.doi.org/10.1016/j.midw.2015.03.015] [PMID: 25912511]

[118]   Togher KL, Treacy E, O'Keeffe GW, Kenny LC. Maternal distress in late pregnancy alters obstetric outcomes and the expression of genes important for placental glucocorticoid signalling. Psychiatry Res 2017; 255: 17-26.
[http://dx.doi.org/10.1016/j.psychres.2017.05.013] [PMID: 28511050]

[119]   Martínez-Paredes JF, Jácome-Pérez N. Depression in pregnancy 2019.
[http://dx.doi.org/10.1016/j.rcpeng.2017.07.002]

[120]   Fitelson E, Kim S, Baker AS, Leight K. Treatment of postpartum depression: clinical, psychological and pharmacological options. Int J Womens Health 2010; 3: 1-14.
[PMID: 21339932]

[121]   Carvalho AF, Sharma MS, Brunoni AR, Vieta E, Fava GA. the safety, tolerability and risks associated with the use of newer generation antidepressant drugs: A critical review of the literature. psychother psychosom 2016; 85(5): 270-88.
[http://dx.doi.org/10.1159/000447034] [PMID: 27508501]

[122]   Creeley CE, Denton LK. Use of Prescribed Psychotropics during Pregnancy: A Systematic Review of Pregnancy, Neonatal, and Childhood Outcomes. Brain Sci 2019; 9(9): 235.
[http://dx.doi.org/10.3390/brainsci9090235] [PMID: 31540060]

[123]   Singal D, Brownell M, Chateau D, Ruth C, Katz LY. Neonatal and childhood neurodevelopmental, health and educational outcomes of children exposed to antidepressants and maternal depression during pregnancy: protocol for a retrospective population-based cohort study using linked administrative data. BMJ Open 2016; 6(11)e013293
[http://dx.doi.org/10.1136/bmjopen-2016-013293] [PMID: 27899401]

[124]   Sit D, Perel JM, Wisniewski SR, Helsel JC, Luther JF, Wisner KL. Mother-infant antidepressant concentrations, maternal depression, and perinatal events. J Clin Psychiatry 2011; 72(7): 994-1001.
[http://dx.doi.org/10.4088/JCP.10m06461] [PMID: 21824458]

[125]   Zakiyah N, ter Heijne LF, Bos JH, Hak E, Postma MJ, Schuiling-Veninga CCM. Antidepressant use during pregnancy and the risk of developing gestational hypertension: a retrospective cohort study. BMC Pregnancy Childbirth 2018; 18(1): 187.
[http://dx.doi.org/10.1186/s12884-018-1825-y] [PMID: 29843629]

[126]   De Vera MA, Bérard A. Antidepressant use during pregnancy and the risk of pregnancy-induced hypertension. Br J Clin Pharmacol 2012; 74(2): 362-9.
[http://dx.doi.org/10.1111/j.1365-2125.2012.04196.x] [PMID: 22435711]

[127]   Flynn HA, O'Mahen HA, Massey L, Marcus S. The impact of a brief obstetrics clinic-based intervention on treatment use for perinatal depression. J Womens Health 2002. diciembre de 2006; 15(10): 1195-204.

[128]   Marcus SM, Flynn HA. Depression, antidepressant medication, and functioning outcomes among pregnant women. Int J Gynaecol Obstet 2008; 100(3): 248-51.
[http://dx.doi.org/10.1016/j.ijgo.2007.09.016] [PMID: 18005968]

[129]   O'Connor E, Senger CA, Henninger ML, Coppola E, Gaynes BN. interventions to prevent perinatal depression. jama 2019; 321(6): 588-601.
[http://dx.doi.org/10.1001/jama.2018.20865] [PMID: 30747970]

[130]   Daley AJ, Foster L, Long G, *et al.* The effectiveness of exercise for the prevention and treatment of antenatal depression: systematic review with meta-analysis. BJOG 2015; 122(1): 57-62.
[http://dx.doi.org/10.1111/1471-0528.12909] [PMID: 24935560]

[131]   Shivakumar G. Exercise improves depressive symptoms during pregnancy. BJOG 2015; 122(1): 63.

[http://dx.doi.org/10.1111/1471-0528.13053] [PMID: 25201178]

[132] Yonkers KA, Wisner KL, Stewart DE, *et al*. The management of depression during pregnancy: a report from the American Psychiatric Association and the American College of Obstetricians and Gynecologists. Gen Hosp Psychiatry 2009; 31(5): 403-13.
[http://dx.doi.org/10.1016/j.genhosppsych.2009.04.003] [PMID: 19703633]

[133] Wisner KL, Gelenberg AJ, Leonard H, Zarin D, Frank E. Pharmacologic treatment of depression during pregnancy. JAMA 1999; 282(13): 1264-9.
[http://dx.doi.org/10.1001/jama.282.13.1264] [PMID: 10517430]

[134] Yonkers KA, Wisner KL, Stowe Z, *et al*. Management of bipolar disorder during pregnancy and the postpartum period. Am J Psychiatry 2004; 161(4): 608-20.
[http://dx.doi.org/10.1176/appi.ajp.161.4.608] [PMID: 15056503]

[135] Briggs , *et al*. Drugs in Pregnancy and Lactation https://www.d.umn.edu/medweb/Modules/OB-Long/RiskFactors.pdf
[http://dx.doi.org/10.1007/978-1-349-13175-4_69]

[136] Briggs GG, Freeman RK, Yaffe SJ. 2008.https://www.ncbi.nlm.nih.gov/pmc/articles/PMC4989726/pdf/10.1258_om.2009.090002.pdf

[137] Sachdeva P, Patel BG, Patel BK. Drug use in pregnancy; a point to ponder! Indian J Pharm Sci 2009; 71(1): 1-7.
[http://dx.doi.org/10.4103/0250-474X.51941] [PMID: 20177448]

[138] Commissioner O of the. Medicine and Pregnancy. FDA [Internet]. 9 de abril de 2019 [citado 14 de agosto de 2021]; Disponible en: 2019.https://www.fda.gov/consumers/free-publication--women/medicine-and-pregnancy

[139] https://chemm.nlm.nih.gov/pregnancycategories.htm

[140] Cohen LS, Altshuler LL, Harlow BL, *et al*. Relapse of major depression during pregnancy in women who maintain or discontinue antidepressant treatment. JAMA 2006; 295(5): 499-507.
[http://dx.doi.org/10.1001/jama.295.5.499] [PMID: 16449615]

[141] Wen SW, Yang Q, Garner P, *et al*. Selective serotonin reuptake inhibitors and adverse pregnancy outcomes. Am J Obstet Gynecol 2006; 194(4): 961-6.
[http://dx.doi.org/10.1016/j.ajog.2006.02.019] [PMID: 16580283]

[142] Malm H, Klaukka T, Neuvonen PJ. Risks associated with selective serotonin reuptake inhibitors in pregnancy. Obstet Gynecol 2005; 106(6): 1289-96.
[http://dx.doi.org/10.1097/01.AOG.0000187302.61812.53] [PMID: 16319254]

[143] Ellfolk M, Malm H. Risks associated with in utero and lactation exposure to selective serotonin reuptake inhibitors (SSRIs). Reprod Toxicol Elmsford N. septiembre de 2010; 30(2): 249-60.

[144] Sie SD, Wennink JMB, van Driel JJ, *et al*. Maternal use of SSRIs, SNRIs and NaSSAs: practical recommendations during pregnancy and lactation. Arch Dis Child Fetal Neonatal Ed 2012; 97(6): F472-6.
[http://dx.doi.org/10.1136/archdischild-2011-214239] [PMID: 23080479]

[145] Huybrechts KF, Palmsten K, Avorn J, *et al*. Antidepressant use in pregnancy and the risk of cardiac defects. N Engl J Med 2014; 370(25): 2397-407.
[http://dx.doi.org/10.1056/NEJMoa1312828] [PMID: 24941178]

[146] Källén B. Neonate characteristics after maternal use of antidepressants in late pregnancy. Arch Pediatr Adolesc Med 2004; 158(4): 312-6.
[http://dx.doi.org/10.1001/archpedi.158.4.312] [PMID: 15066868]

[147] Yaris F, Kadioglu M, Kesim M, Ulku C, Yaris E, Kalyoncu NI, *et al*. Newer antidepressants in pregnancy: prospective outcome of a case series 2004.
[http://dx.doi.org/10.1016/j.reprotox.2004.07.004]

[148] Kesim M, Yaris F, Kadioglu M, Yaris E, Kalyoncu NI, Ulku C. Mirtazapine use in two pregnant women: Is it safe? Teratology 2002; 66(5): 204.
[http://dx.doi.org/10.1002/tera.10095] [PMID: 12397626]

[149] Smit M, Dolman KM, Honig A. Mirtazapine in pregnancy and lactation – A systematic review. Eur Neuropsychopharmacol 2016; 26(1): 126-35.
[http://dx.doi.org/10.1016/j.euroneuro.2015.06.014] [PMID: 26631373]

[150] Sokolover N, Merlob P, Klinger G. Neonatal recurrent prolonged hypothermia associated with maternal mirtazapine treatment during pregnancy. J Popul Ther Clin Pharmacol 2008; 15(2): e188-90.
[PMID: 18515920]

[151] Louik C, Kerr S, Mitchell AA. First-trimester exposure to bupropion and risk of cardiac malformations. Pharmacoepidemiol Drug Saf 2014; 23(10): 1066-75.
[http://dx.doi.org/10.1002/pds.3661] [PMID: 24920293]

[152] ACOG Practice Bulletin: Clinical management guidelines for obstetrician-gynecologists number 92, April 2008 (replaces practice bulletin number 87, November 2007). Use of psychiatric medications during pregnancy and lactation. Obstet Gynecol 2008; 111(4): 1001-20.
[PMID: 18378767]

[153] Wald MF, Muzyk AJ, Clark D. Bipolar Depression. Psychiatr Clin North Am 2016; 39(1): 57-74.
[http://dx.doi.org/10.1016/j.psc.2015.10.002] [PMID: 26876318]

[154] Björkstedt SM, Kautiainen H, Tuomi U, et al. Maternal use of sedative drugs and its effects on pregnancy outcomes: a Finnish birth cohort study. Sci Rep 2021; 11(1): 4467.
[http://dx.doi.org/10.1038/s41598-021-84151-7] [PMID: 33627788]

[155] Kendell RE, Chalmers JC, Platz C. Epidemiology of puerperal psychoses. Br J Psychiatry 1987; 150(5): 662-73.
[http://dx.doi.org/10.1192/bjp.150.5.662] [PMID: 3651704]

[156] Kupfer DJ, Frank E. Relapse in recurrent unipolar depression. Am J Psychiatry 1987; 144(1): 86-8.
[http://dx.doi.org/10.1176/ajp.144.1.86] [PMID: 3799845]

[157] Lewis-Hall F, Ed. Psychiatric illness in women: emerging treatments and research 1st ed., 2002.

[158] Seyfried LS, Marcus SM. Postpartum mood disorders. Int Rev Psychiatry 2003; 15(3): 231-42.
[http://dx.doi.org/10.1080/0954026031000136857] [PMID: 15276962]

[159] Field T. Prenatal depression effects on early development: A review. Infant Behav Dev 2011; 34(1): 1-14.
[http://dx.doi.org/10.1016/j.infbeh.2010.09.008] [PMID: 20970195]

[160] Wisner KL, Chambers C, Sit DKY. Postpartum Depression. JAMA 2006; 296(21): 2616-8.
[http://dx.doi.org/10.1001/jama.296.21.2616] [PMID: 17148727]

[161] Goodman JH, Guarino A, Chenausky K, et al. CALM Pregnancy: results of a pilot study of mindfulness-based cognitive therapy for perinatal anxiety. Arch Women Ment Health 2014; 17(5): 373-87.
[http://dx.doi.org/10.1007/s00737-013-0402-7] [PMID: 24449191]

[162] Palagini L, Maria Bruno R, Gemignani A, Baglioni C, Ghiadoni L, Riemann D. Sleep loss and hypertension: a systematic review. Curr Pharm Des 2013; 19(13): 2409-19.
[http://dx.doi.org/10.2174/1381612811319130009] [PMID: 23173590]

[163] Cappuccio FP, D'Elia L, Strazzullo P, Miller MA. Quantity and quality of sleep and incidence of type 2 diabetes: a systematic review and meta-analysis. Diabetes Care 2010; 33(2): 414-20.
[http://dx.doi.org/10.2337/dc09-1124] [PMID: 19910503]

[164] Mellor R, Chua SC, Boyce P. Antenatal depression: an artefact of sleep disturbance? Arch Women Ment Health 2014; 17(4): 291-302.
[http://dx.doi.org/10.1007/s00737-014-0427-6] [PMID: 24793592]

[165] Baglioni C, Battagliese G, Feige B, *et al.* Insomnia as a predictor of depression: A meta-analytic evaluation of longitudinal epidemiological studies. J Affect Disord 2011; 135(1-3): 10-9.
[http://dx.doi.org/10.1016/j.jad.2011.01.011] [PMID: 21300408]

[166] Hertenstein E, Feige B, Gmeiner T, *et al.* Insomnia as a predictor of mental disorders: A systematic review and meta-analysis. Sleep Med Rev 2019; 43: 96-105.
[http://dx.doi.org/10.1016/j.smrv.2018.10.006] [PMID: 30537570]

[167] Pigeon WR, Bishop TM, Krueger KM. Insomnia as a Precipitating Factor in New Onset Mental Illness: a Systematic Review of Recent Findings. Curr Psychiatry Rep 2017; 19(8): 44.
[http://dx.doi.org/10.1007/s11920-017-0802-x] [PMID: 28616860]

[168] Gruber R, Cassoff J. The interplay between sleep and emotion regulation: conceptual framework empirical evidence and future directions. Curr Psychiatry Rep 2014; 16(11): 500.
[http://dx.doi.org/10.1007/s11920-014-0500-x] [PMID: 25200984]

[169] Palmer CA, Alfano CA. Sleep and emotion regulation: An organizing, integrative review. Sleep Med Rev 2017; 31: 6-16.
[http://dx.doi.org/10.1016/j.smrv.2015.12.006] [PMID: 26899742]

[170] Watling J, Pawlik B, Scott K, Booth S, Short MA. Sleep Loss and Affective Functioning: More Than Just Mood. Behav Sleep Med 2017; 15(5): 394-409.
[http://dx.doi.org/10.1080/15402002.2016.1141770] [PMID: 27158937]

[171] Reddy R, Palmer CA, Jackson C, Farris SG, Alfano CA. Impact of sleep restriction versus idealized sleep on emotional experience, reactivity and regulation in healthy adolescents. J Sleep Res 2017; 26(4): 516-25.
[http://dx.doi.org/10.1111/jsr.12484] [PMID: 27976447]

[172] Rohr CS, Dreyer FR, Aderka IM, *et al.* Individual differences in common factors of emotional traits and executive functions predict functional connectivity of the amygdala. Neuroimage 2015; 120: 154-63.
[http://dx.doi.org/10.1016/j.neuroimage.2015.06.049] [PMID: 26108101]

[173] Galderisi S, Heinz A, Kastrup M, Beezhold J, Sartorius N. Toward a new definition of mental health. World Psychiatry 2015; 14(2): 231-3.
[http://dx.doi.org/10.1002/wps.20231] [PMID: 26043341]

[174] McEwen BS. Protective and damaging effects of stress mediators: central role of the brain. Dialogues Clin Neurosci 2006; 8(4): 367-81.
[http://dx.doi.org/10.31887/DCNS.2006.8.4/bmcewen] [PMID: 17290796]

[175] McEwen BS, Bowles NP, Gray JD, *et al.* Mechanisms of stress in the brain. Nat Neurosci 2015; 18(10): 1353-63.
[http://dx.doi.org/10.1038/nn.4086] [PMID: 26404710]

[176] Galderisi S, Heinz A, Kastrup M, Beezhold J, Sartorius N. A proposed new definition of mental health. Psychiatr Pol 2017; 51(3): 407-11.
[http://dx.doi.org/10.12740/PP/74145] [PMID: 28866712]

[177] Nodine PM, Matthews EE. Common sleep disorders: management strategies and pregnancy outcomes. J Midwifery Womens Health 2013; 58(4): 368-77.
[http://dx.doi.org/10.1111/jmwh.12004] [PMID: 23855316]

[178] Palagini L, Gemignani A, Banti S, Manconi M, Mauri M, Riemann D. Chronic sleep loss during pregnancy as a determinant of stress: impact on pregnancy outcome. Sleep Med 2014; 15(8): 853-9.
[http://dx.doi.org/10.1016/j.sleep.2014.02.013] [PMID: 24994566]

[179] Swanson LM, Arnedt JT, Rosekind MR, Belenky G, Balkin TJ, Drake C. Sleep disorders and work performance: findings from the 2008 National Sleep Foundation Sleep in America poll. J Sleep Res 2011; 20(3): 487-94.
[http://dx.doi.org/10.1111/j.1365-2869.2010.00890.x] [PMID: 20887396]

[180] Balkin TJ, Belenky G, Drake C, Rosa R, Rosekind M. Sleep in America poll: summary of findings 2008.

[181] Elek SM, Hudson DB, Fleck MO. Expectant parents' experience with fatigue and sleep during pregnancy. Birth 1997; 24(1): 49-54.
[http://dx.doi.org/10.1111/j.1523-536X.1997.tb00336.x] [PMID: 9271967]

[182] Hutchison BL, Stone PR, McCowan LME, Stewart AW, Thompson JMD, Mitchell EA. A postal survey of maternal sleep in late pregnancy. BMC Pregnancy Childbirth 2012; 12(1): 144.
[http://dx.doi.org/10.1186/1471-2393-12-144] [PMID: 23228137]

[183] Mindell JA, Jacobson BJ. Sleep disturbances during pregnancy. J Obstet Gynecol Neonatal Nurs 2000; 29(6): 590-7.
[http://dx.doi.org/10.1111/j.1552-6909.2000.tb02072.x] [PMID: 11110329]

[184] Hertz G, Fast A, Feinsilver SH, Albertario CL, Schulman H, Fein AM. Sleep in normal late pregnancy. Sleep 1992; 15(3): 246-51.
[http://dx.doi.org/10.1093/sleep/15.3.246] [PMID: 1621025]

[185] Waters M, Lee KA. Differences between primigravidae and multigravidae mothers in sleep disturbances, fatigue, and functional status. J Nurse Midwifery 1996; 41(5): 364-7.
[http://dx.doi.org/10.1016/S0091-2182(96)00049-3] [PMID: 8916676]

[186] Greenwood KM, Hazendonk KM. Self-reported sleep during the third trimester of pregnancy. Behav Sleep Med 2004; 2(4): 191-204.
[http://dx.doi.org/10.1207/s15402010bsm0204_2] [PMID: 15600055]

[187] Mindell JA, Cook RA, Nikolovski J. Sleep patterns and sleep disturbances across pregnancy. Sleep Med 2015; 16(4): 483-8.
[http://dx.doi.org/10.1016/j.sleep.2014.12.006] [PMID: 25666847]

[188] Facco FL, Kramer J, Ho KH, Zee PC, Grobman WA. Sleep disturbances in pregnancy. Obstet Gynecol 2010; 115(1): 77-83.
[http://dx.doi.org/10.1097/AOG.0b013e3181c4f8ec] [PMID: 20027038]

[189] Oyiengo D, Louis M, Hott B, Bourjeily G. Sleep disorders in pregnancy. Clin Chest Med 2014; 35(3): 571-87.
[http://dx.doi.org/10.1016/j.ccm.2014.06.012] [PMID: 25156772]

[190] Tomfohr LM, Buliga E, Letourneau NL, Campbell TS, Giesbrecht GF. Trajectories of Sleep Quality and Associations with Mood during the Perinatal Period. Sleep 2015; 38(8): 1237-45.
[http://dx.doi.org/10.5665/sleep.4900] [PMID: 25845691]

[191] Skouteris H, Germano C, Wertheim EH, Paxton SJ, Milgrom J. Sleep quality and depression during pregnancy: a prospective study. J Sleep Res 2008; 17(2): 217-20.
[http://dx.doi.org/10.1111/j.1365-2869.2008.00655.x] [PMID: 18482110]

[192] Okun ML, Schetter CD, Glynn LM. Poor sleep quality is associated with preterm birth. Sleep 2011; 34(11): 1493-8.
[http://dx.doi.org/10.5665/sleep.1384] [PMID: 22043120]

[193] August E, Biroscak B, Rahman S, Bruder K, Whiteman V, Salihu H. Systematic review on sleep disorders and obstetric outcomes: scope of current knowledge. Am J Perinatol 2012; 30(4): 323-34.
[http://dx.doi.org/10.1055/s-0032-1324703] [PMID: 22893551]

[194] Naghi I, Keypour F, Ahari SB, Tavalai SA, Khak M. Sleep disturbance in late pregnancy and type and duration of labour. J Obstet Gynaecol 2011; 31(6): 489-91.
[http://dx.doi.org/10.3109/01443615.2011.579196] [PMID: 21823845]

[195] Sharma SK, Nehra A, Sinha S, *et al.* Sleep disorders in pregnancy and their association with pregnancy outcomes: a prospective observational study. Sleep Breath 2016; 20(1): 87-93.
[http://dx.doi.org/10.1007/s11325-015-1188-9] [PMID: 25957617]

[196] Ugur MG, Boynukalin K, Atak Z, Ustuner I, Atakan R, Baykal C. Sleep disturbances in pregnant patients and the relation to obstetric outcome. Clin Exp Obstet Gynecol 2012; 39(2): 214-7. [PMID: 22905467]

[197] Zafarghandi N, Hadavand S, Davati A, Mohseni SM, Kimiaiimoghadam F, Torkestani F. The effects of sleep quality and duration in late pregnancy on labor and fetal outcome. J Matern Fetal Neonatal Med 2012; 25(5): 535-7. [http://dx.doi.org/10.3109/14767058.2011.600370] [PMID: 21827377]

[198] Spiegel K, Knutson K, Leproult R, Tasali E, Van Cauter E. Sleep loss: a novel risk factor for insulin resistance and Type 2 diabetes. J Appl Physiol Bethesda Md 1985. 2005; 9(5): 2008-19.

[199] Copinschi G, Leproult R, Spiegel K. The important role of sleep in metabolism. Front Horm Res 2014; 42: 59-72. [http://dx.doi.org/10.1159/000358858] [PMID: 24732925]

[200] Reutrakul S, Van Cauter E. Interactions between sleep, circadian function, and glucose metabolism: implications for risk and severity of diabetes. Ann N Y Acad Sci 2014; 1311(1): 151-73. [http://dx.doi.org/10.1111/nyas.12355] [PMID: 24628249]

[201] Riemann D, Baglioni C, Bassetti C, *et al.* European guideline for the diagnosis and treatment of insomnia. J Sleep Res 2017; 26(6): 675-700. [http://dx.doi.org/10.1111/jsr.12594] [PMID: 28875581]

[202] Qaseem A, Kansagara D, Forciea MA, Cooke M, Denberg TD. Management of Chronic Insomnia Disorder in Adults: A Clinical Practice Guideline From the American College of Physicians. Ann Intern Med 2016; 165(2): 125-33. [http://dx.doi.org/10.7326/M15-2175] [PMID: 27136449]

[203] Sateia MJ, Buysse DJ, Krystal AD, Neubauer DN, Heald JL. Clinical Practice Guideline for the Pharmacologic Treatment of Chronic Insomnia in Adults: An American Academy of Sleep Medicine Clinical Practice Guideline. J Clin Sleep Med 2017; 13(2): 307-49. [http://dx.doi.org/10.5664/jcsm.6470] [PMID: 27998379]

[204] Ballesio A, Aquino MRJV, Feige B, *et al.* The effectiveness of behavioural and cognitive behavioural therapies for insomnia on depressive and fatigue symptoms: A systematic review and network meta-analysis. Sleep Med Rev 2018; 37: 114-29. [http://dx.doi.org/10.1016/j.smrv.2017.01.006] [PMID: 28619248]

[205] Wu JQ, Appleman ER, Salazar RD, Ong JC. Cognitive Behavioral Therapy for Insomnia Comorbid With Psychiatric and Medical Conditions. JAMA Intern Med 2015; 175(9): 1461-72. [http://dx.doi.org/10.1001/jamainternmed.2015.3006] [PMID: 26147487]

[206] Kruisbrink M, Robertson W, Ji C, Miller MA, Geleijnse JM, Cappuccio FP. Association of sleep duration and quality with blood lipids: a systematic review and meta-analysis of prospective studies. BMJ Open 2017; 7(12)e018585 [http://dx.doi.org/10.1136/bmjopen-2017-018585] [PMID: 29247105]

[207] Cappuccio FP, D'Elia L, Strazzullo P, Miller MA. Sleep duration and all-cause mortality: a systematic review and meta-analysis of prospective studies. Sleep 2010; 33(5): 585-92. [http://dx.doi.org/10.1093/sleep/33.5.585] [PMID: 20469800]

[208] Trauer JM, Qian MY, Doyle JS, Rajaratnam SMW, Cunnington D. Cognitive Behavioral Therapy for Chronic Insomnia. Ann Intern Med 2015; 163(3): 191-204. [http://dx.doi.org/10.7326/M14-2841] [PMID: 26054060]

[209] Johann A, Baglioni C, Hertenstein E, Riemann D, Spiegelhalder K. Prävention psychischer Störungen durch kognitive Verhaltenstherapie bei Insomnie 2015. [http://dx.doi.org/10.1007/s11818-015-0008-6]

[210] Shi Z, MacBeth A. The Effectiveness of Mindfulness-Based Interventions on Maternal Perinatal Mental Health Outcomes: a Systematic Review. Mindfulness 2017; 8(4): 823-47.

[http://dx.doi.org/10.1007/s12671-016-0673-y] [PMID: 28757900]

[211]   Duarte R, Lloyd A, Kotas E, Andronis L, White R. Are acceptance and mindfulness-based interventions 'value for money'? Evidence from a systematic literature review. Br J Clin Psychol 2019; 58(2): 187-210.
[http://dx.doi.org/10.1111/bjc.12208] [PMID: 30499217]

[212]   Casey P, Cowan PA, Cowan CP, Draper L, Mwamba N, Hewison D. Parents as Partners: A U.K. Trial of a U.S. Couples-Based Parenting Intervention For At-Risk Low-Income Families. Fam Process 2017; 56(3): 589-606.
[http://dx.doi.org/10.1111/famp.12289] [PMID: 28439899]

[213]   Kabat-Zinn J. Mindfulness-based interventions in context: Past, present, and future. Clin Psychol Sci Pract 2003; 10(2): 144-56.
[http://dx.doi.org/10.1093/clipsy.bpg016]

[214]   Kabat-Zinn J. Full catastrophe living: using the wisdom of your body and mind to face stress, pain, and illness 2013.

[215]   Brown KW, Weinstein N, Creswell JD. Trait mindfulness modulates neuroendocrine and affective responses to social evaluative threat. Psychoneuroendocrinology 2012; 37(12): 2037-41.
[http://dx.doi.org/10.1016/j.psyneuen.2012.04.003] [PMID: 22626868]

[216]   Tomfohr LM, Pung MA, Mills PJ, Edwards K. Trait mindfulness is associated with blood pressure and interleukin-6: exploring interactions among subscales of the Five Facet Mindfulness Questionnaire to better understand relationships between mindfulness and health. J Behav Med 2015; 38(1): 28-38.
[http://dx.doi.org/10.1007/s10865-014-9575-4] [PMID: 24888477]

[217]   Ede DE, Walter FA, Hughes JW. Exploring How Trait Mindfulness Relates to Perceived Stress and Cardiovascular Reactivity. Int J Behav Med 2020; 27(4): 415-25.
[http://dx.doi.org/10.1007/s12529-020-09871-y] [PMID: 32144687]

[218]   Creswell JD, Pacilio LE, Lindsay EK, Brown KW. Brief mindfulness meditation training alters psychological and neuroendocrine responses to social evaluative stress. Psychoneuroendocrinology 2014; 44: 1-12.
[http://dx.doi.org/10.1016/j.psyneuen.2014.02.007] [PMID: 24767614]

[219]   Epel E, Daubenmier J, Moskowitz JT, Folkman S, Blackburn E. Can meditation slow rate of cellular aging? Cognitive stress, mindfulness, and telomeres. Ann N Y Acad Sci 2009; 1172(1): 34-53.
[http://dx.doi.org/10.1111/j.1749-6632.2009.04414.x] [PMID: 19735238]

[220]   Pascoe MC, Thompson DR, Jenkins ZM, Ski CF. Mindfulness mediates the physiological markers of stress: Systematic review and meta-analysis. J Psychiatr Res 2017; 95: 156-78.
[http://dx.doi.org/10.1016/j.jpsychires.2017.08.004] [PMID: 28863392]

[221]   Nykliček I, Mommersteeg PMC, Van Beugen S, Ramakers C, Van Boxtel GJ. Mindfulness-based stress reduction and physiological activity during acute stress: a randomized controlled trial. Health Psychol Off J Div Health Psychol Am Psychol Assoc 2013; 32(10): 1110-3.

[222]   Manigault AW, Shorey RC, Decastro G, et al. Standardized stress reduction interventions and blood pressure habituation: Secondary results from a randomized controlled trial. Health Psychol 2021; 40(3): 196-206.
[http://dx.doi.org/10.1037/hea0000954] [PMID: 33630641]

[223]   Anderson JW, Liu C, Kryscio RJ. Blood pressure response to transcendental meditation: a meta-analysis. Am J Hypertens 2008; 21(3): 310-6.
[http://dx.doi.org/10.1038/ajh.2007.65] [PMID: 18311126]

[224]   Dickinson HO, Campbell F, Beyer FR, et al. Relaxation therapies for the management of primary hypertension in adults: a Cochrane review. J Hum Hypertens 2008; 22(12): 809-20.
[http://dx.doi.org/10.1038/jhh.2008.65] [PMID: 18548088]

[225]   Carlson LE, Garland SN. Impact of mindfulness-based stress reduction (MBSR) on sleep, mood, stress

and fatigue symptoms in cancer outpatients. Int J Behav Med 2005; 12(4): 278-85.
[http://dx.doi.org/10.1207/s15327558ijbm1204_9] [PMID: 16262547]

[226] Beddoe AE, Lee KA, Weiss SJ, Powell Kennedy H, Yang CPP. Effects of mindful yoga on sleep in pregnant women: a pilot study. Biol Res Nurs 2010; 11(4): 363-70.
[http://dx.doi.org/10.1177/1099800409356320] [PMID: 20338897]

[227] Hughes A, Williams M, Bardacke N, Duncan LG, Dimidjian S, Goodman SH. Mindfulness approaches to childbirth and parenting. Br J Midwifery 2009; 17(10): 630-5.
[http://dx.doi.org/10.12968/bjom.2009.17.10.44470] [PMID: 24307764]

[228] Warriner S, Crane C, Dymond M, Krusche A. An evaluation of mindfulness-based childbirth and parenting courses for pregnant women and prospective fathers/partners within the UK NHS (MBCP--NHS). Midwifery 2018; 64: 1-10.
[http://dx.doi.org/10.1016/j.midw.2018.05.004] [PMID: 29843001]

[229] Botha E, Gwin T, Purpora C. The effectiveness of mindfulness based programs in reducing stress experienced by nurses in adult hospital settings: a systematic review of quantitative evidence protocol. JBI Database Syst Rev Implement Reports 2015; 13(10): 21-9.
[http://dx.doi.org/10.11124/jbisrir-2015-2380] [PMID: 26571279]

[230] Khoury B, Sharma M, Rush SE, Fournier C. Mindfulness-based stress reduction for healthy individuals: A meta-analysis. J Psychosom Res 2015; 78(6): 519-28.
[http://dx.doi.org/10.1016/j.jpsychores.2015.03.009] [PMID: 25818837]

[231] Spinelli C, Wisener M, Khoury B. Mindfulness training for healthcare professionals and trainees: A meta-analysis of randomized controlled trials. J Psychosom Res 2019; 120: 29-38.
[http://dx.doi.org/10.1016/j.jpsychores.2019.03.003] [PMID: 30929705]

[232] Dunn C, Hanieh E, Roberts R, Powrie R. Mindful pregnancy and childbirth: effects of a mindfulness-based intervention on women's psychological distress and well-being in the perinatal period. Arch Women Ment Health 2012; 15(2): 139-43.
[http://dx.doi.org/10.1007/s00737-012-0264-4] [PMID: 22382281]

[233] Guardino CM, Dunkel Schetter C, Bower JE, Lu MC, Smalley SL. Randomised controlled pilot trial of mindfulness training for stress reduction during pregnancy. Psychol Health 2014; 29(3): 334-49.
[http://dx.doi.org/10.1080/08870446.2013.852670] [PMID: 24180264]

[234] Pan WL, Gau ML, Lee TY, Jou HJ, Liu CY, Wen TK. Mindfulness-based programme on the psychological health of pregnant women. Women Birth 2019; 32(1): e102-9.
[http://dx.doi.org/10.1016/j.wombi.2018.04.018] [PMID: 29752225]

[235] Li AW, Goldsmith C-AW. The effects of yoga on anxiety and stress. Altern Med Rev 2012; 17(1): 21-35.
[PMID: 22502620]

[236] Vieten C, Astin J. Effects of a mindfulness-based intervention during pregnancy on prenatal stress and mood: results of a pilot study. Arch Women Ment Health 2008; 11(1): 67-74.
[http://dx.doi.org/10.1007/s00737-008-0214-3] [PMID: 18317710]

[237] Woolhouse H, Mercuri K, Judd F, Brown SJ. Antenatal mindfulness intervention to reduce depression, anxiety and stress: a pilot randomised controlled trial of the MindBabyBody program in an Australian tertiary maternity hospital. BMC Pregnancy Childbirth 2014; 14(1): 369.
[http://dx.doi.org/10.1186/s12884-014-0369-z] [PMID: 25343848]

[238] Duncan LG, Bardacke N. Mindfulness-Based Childbirth and Parenting Education: Promoting Family Mindfulness During the Perinatal Period. J Child Fam Stud 2010; 19(2): 190-202.
[http://dx.doi.org/10.1007/s10826-009-9313-7] [PMID: 20339571]

[239] Lönnberg G, Jonas W, Unternaehrer E, Bränström R, Nissen E, Niemi M. Effects of a mindfulness based childbirth and parenting program on pregnant women's perceived stress and risk of perinatal depression–Results from a randomized controlled trial. J Affect Disord 2020; 262: 133-42.

[http://dx.doi.org/10.1016/j.jad.2019.10.048] [PMID: 31733457]

[240] Dhillon A, Sparkes E, Duarte RV. Mindfulness-Based Interventions During Pregnancy: a Systematic Review and Meta-analysis. Mindfulness 2017; 8(6): 1421-37.
[http://dx.doi.org/10.1007/s12671-017-0726-x] [PMID: 29201244]

[241] Byrne J, Hauck Y, Fisher C, Bayes S, Schutze R. Effectiveness of a Mindfulness-Based Childbirth Education pilot study on maternal self-efficacy and fear of childbirth. J Midwifery Womens Health 2014; 59(2): 192-7.
[http://dx.doi.org/10.1111/jmwh.12075] [PMID: 24325752]

[242] Epel ES, Puterman E, Lin J, Blackburn E, Lazaro A, Mendes WB. Wandering Minds and Aging Cells. Clin Psychol Sci 2013; 1(1): 75-83.
[http://dx.doi.org/10.1177/2167702612460234]

[243] Astin JA. Stress reduction through mindfulness meditation. Effects on psychological symptomatology, sense of control, and spiritual experiences. Psychother Psychosom 1997; 66(2): 97-106.
[http://dx.doi.org/10.1159/000289116] [PMID: 9097338]

[244] Hofmann SG, Sawyer AT, Witt AA, Oh D. The effect of mindfulness-based therapy on anxiety and depression: A meta-analytic review. J Consult Clin Psychol 2010; 78(2): 169-83.
[http://dx.doi.org/10.1037/a0018555] [PMID: 20350028]

[245] Vásquez-Dextre ER. Mindfulness: Conceptos generales, psicoterapia y aplicaciones clínicas. Rev Neuropsiquiatr 2016; 79(1): 42-51.
[http://dx.doi.org/10.20453/rnp.v79i1.2767]

[246] Pérez MA, Botella L. Conciencia plena (mindfulness) y psicoterapia: concepto, evaluación y aplicaciones clínicas. Rev Psicoter 2006; 17(66/67): 77-120.
[http://dx.doi.org/10.33898/rdp.v17i66/67.907]

[247] M. Simón V. Mindfulness y neurobiología. Rev Psicoter 2006; 17(66/67): 5-30.
[http://dx.doi.org/10.33898/rdp.v17i66/67.905]

[248] Siegel RD, Germer CK, Olendzki A. 2009.http://link.springer.com/10.1007/978-0-387-09593-6_2

[249] Hervás G, Cebolla A, Soler J. Intervenciones psicológicas basadas en mindfulness y sus beneficios: estado actual de la cuestión. Clin Salud 2016; 27(3): 115-24.
[http://dx.doi.org/10.1016/j.clysa.2016.09.002]

[250] Miró MT, Perestelo-Pérez L, Ramos JP, Rivero A, González M, de la Fuente JA, *et al.* Eficacia de los tratamientos psicológicos basados en mindfulness para los trastornos de ansiedad y depresión  una revisión sistemática. Rev Psicopatol Psicol Clin 2011; 16(1): 1-16.
[http://dx.doi.org/10.5944/rppc.vol.16.num.1.2011.10347]

[251] Khoury B, Lecomte T, Fortin G, *et al.* Mindfulness-based therapy: A comprehensive meta-analysis. Clin Psychol Rev 2013; 33(6): 763-71.
[http://dx.doi.org/10.1016/j.cpr.2013.05.005] [PMID: 23796855]

[252] Reiner K, Tibi L, Lipsitz JD. Do mindfulness-based interventions reduce pain intensity? A critical review of the literature. Pain Med 2013; 14(2): 230-42.
[http://dx.doi.org/10.1111/pme.12006] [PMID: 23240921]

[253] Baer RA. Mindfulness training as a clinical intervention: A conceptual and empirical review. Clin Psychol Sci Pract 2003; 10(2): 125-43.
[http://dx.doi.org/10.1093/clipsy.bpg015]

[254] Dimidjian S, Goodman SH, Felder JN, Gallop R, Brown AP, Beck A. An open trial of mindfulness-based cognitive therapy for the prevention of perinatal depressive relapse/recurrence. Arch Women Ment Health 2015; 18(1): 85-94.
[http://dx.doi.org/10.1007/s00737-014-0468-x] [PMID: 25298253]

[255] Dimidjian S, Goodman SH, Felder JN, Gallop R, Brown AP, Beck A. Staying well during pregnancy

and the postpartum: A pilot randomized trial of mindfulness-based cognitive therapy for the prevention of depressive relapse/recurrence. J Consult Clin Psychol 2016; 84(2): 134-45.
[http://dx.doi.org/10.1037/ccp0000068] [PMID: 26654212]

[256]   Staneva A, Bogossian F, Pritchard M, Wittkowski A. The effects of maternal depression, anxiety, and perceived stress during pregnancy on preterm birth: A systematic review. Women Birth 2015; 28(3): 179-93.
[http://dx.doi.org/10.1016/j.wombi.2015.02.003] [PMID: 25765470]

[257]   Evans S. Review: mindfulness-based therapies effective for anxiety and depression. Evid Based Ment Health 2011; 13(4): 116.
[http://dx.doi.org/10.1136/ebmh1094] [PMID: 21036978]

[258]   Hölzel BK, Carmody J, Evans KC, *et al.* Stress reduction correlates with structural changes in the amygdala. Soc Cogn Affect Neurosci 2010; 5(1): 11-7.
[http://dx.doi.org/10.1093/scan/nsp034] [PMID: 19776221]

[259]   Roozendaal B, McEwen BS, Chattarji S. Stress, memory and the amygdala. Nat Rev Neurosci 2009; 10(6): 423-33.
[http://dx.doi.org/10.1038/nrn2651] [PMID: 19469026]

[260]   Liu WZ, Zhang WH, Zheng ZH, *et al.* Identification of a prefrontal cortex-to-amygdala pathway for chronic stress-induced anxiety. Nat Commun 2020; 11(1): 2221.
[http://dx.doi.org/10.1038/s41467-020-15920-7] [PMID: 32376858]

[261]   Zhang JY, Liu TH, He Y, *et al.* Chronic Stress Remodels Synapses in an Amygdala Circuit–Specific Manner. Biol Psychiatry 2019; 85(3): 189-201.
[http://dx.doi.org/10.1016/j.biopsych.2018.06.019] [PMID: 30060908]

[262]   Lautarescu A, Craig MC, Glover V. Prenatal stress: Effects on fetal and child brain development. Int Rev Neurobiol 2020; 150: 17-40.
[http://dx.doi.org/10.1016/bs.irn.2019.11.002] [PMID: 32204831]

[263]   Humphreys KL, Camacho MC, Roth MC, Estes EC. Prenatal stress exposure and multimodal assessment of amygdala–medial prefrontal cortex connectivity in infants. Dev Cogn Neurosci 2020; 46100877
[http://dx.doi.org/10.1016/j.dcn.2020.100877] [PMID: 33220629]

[264]   Shin LM, Rauch SL, Pitman RK. Amygdala, medial prefrontal cortex, and hippocampal function in PTSD. Ann N Y Acad Sci 2006; 1071(1): 67-79.
[http://dx.doi.org/10.1196/annals.1364.007] [PMID: 16891563]

[265]   Frewen PA, Evans EM, Maraj N, Dozois DJA, Partridge K. Letting Go: Mindfulness and Negative Automatic Thinking. Cognit Ther Res 2008; 32(6): 758-74.
[http://dx.doi.org/10.1007/s10608-007-9142-1]

[266]   Talge NM, Neal C, Glover V. Antenatal maternal stress and long-term effects on child neurodevelopment: how and why? J Child Psychol Psychiatry 2007; 48(3-4): 245-61.
[http://dx.doi.org/10.1111/j.1469-7610.2006.01714.x] [PMID: 17355398]

[267]   Salmon P, Lush E, Jablonski M, Sephton SE. Yoga and Mindfulness: Clinical Aspects of an Ancient Mind/Body Practice. Cognit Behav Pract 2009; 16(1): 59-72.
[http://dx.doi.org/10.1016/j.cbpra.2008.07.002]

[268]   Garland EL, Roberts-Lewis A, Tronnier CD, Graves R, Kelley K. Mindfulness-Oriented Recovery Enhancement versus CBT for co-occurring substance dependence, traumatic stress, and psychiatric disorders: Proximal outcomes from a pragmatic randomized trial. Behav Res Ther 2016; 77: 7-16.
[http://dx.doi.org/10.1016/j.brat.2015.11.012] [PMID: 26701171]

[269]   Ong JC, Shapiro SL, Manber R. Combining mindfulness meditation with cognitive-behavior therapy for insomnia: a treatment-development study. Behav Ther 2008; 39(2): 171-82.
[http://dx.doi.org/10.1016/j.beth.2007.07.002] [PMID: 18502250]

[270] Ong JC, Shapiro SL, Manber R. Mindfulness meditation and cognitive behavioural therapy for insomnia: a naturalistic 12-month follow-up. Explore N Y N. febrero de 2009; 5(1): 30-6.

[271] Martires J, Zeidler M. The value of mindfulness meditation in the treatment of insomnia. Curr Opin Pulm Med 2015; 21(6): 547-52.
[http://dx.doi.org/10.1097/MCP.0000000000000207] [PMID: 26390335]

[272] Kennett L, Bei B, Jackson ML. A Randomized Controlled Trial to Examine the Feasibility and Preliminary Efficacy of a Digital Mindfulness-Based Therapy for Improving Insomnia Symptoms. Mindfulness 2021; 12(10): 2460-72.
[http://dx.doi.org/10.1007/s12671-021-01714-5] [PMID: 34377217]

[273] Felder JN, Laraia B, Coleman-Phox K, *et al.* Poor Sleep Quality, Psychological Distress, and the Buffering Effect of Mindfulness Training During Pregnancy. Behav Sleep Med 2018; 16(6): 611-24.
[http://dx.doi.org/10.1080/15402002.2016.1266488] [PMID: 28060531]

[274] Vieten C, Laraia BA, Kristeller J, *et al.* The mindful moms training: development of a mindfulness-based intervention to reduce stress and overeating during pregnancy. BMC Pregnancy Childbirth 2018; 18(1): 201.
[http://dx.doi.org/10.1186/s12884-018-1757-6] [PMID: 29859038]

[275] Epel E, Laraia B, Coleman-Phox K, *et al.* Effects of a Mindfulness-Based Intervention on Distress, Weight Gain, and Glucose Control for Pregnant Low-Income Women: A Quasi-Experimental Trial Using the ORBIT Model. Int J Behav Med 2019; 26(5): 461-73.
[http://dx.doi.org/10.1007/s12529-019-09779-2] [PMID: 30993601]

[276] Narendran S, Nagarathna R, Narendran V, Gunasheela S, Nagendra HRR. Efficacy of yoga on pregnancy outcome. J Altern Complement Med N Y N. abril de 2005; 11(2): 237-44.

[277] Fields N. Yoga: empowering women to give birth. Pract Midwife 2008; 11(5): 30-2.
[PMID: 18540506]

[278] Sharma M, Branscum P. Yoga interventions in pregnancy: a qualitative review. J Altern Complement Med N Y N. abril de 2015; 21(4): 208-16.

[279] Wadhwa Y, Alghadir AH, Iqbal ZA. Effect of Antenatal Exercises, Including Yoga, on the Course of Labor, Delivery and Pregnancy: A Retrospective Study. Int J Environ Res Public Health 2020; 17(15): 5274.
[http://dx.doi.org/10.3390/ijerph17155274] [PMID: 32707830]

[280] Bauer I, Hartkopf J, Kullmann S, *et al.* Spotlight on the fetus: how physical activity during pregnancy influences fetal health: a narrative review. BMJ Open Sport Exerc Med 2020; 6(1)e000658
[http://dx.doi.org/10.1136/bmjsem-2019-000658] [PMID: 32206341]

[281] Skovbjerg S, Birk D, Bruggisser S, Wolf ALA, Fjorback L. Mindfulness-based stress reduction adapted to pregnant women with psychosocial vulnerabilities—a protocol for a randomized feasibility study in a Danish hospital-based outpatient setting. Pilot Feasibility Stud 2021; 7(1): 118.
[http://dx.doi.org/10.1186/s40814-021-00860-w] [PMID: 34082839]

[282] Zhang JY, Cui YX, Zhou YQ, Li YL. Effects of mindfulness-based stress reduction on prenatal stress, anxiety and depression. Psychol Health Med 2019; 24(1): 51-8.
[http://dx.doi.org/10.1080/13548506.2018.1468028] [PMID: 29695175]

[283] Tomfohr-Madsen LM, Campbell TS, Giesbrecht GF, *et al.* Mindfulness-based cognitive therapy for psychological distress in pregnancy: study protocol for a randomized controlled trial. Trials 2016; 17(1): 498.
[http://dx.doi.org/10.1186/s13063-016-1601-0] [PMID: 27737714]

[284] Zemestani M, Fazeli Nikoo Z. Effectiveness of mindfulness-based cognitive therapy for comorbid depression and anxiety in pregnancy: a randomized controlled trial. Arch Women Ment Health 2020; 23(2): 207-14.
[http://dx.doi.org/10.1007/s00737-019-00962-8] [PMID: 30982086]

[285] Luberto CM, Park ER, Goodman JH. Postpartum Outcomes and Formal Mindfulness Practice in Mindfulness-Based Cognitive Therapy for Perinatal Women. Mindfulness 2018; 9(3): 850-9.
[http://dx.doi.org/10.1007/s12671-017-0825-8] [PMID: 30079120]

[286] Miklowitz DJ, Semple RJ, Hauser M, Elkun D, Weintraub MJ, Dimidjian S. Mindfulness-Based Cognitive Therapy for Perinatal Women with Depression or Bipolar Spectrum Disorder. Cognit Ther Res 2015; 39(5): 590-600.
[http://dx.doi.org/10.1007/s10608-015-9681-9] [PMID: 32063660]

[287] Faramarzi M, Yazdani S, Barat S. A RCT of psychotherapy in women with nausea and vomiting of pregnancy. Hum Reprod 2015; 30(12)dev248
[http://dx.doi.org/10.1093/humrep/dev248] [PMID: 26466913]

[288] Conley CS, Shapiro JB, Kirsch AC, Durlak JA. A meta-analysis of indicated mental health prevention programs for at-risk higher education students. J Couns Psychol 2017; 64(2): 121-40.
[http://dx.doi.org/10.1037/cou0000190] [PMID: 28277730]

[289] Goldberg SB, Tucker RP, Greene PA, *et al.* Mindfulness-based interventions for psychiatric disorders: A systematic review and meta-analysis. Clin Psychol Rev 2018; 59: 52-60.
[http://dx.doi.org/10.1016/j.cpr.2017.10.011] [PMID: 29126747]

[290] O'Hara MW, McCabe JE. Postpartum depression: current status and future directions. Annu Rev Clin Psychol 2013; 9(1): 379-407.
[http://dx.doi.org/10.1146/annurev-clinpsy-050212-185612] [PMID: 23394227]

[291] Veringa IK, de Bruin EI, Bardacke N, *et al.* 'I've Changed My Mind', Mindfulness-Based Childbirth and Parenting (MBCP) for pregnant women with a high level of fear of childbirth and their partners: study protocol of the quasi-experimental controlled trial. BMC Psychiatry 2016; 16(1): 377.
[http://dx.doi.org/10.1186/s12888-016-1070-8] [PMID: 27821151]

[292] Kabat-Zinn J. An outpatient program in behavioral medicine for chronic pain patients based on the practice of mindfulness meditation: Theoretical considerations and preliminary results. Gen Hosp Psychiatry 1982; 4(1): 33-47.
[http://dx.doi.org/10.1016/0163-8343(82)90026-3] [PMID: 7042457]

[293] Piet J, Hougaard E. The effect of mindfulness-based cognitive therapy for prevention of relapse in recurrent major depressive disorder: A systematic review and meta-analysis. Clin Psychol Rev 2011; 31(6): 1032-40.
[http://dx.doi.org/10.1016/j.cpr.2011.05.002] [PMID: 21802618]

[294] https://www.nice.org.uk/guidance/cg90

[295] Chiesa A, Serretti A. Mindfulness based cognitive therapy for psychiatric disorders: a systematic review and meta-analysis 2011.
[http://dx.doi.org/10.1016/j.psychres.2010.08.011]

[296] Fjorback LO, Arendt M, Ørnbøl E, Fink P, Walach H. Mindfulness-Based Stress Reduction and Mindfulness-Based Cognitive Therapy - a systematic review of randomized controlled trials. Acta Psychiatr Scand 2011; 124(2): 102-19.
[http://dx.doi.org/10.1111/j.1600-0447.2011.01704.x] [PMID: 21534932]

[297] Strauss C, Cavanagh K, Oliver A, Pettman D. Mindfulness-Based Interventions for People Diagnosed with a Current Episode of an Anxiety or Depressive Disorder: A Meta-Analysis of Randomised Controlled Trials. 2014.
[http://dx.doi.org/10.1371/journal.pone.0096110]

[298] Vøllestad J, Nielsen MB, Nielsen GH. Mindfulness- and acceptance-based interventions for anxiety disorders: A systematic review and meta-analysis. Br J Clin Psychol 2012; 51(3): 239-60.
[http://dx.doi.org/10.1111/j.2044-8260.2011.02024.x] [PMID: 22803933]

[299] Muzik M, Hamilton SE, Lisa Rosenblum K, Waxler E, Hadi Z. Mindfulness yoga during pregnancy for psychiatrically at-risk women: Preliminary results from a pilot feasibility study. Complement Ther

Clin Pract 2012; 18(4): 235-40.
[http://dx.doi.org/10.1016/j.ctcp.2012.06.006] [PMID: 23059438]

[300] Matvienko-Sikar K, Dockray S. Effects of a novel positive psychological intervention on prenatal stress and well-being: A pilot randomised controlled trial. Women Birth 2017; 30(2): e111-8.
[http://dx.doi.org/10.1016/j.wombi.2016.10.003] [PMID: 27810284]

[301] Muthukrishnan S, Jain R, Kohli S, Batra S. Effect of Mindfulness Meditation on Perceived Stress Scores and Autonomic Function Tests of Pregnant Indian Women. J Clin Diagn Res 2016; 10(4): CC05-8.
[http://dx.doi.org/10.7860/JCDR/2016/16463.7679] [PMID: 27190795]

[302] Astin JA, Berman BM, Bausell B, Lee W-L, Hochberg M, Forys KL. The efficacy of mindfulness meditation plus Qigong movement therapy in the treatment of fibromyalgia: a randomized controlled trial. J Rheumatol 2003; 30(10): 2257-62.
[PMID: 14528526]

[303] Agampodi T, Katumuluwa S, Pattiyakumbura T, Rankaduwa N, Dissanayaka T, Agampodi S. Feasibility of incorporating mindfulness based mental health promotion to the pregnancy care program in Sri Lanka: a pilot study. F1000 Res 2018; 7: 1850.
[http://dx.doi.org/10.12688/f1000research.17049.1] [PMID: 32226605]

SUBJECT INDEX

Eugenio Daniel Martinez-Hurtado, Monica Sanjuan-Alvarez & Marta Chacon-Castillo (Eds.)
All rights reserved-© 2022 Bentham Science Publishers

www.ingramcontent.com/pod-product-compliance
Lightning Source LLC
Chambersburg PA
CBHW080018240326
41598CB00075B/74